Communication Solutions *for* Older Students

Assessment and Intervention Strategies

Vicki Lord Larson, PhD
Nancy L. McKinley, MS

Thinking Publications • **Eau Claire, Wisconsin**

10   09   08   07   06   05   04   03   8   7   6   5   4   3   2   1

Library of Congress Cataloging-in-Publication Data

Larson, Vicki Lord.
   Communication solutions for older students : assessment and intervention strategies /
Vicki Lord Larson, Nancy L. McKinley
     p. cm.
   Includes bibliographical references and index.
   ISBN 1-888222-99-9
    1. Communicative disorders in adolescence. I. McKinley, Nancy L. II. Title.

RJ496.C67L373 2003
616.85'5'00835—dc21

                   2003040209

Printed in the United States of America
Cover design by Debbie Olson

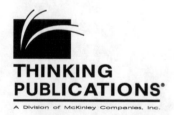

THINKING
PUBLICATIONS®
A Division of McKinley Companies, Inc.

424 Galloway Street • Eau Claire, WI 54703
715.832.2488 • Fax 715.832.9082
Email: custserv@ThinkingPublications.com

COMMUNICATION SOLUTIONS THAT CHANGE LIVES®

To James R. Larson
husband, best friend, and soulmate

To Michael P. McKinley
husband, mentor, business partner, and best friend

List of Tables

Communication Solutions
for Older Students

Foreword

No professional educator would set out to squander human potential, yet that is exactly what we do every day that we fail to serve youth and adolescents with communication disorders. Speech language pathologists (SLPs) and other educators have not done enough for older students with language disorders. This is the message, loud and strong, in *Communication Solutions for Older Students.* Authors Vicki Lord Larson and Nancy L. McKinley use the same clear, clean prose of their popular *Language Disorders in Older Students* to present useful assessments and interventions for adolescents. However, this newest release is vastly expanded and reorganized from 8 chapters to 15. They have added entire chapters on such current issues as cultural/linguistic diversity, concomitant problems, and efficacy of services. In the latter chapter, they bravely tackle the big issues of effectiveness of interventions and the likelihood of beneficial results, asking how do you know it works?

There is a strong rationale for speech-language pathologists to serve older students. Position papers from the American Speech-Language-Hearing Association (ASHA) in the last five years have clearly included "youth and adolescents" or "older students" in their titles. Support is needed for students who do not acquire formal operational skills during their cognitive development. They barely make it through elementary school; they drop out of high school. Does it cost too much to support these students in high school? It is clear that it costs society much more to help them later as adults who cannot hold a job, fail at personal relationships, turn to crime, or are incarcerated.

Having known these outstanding authors for many years, I was gratified to recognize that their new informative text about language disorders in youth had "moved up a notch." Their new Chapter 1, for example, is personal, emotional, and intense. They tell us plainly why we simply must care about the topics they present. I especially liked the new organizational sidebars that target the key issues. Elkind's (1974, 1978, 2000) descriptions of imaginary audience and personal fables come to life in this format. This is what adolescents are struggling with. Add a language disability to the mix and it gets even more complex. These cohesive text elements arrest the attention of both the busy clinician in today's schools and private practices and the university student preparing for our discipline.

Another example of updating in this state-of-the-art text is the expanded definition of reading and writing. The information reflects the scientifically based reading research (SBRR) referred to in all of the current literature on reading and literacy. It is highly relevant for adolescents with language disorders. An entirely new section on spelling and its relationship to phonemic awareness conveniently brings the current research in the field to the clinician for immediate use. Reading is a grapheme-to-phoneme process, using distinctive features. Spelling is a phoneme-to-grapheme process, using letter combinations. There are approximately 40 distinctive features in

English, and 70 letter combinations to represent those features. Thus, it is considerably easier to read English than to spell it! Many clinicians are not aware of that. When high school students cannot read fluently, no one is teaching them the skills any longer. Reading is not taught in high school. If you missed it in the younger grades, you can't go back home again. Most times, it is the SLP who is teaching reading, spelling, and literacy at the secondary level. We must know what it is and how to do it. This includes both functional literacy (how to decode words) and critical literacy (what the words mean). Both aspects are required in high school. The debates about top-down vs. bottom-up reading philosophies don't attract much attention in high school. Every educator who is making a contribution is on a "what works" trajectory to try to make a difference while there are still a few years, or months, or days left in school.

Speech-language pathologists and professionals in other related services are always in search of new, better, faster, more discriminating assessments for older students. Larson and McKinley are keenly aware of this need and offer a robust Chapter 9 on assessment followed by Chapter 10, which provides dynamic directed tasks. They recognize that older students have a "style" of learning that we don't see in younger students, as well as emotional intelligence, social skills, and discourse abilities and disabilities. An age-appropriate method of analyzing language samples is noteworthy. Most practitioners and faculty are unaware of the list of 38 norm-referenced tests of adolescent language that this text offers. This text also comes out strongly against the cognitive discrepancy model of assessment and eligibility for speech and language services. The authors, along with countless other clear thinkers in the field, assert that students can benefit from speech and language services even though they have cognitive deficits. Their recommended services are based on an intervention strategies approach using mediated learning and focusing on meta-abilities.

We should not be seeking ways to avoid supporting students; we should be seeking ways to provide more service to them. Somehow that idea has been lost in the last decade of streamlining what the speech-language pathologist does and stands for in education. Secondary school is the last chance for many of these students—There is no safety net. They will fall. We must be there for them.

Larson and McKinley give us the tools to be better clinicians, and then challenge us to be equally passionate about how and when we use these tools to help adolescents. The characteristics and academic expectations of older school-age students with language disorders are the more exciting frontiers for today's SLP. The speech-language pathologist must become a stronger voice for our youth in today's schools. Given the strength of this text, and the will of these authors, we can do no less.

Judy K. Montgomery, PhD, CCC-SLP
Professor, Special Education and Literacy
School of Education, Chapman University, Orange, CA
Former President, American Speech-Language-Hearing Association

Preface

When the two of us tackled the topic of serving older students with language disorders in the early 1980s, little did we realize it would become a lifelong passion. The flame was lit by graduate students from our Communication Disorders program at the University of Wisconsin—Eau Claire after they embarked on their first jobs, which happened to be at the secondary level. They had some very negative feedback in response to our university's program: No one had prepared them to work with adolescents. And they were right. Our curriculum was devoid of information between childhood and adulthood. (And anyone working with that age group knows that merely blending assessment and intervention information on children and adults, then extrapolating what to do for adolescents doesn't work.)

We began searching for information on older students in related disciplines, notably learning disabilities, psychology, and special education. We scrutinized data on at-risk students, incarcerated youth, and college students with learning disabilities for their relationships to language disorders. In pursuit of learning what worked and what didn't, we interviewed speech-language pathologists who worked with adolescents struggling with the communication demands of academic and social situations. Together, these sources became our initial knowledge base of how to serve older students with language disorders.

The flame lit by our graduate students became fully ignited when we began presenting workshops on working with older students. We discovered that many speech-language pathologists were clamoring for information on this topic. As we began to travel around the country, opportunities for consulting with specific programs and agencies surfaced. Few jobs were more gratifying to us than helping a secondary-level speech-language program turn the corner from one that students avoided to one that students appreciated for teaching them the communication skills needed for lifelong success.

Over the past 20 years, we have written three books on the topic of older students: *Adolescent's Communication: Development and Disorders* (1983), *Communication Assessment and Intervention Strategies for Adolescents* (1987), and *Language Disorders in Older Students* (1995). As our study and thinking on the topic evolved over the decades, we adjusted the content in each book accordingly. Sometimes people in our audiences ask about information that appeared only in our original book back in 1983, explaining how they still use this information today. Comments like these are what fueled this current text, *Communication Solutions for Older Students*, in which we've blended classic information from our past three books with current best practices.

As we have matured the last 20 years, so, too, has the topic of serving older students with communication disorders. We are happy to report that journals in the discipline now feature articles that encompass this age group, and occasionally whole issues of journals (e.g., *Clinical Linguistics and Phonetics, 12(3)* in 1998 and *Seminars in Speech-Language Pathology,* (in press) are devoted to the topic. In addition, a growing number of books, tests, and intervention materials have been published, especially since 1990.

Even with these advances, the number of university classes that address this topic remains disappointingly low. It is our hope that *Communication Solutions for Older Students* can:

- Teach university students the basic set of skills so desperately needed when serving older students

- Serve as a solid reference tool for any professional already working with students from ages 9–19

- Provide guidance to supervisors, administrators, and policy makers for why services are so essential for older students with language disorders, and how best to address their needs

In whatever capacity this book can serve you, may it prove instrumental in the quality of services delivered to older students in your community.

No book is ever written in isolation; a number of individuals assisted us in developing and improving this book. A special thank-you to Linda Schreiber for her conscientious approach to clarifying content; to Sarah Thurs for her incredible editing skills that improved the content, format, and mechanics of our writing; to Debbie Olson for her visual sensitivity to structuring the tables, sidebars, and appendices; to Dannelle Cheng for her cheerful assistance in securing permissions and retrieving references; to Jan Carroll for her honors of indexing; to Joyce Olson for sharing her expertise on educational law; to Linda Revak for photographing adolescents in typical school, home, and community situations; and to the adolescents who were willing to be photographed. A special thank-you, too, to the university professors and practicing clinicians who provided feedback to us on our previous textbooks, thus allowing us to select best practices and to expand content in areas such as written communication and emotional intelligence. Finally, we owe a special recognition to all the 9- to 19-year-olds who have interacted with us over the years who have taught us about this developmental period and the ways in which communication skills make a difference in improving academic progress, personal-social interactions, and vocational potential.

1

Introduction

Communication Solutions for Older Students: Assessment and Intervention Strategies highlights the best practices from our three previous textbooks on adolescents: *Adolescents' Communication: Development and Disorders* (Boyce and Larson, 1983), *Communication Assessment and Intervention Strategies for Adolescents* (Larson and McKinley, 1987), and *Language Disorders in Older Students* (Larson and McKinley, 1995) and incorporates the most current information on serving older students with language and literacy disorders (i.e., problems in thinking, listening, speaking, reading and/or writing). Thus, *Communication Solutions for Older Students* is our most comprehensive textbook on:

- Oral and written communication development and disorders,

- Assessment and intervention strategies

- Transition issues for older students ages 9 to 19

Language disorder is a term we use throughout this text. We concur with the ASHA (1993) definition of *language disorder* as "impaired comprehension and/or use of spoken, written and/or other symbol systems. The disorder may involve (1) the form of language (phonology, morphology, syntax), (2) the content of language (semantics), and/or (3) the function of language in communication (pragmatics) in any combination" (p. 40). Reference is also made to communication disorders, a broader term than language disorder, in numerous sections. "A communication disorder is an impairment in the ability to receive, send, process, and comprehend concepts or verbal, nonverbal and graphic symbol systems" (ASHA, 1993, p. 40). The latter term is used when the information presented holds true for older students who present with problems instead of or in addition to a language disorder (e.g., executive function impairments, speech disorders, hearing impairments, or social communication deficits).

Communication Solutions
for Older Students

The book is divided into four parts with several chapters in each part. Each chapter begins with a list of goals for the chapter and concludes with points of discussion and suggested readings. We recommend that you discuss the questions among yourselves and pursue the selected readings for more in-depth coverage of the topic. There are 24 appendixes, which feature numerous practical clinical forms or applications, many to be used as assessment and intervention protocols with older students. All these forms are on the accompanying CD-ROM and easily reprintable. Each of the four parts of the book will now be summarized as to the pertinent content in each of the chapters.

Part I: Adolescent Development— Normal and Disordered consists of seven chapters, which present an overview of the theoretical underpinnings of adolescence; normal developmental milestones in terms of physical, psychological, and cognitive skills; oral and written language; and nonverbal communication. In addition, there are chapters on communication parameters in culturally and linguistically diverse populations, the nature of language disorders in older students, and a discussion of frequent concomitant problems that older students with language disorders may face. Part I serves as an overview of, as well as the foundation for, the rest of the book. It is up to your discretion as to whether this section of the book needs to be read before proceeding to learning more about assessment and intervention. We provide this caveat: Because

of the critical nature this information plays for the parts of the book that follow, we urge you to read Part I either to review or to update your current knowledge of the topic.

Chapter 1: Adolescence—An Overview provides insights on what adolescence is and defines *adolescence* as the period between 10 and 19 years of age. The theories of adolescence reviewed are those that have been espoused during the 20th century and into the 21st century. A review of the biological, anthropological, sociological, and psychological theories of adolescence is presented. Over the decades, four psychological theories—psychoanalytic, field, social learning, and stage theory—have predominated. Of these, the most pertinent has been stage theory, as it provides a framework for general, identity, cognitive, and moral development. We provide a summary of the various theories by comparing and contrasting them to one another and then noting how the reader might cope with these different theories of adolescence. Selecting precepts from a variety of theories to develop a more comprehensive synthesized perspective is what we emphasize. We strongly subscribe to the notion that nothing is as practical as a good theory to provide a rationale for why, what, and how we conduct ourselves in research and provide clinical services.

Chapter 2: Developmental Milestones during Adolescence provides an overview of normal physical and psychological development. Physical development is characterized by rapid changes during early adolescence, more modest changes during middle adolescence, and fewer changes during late adolescence. Adolescents' physical development is incomplete without acknowledging its interaction with psychological development. Psychological developmental principles of dividing adolescence into early, middle, and late are highlighted in terms of characteristics of the three stages and developmental tasks of normal adolescence. Cognitive development includes Piagetian, inductive and deductive reasoning, and Benjamin Bloom et al.'s (1956) taxonomy. Concept development of older students is noted, especially in the flexible nature of the adolescent's ability to shift back and forth between abstract-categorical and perceptual orientations. Critical thinking is noted as the ability to evaluate one's own thinking, and bipolar parameters that should be used to evaluate the quality of thinking are presented. Regardless of the approach used to evaluate cognitive development during adolescence, it should be noted that both quantitative and qualitative differences occur.

Chapter 3: Oral and Nonverbal Communication Development enumerates the comparisons of early to later language development. It is demonstrated and emphasized that language continues to grow throughout adolescence both quantitatively and qualitatively. Oral communication development in terms of both comprehension (listening) and production (speaking) of language is described. Listening is the skill that people use the most, yet it is the least taught in the educational system. Production

of linguistic features or speaking includes Loban's 13-year longitudinal study data to note the changes from grades 1 to 12. Normal discourse skills of conversation, narration, expository text, persuasion, and negotiation are defined, and major normal development characteristics are presented. The chapter also presents nonverbal communication development into the adolescent years. These normal developmental language, discourse, and nonverbal features serve as a foundation to provide baseline data to make decisions about when an older student's language is disordered.

Chapter 4: Literacy Development provides definitions of reading, writing, and spelling. Normal developmental trends in older students are discussed. Writing skills continue to develop into late adolescence and adult years. Perfecting the writing process of prewriting or planning, writing or drafting composition, and postwriting or revising/editing is a lifelong pursuit. Also, the skills needed to take adequate notes are presented since this skill is critical to being successful in gaining knowledge from classroom lectures. Reading skills that are needed to be successful when decoding unknown printed words—including phonological skills, synthesis, attention, auditory perceptual skills, knowledge of morphological rules, sequential memory, and visual perceptual memory—are presented. Likewise, skills required for reading with comprehension—including attention, syntax, semantics, memory, imagery, pragmatics, and higher level cognitive skills—are noted. Stages of spelling development from ages 1 to 12 years of age are described. The importance of spelling to word knowledge, reading, and writing is emphasized. Chapters 3 and 4 are closely intertwined since it has been established that there is an interrelationship between oral and written language. Also, like oral language, written language continues to emerge throughout adolescence.

Chapter 5: Communication in Culturally and Linguistically Diverse Populations provides pertinent statistics on cultural and linguistic diversity within the United States, especially as they relate to older students. Knowledge about culturally and linguistically diverse populations is critical for professionals because they must differentiate between a student with a language difference and a language disorder. A language difference is a rule-governed language code or system that is different from Standard American English (SAE) but that meets the norms of the individual's primary linguistic community. A series of tables presents linguistic and pragmatic features of various cultural populations, such as African Americans, Native Americans, Asian Americans, and Hispanic Americans.

Chapter 6: Language Disorders in Older Students cites the prevalence of communication disorders in adolescents in schools and juvenile detention facilities. A table provides an overview of the types of characteristic expectations and problems experienced by older students with language disorders,

across the areas of cognition, metalinguistics, comprehension and production of linguistic features, discourse, nonverbal communication, reading, and writing. Deficits within each of these areas are noted to provide data on what problems are likely to occur in the older student with a language disorder.

Chapter 7: Frequent Concomitant Problems with Language Disorders discusses the types of problems likely to co-occur with language disorders: Traumatic Brain Injury; Attention Deficit Disorders; fetal alcohol syndrome, learning disabilities, and autism. Many students who have language disorders also are youth-at-risk. They are at-risk for dropping out of school or for being unprepared to enter the workforce. A review of the literature reveals that many students with language disorders have lifelong language problems. Professionals refer to this phenomenon as a "continuum of failure." Various researchers have noted that there is a continuum of language disorders that initially is seen in oral language and eventually is revealed in written language or in both oral and written language (Aram, Ekelman, and Nation, 1984; Aram and Hall, 1989; C.J. Johnston, Beitchman, Young, Atkinson, Wilson, et al., 1999; Stothard, Snowling, Bishop, Chipchase, and Kaplan, 1998). It is apparent that most children do not outgrow their language problems and that they persist into the adolescent years and beyond.

Part II: Language Assessment of Adolescents consists of three chapters. These chapters provide an overview of assessment as a dynamic process, a discussion of the specific behaviors (what to assess) and procedures (how to assess), and a presentation of how to use directed tasks to assess specific behaviors and skills.

Chapter 8: Assessment—A Comprehensive Process begins with a definition and overview of the assessment process. A comprehensive/holistic model is outlined consisting of five facets: descriptive, authentic, dynamic, student-centered, and multidimensional. The multidimensional aspect of assessment includes assessing the educational and environmental systems. It is critical to note that all problems may not be located in the student. The educational (e.g., teacher language, selected curriculum variables) or environmental (family constellation or peer group) systems may be the culprit. Within this chapter is also a discussion of assessment issues as they relate to a pluralistic society. Issues such as assessing communication dimensions using ethnographic methods, differentiating between a language difference and disorder, and determining when and how to use trained interpreters, to name only a few, are covered. A sample of standardized multicultural tests is provided.

Chapter 9: Procedures for Direct Assessment presents a comprehensive review of what behaviors to assess and how to assess those behaviors. More specifically, a discussion ensues on what aspects of language skills need to be assessed, such as history of thinking, listening, speaking, reading and writing intervention; learning style;

emotional intelligence; social skills; cognition; linguistic features; discourse areas of conversations, narrations, and expository test; reading and writing; meta-abilities; and nonverbal communication. Two overriding procedures are used to provide insight on how to go about assessing the various components listed under what to assess: informal and formal assessment protocols. Informal procedures include using a case history form, interviews, questionnaires, checklists, rubrics, and portfolios, as well as gathering discourse samples (conversations, narrations, and expository text). Both spoken and written samples using semistructured procedures should be collected, analyzed, and interpreted. Formal assessment or standardized tests are presented, and a list of parameters to critique standardized tests is provided.

Chapter 10: Directed Tasks for Assessment presents a series of procedures that utilize dynamic assessment principles in which the emphasis is on the process the student goes through, rather than on the product or outcome. Eight directed tasks are provided: problem solving, organization, giving/getting directions, informational listening, critical listening, question asking and answering, topic management, and textbook analysis. Each of these directed tasks is presented using this format: administrative steps, analysis procedures, and interpretation guidelines. Directed tasks should be used to supplement, not supplant, other assessment procedures.

Communication Solutions
for Older Students

Part III: Language Intervention with Adolescents has three chapters, which focus on service delivery models for older students, general intervention considerations, and specific intervention methods. Collectively these chapters provide a framework for working with older students who have language disorders.

Chapter 11: Service Delivery Models and Issues contains a rationale for providing speech-language services to older students. This rationale can be used with school board members, district administrators, and all taxpayers to convince them of the need for and efficacy of services delivered to older students. A continuum of service delivery models is presented; we maintain that one or more of these models should be used. The selection of a given delivery model is contingent on the need of the student. The chapter provides considerable detail about the comprehensive delivery model for secondary-level students that we constructed, which consists of six components: information dissemination, identification, assessment, program planning, intervention, and follow-up. In addition, the chapter presents indirect service delivery models that show how to work within the educational and environmental systems to change these systems, as opposed to working with the student directly. Modifications of the educational system consists of such aspects as noting the organization of curriculum materials, modifying the teacher's language within the classroom context, restructuring the written language of the textbooks and other printed materials, and using peer tutors. Modifications of the environmental system consist of noting the oral language of others in the student's environment, analyzing the structure of the learning environment outside of school, and determining the attitudes and feeling of those in the student's surroundings.

Chapter 12: Overview of Intervention with Older Students presents an overview of general principles to be used in any given language session with the student. The general intervention principles to note with the older student are to determine the purpose of intervention; establish responsibility for the communication disorder; be prepared to counsel about the communication problems; adjust to the social-cognitive development level of the student; be cognizant of adult learning theory (e.g., active learning remains within one's repertoire far longer than passive learning); establish ground rules for intervention sessions; and hold a class meeting time that includes self-reports, issues, and compliments. The chapter goes on to discuss what to teach by providing an extensive list of potential goals in areas such as thinking, listening, reading, and writing. How to intervene using such principles as mediation and bridging, which are part of mediated learning experiences, is described. Enhancing listening, speaking, reading, and writing is also discussed in some length.

Chapter 13: Specific Intervention Methods lists a number of specific activities that can be selected depending on the student's needs. These activities consist of referential communication, narrative story-telling, expository discourse, word-finding, emotional intelligence enhancement, and social skills. Each of these specific intervention methods includes within them the procedures, materials, areas of emphasis, bridging questions, and strategies to mediate. Particularly noteworthy is the section on emotional intelligence that provides the 5 dimensions and 25 competencies needed to be developed to be proficient in this area, as well as prepared to be successful in school and at work.

Part IV: Transitions of Adolescents consists of two chapters. These chapters provide information on how adolescents must transition into the future and how, as professionals, we must be ever conscious about our evolving roles and the efficacy of our services.

Chapter 14: Transitions to the Future conveys information about transition points in the student's life: elementary to middle school, middle school to high school, and high school to postsecondary life. The chapter describes school-to-work issues as they relate to employment options and to society's old vs. new economy within the information age. Likewise, since some older students with language disorders will go on to postsecondary education, it is important to note the type of transition planning needed, legal accommodations available, and the guide-lines for success in the postsecondary educational system.

Chapter 15: Merging the Futures explains the evolving roles of speech-language pathologists and contrasting generational viewpoints as they impact the scope and practice of the discipline. A survey conducted through the decades summarizes changes in personal preparation related to speech-language services for older students. Also discussed are the issues surrounding both the efficacy and effectiveness of services. A call to action is reiterated so that adolescents with language disorders do not continue to be unserved and underserved, thus wasting an enormous amount of human resources, which are needed if the United States—or any nation—is to compete in the global society.

The *appendixes* provide a wealth of practical tools and forms that are appropriate to use with older students. Some forms are intended to be used by the students themselves, and others are for those who serve them. All appendixes may be duplicated for clinical use with individual students and can easily be printed from the accompanying CD-ROM. It is our hope that by combining such practical resource materials, along with the depth of information in individual chapters to support them, *Communication Solutions for Older Students* can serve as an exemplary text for students and a much-used reference for practicing professionals.

Adolescent Development—
Normal and Disordered

Chapter 1

Adolescence—An Overview

Goals

- Define *adolescence*
- Describe theories of adolescence
- Present a theory of adolescence as it relates to older students with language disorders

Many older students between the ages of 9 and 19 with communication disorders remain undetected, unserved, or underserved and thus unable to realize their human potential (Boyce and Larson, 1983; Ehren, 2002b; Larson and McKinley, 1985a, 1987, 1995; Larson, McKinley, and Boley, 1993; McKinley and Larson, 1985). The financial and psychological costs to society and to the individual are astronomical. We believe that speech-language pathologists and related professionals can help stem these high costs when they understand youth with language disorders and how to best serve their needs.

The focus of our book is primarily on older students who are in the period called adolescence, though we include some information also applicable to preadolescents (approximately ages 9–11) and some to youth past the age of 19. Please note that we use the terms *older students* and *youth* interchangeably throughout this text and that these terms include those in preadolescence as well as those in adolescence.

Definitions of *Adolescence*

Adolescence, derived from the Latin word *adolescere*, means "to grow into maturity"

11

(Turner and Helms, 1979). Adolescents are maturing both biologically and psychologically. They are establishing their identities, making career choices, learning how to think about their thinking, and realizing the potential of adult communication.

The World Health Organization's (WHO's) description of adolescence is well formulated, with recognition of the overlapping definitions of *adolescents, youth,* and *young people.* To eliminate confusion regarding these definitions, WHO (n.d.) distinguished the terms like this:

- Adolescence = 10–19 years
- Youth = 15–24 years
- Young people = 10–24 years

Numerous additional definitions of *adolescence* can be found in the literature: a transitional period between childhood and adulthood (Hartzell, 1984; Lewin, 1939; Turner and Helms, 1979; Whitmire, 2000); a rite of passage into adulthood (Kett, 1977); a time of identity crisis and psychosocial moratorium (Erikson, 1968); a coming of age (Freeman, 1983; Mead, 1950); and the age of commitment and a move toward interdependence (Konopka, 1973). At the root of each of these definitions is the heated debate on whether adolescence is a biological developmental stage or is a sociologically determined developmental period, and thus a product of Western culture (Konopka, 1971). Elder (1975) emphasized that adolescence must be discussed from a sociohistorical perspective (i.e., relative to the current decade or to a specific moment in time). For example, an adolescent growing up in a WWII concentration camp had a very different adolescent experience than one growing up in the United States in a middle-class family today. Furthermore, these same adolescents in the United States today are having a very different experience than those in countries without child labor laws. Thus, adolescents' experiences vary with social, cultural, and historical parameters.

Adolescence as a Developmental Period

We view adolescence, as Lipsitz (1980) and Sheehy (1995) did, as just one of the developmental periods within a person's overall life cycle. Adolescents must be perceived first as unique individuals and second as people going through a period of development called *adolescence.* Adolescence involves biological, sociological, and psychological aspects, and each interacts with the others. No single aspect is sufficient to explain adolescence, but all are necessary; collectively, they may describe adolescence (Lipsitz, 1980).

Biologically, adolescence spans the years between the onset of puberty and the completion of bone growth (Lipsitz, 1980). These rapid bodily changes profoundly affect how adolescents perceive themselves and communicate with others.

Sociologically, adolescence is influenced by cultural values, attitudes, and beliefs, as well as by socioeconomic class and Western society's laws on compulsory education, child labor, and juvenile proceedings (Bakan, 1971). Most societies use functional criteria (e.g., the ability to support oneself) or status criteria (e.g., the acquisition of voting rights) to mark the end of adolescence. These sociocultural dimensions influence society's tolerance range for what is the appropriate time length for "typical adolescence." The more sophisticated a society's technology, the more prolonged the period of adolescence (Eisenberg, 1965).

Psychologically, adolescents attain the ability to think at an abstract level (Inhelder and Piaget, 1958) and to establish a personal identity (Erikson, 1968). Thus, this is a time of accelerated cognitive growth (Alley and Deshler, 1979; H. Epstein, 1978) and of personality formation (Ferguson, 1970). Both of these domains continue to evolve in later stages of adulthood, but at a lesser rate.

The critical aspect of a definition of *adolescence* is that it emphasizes an interrelationship among biological, sociocultural, and psychological dimensions. For example, as people mature physically and thus sexually, they learn, through their culture and social class, a specific sex role, which in turn is made a part of their personality—or it is rejected and may result in some psychological confusion.

In summary, we believe that any cohesive definition of *adolescence* must accommodate the fact that adolescence as a developmental period is constantly changing, contingent on the sociocultural environment and on the function of time. Whitmire (2000) viewed adolescence "as a bridge between childhood and adulthood, qualitatively different from the two life stages that it joins, with its own unique set of interdependent cognitive, linguistic, and social developmental goals" (p. 2).

To select and appropriately apply assessment and intervention procedures for older students with language disorders, speech-language pathologists must understand normal developmental milestones and theories of adolescence. This knowledge will allow such professionals to recognize how the student with a language disorder is similar to or different from an adolescent without a language disorder. To serve as a foundation for making wise decisions about assessment outcomes and intervention protocols, a brief overview of theories of adolescence is presented, followed by more specific data on physical, psychological, and language/cognitive/communication development.

Theories of Adolescence

Knowles; Holton, III; and Swanson (1998) isolate the most salient features of a theory when they state, "A theory is a comprehensive, coherent, and internally consistent system of ideas about a set of phenomena" (p. 10). A theory should unify, relate, and explain diverse phenomena that were previously viewed as separate, unrelated, and unaccountable (Eisner, 1965). Theories provide an explanation of phenomena and guidelines for action (Knowles et al., 1998). In communication sciences and disorders, theories should provide the framework on which procedures are based. In summary, a theory provides a basis for action, a rationale for practice, and a road map for exploring unfamiliar terrain.

In communication sciences

and disorders, theories

should provide the

framework on which

procedures are based.

A number of theorists have contributed to professionals' knowledge of adolescence. How these theorists affect speech-language pathologists' work with adolescents who have language disorders is discussed later in this chapter.

After considering various theories of adolescence, Muuss (1975) isolated the following theoretical viewpoints: biological, anthropological, sociological, and psychological. These major theoretical positions and their theorists or significant contributors are presented in Table 1.1 Each of these theoretical positions has influenced how adolescents are currently viewed. We present in the sections that follow a summary of each of these theories and their implications for educators and clinicians.

Biological Theory

In 1904, Hall perceived adolescence as a period of "sturm und drang" (storm and stress), a myth that remains to the present day. Hall's (1904) recapitulation theory presented adolescence as a genetically predetermined time that corresponds to a turbulent transitional stage in the human race. Today, many people continue to view adolescence as "turbulent" and "transitional," due mainly to the major physiological changes that adolescents experience. Research has not borne out this "storm and stress" period except in a minority of adolescents (Glover, 1999).

According to Hall's (1904) biological theory, environmental influences are limited by a biological clock. P. Miller (1989) stated that the main message of the biological theory for professionals is "that they should be sensitive to when all children as individuals, directed by their own innate growth potential, have reached a state of readiness for acquiring new behaviors...or concepts...via training" (p. 18).

Anthropological Theories

Anthropologists (Benedict, 1954; Mead, 1950) have argued that adolescence is culturally determined. According to Benedict (1954), growth is a gradual, continuous process from infantile dependence to adult independence, unless altered by the culture. The implication in Benedict's and in Mead's work is that Western society has created a

Table 1.1

Theories of Adolescence

Theoretical Viewpoint	Theorist(s)/Significant Contributor(s)	
Biological	Hall (1904)	
Anthropological	Benedict (1954)	Mead (1950)
Sociological	Davis (1944)	Havighurst (1953)
Psychological		
Central European Theories	Kretschmer (1951) Remplein (1956) Zeller (1952)	Kroh (1944) Spranger (1955)
Psychoanalytic Theory	A. Freud (1948) Rank (1936)	S. Freud (1953)
Field Theory	Lewin (1939)	
Social Learning Theory	Bandura and Walters (1963)	N. Miller and Dollard (1941)
Stage Theories		
General Development	Gesell, Ilg, and Ames (1956)	Mitchell (1979)
Identity Development	Erikson (1968)	
Cognitive Development *Piagetian*	Elkind (1974, 1978, 2000) Inhelder and Piaget (1958)	Reuven Feuerstein (1979, 1980) Piaget (1952, 1970)
Information-Processing	Case (1984, 1985) Sternberg (1985)	Fischer (1980)
Moral Development	Kohlberg (1975)	

Sources: Larson and McKinley (1995); Muuss (1975)

phenomenon called *adolescence* and has decreed that this time is filled with stress and turmoil.

An anthropological perspective emphasizes the need to take a more multicultural perspective on adolescent development. According to this theory, educators need to account for and accommodate differences in each adolescent's culture as educational/clinical assessment and intervention strategies are developed.

Sociological Theories

In contrast with the biologists and anthropologists, sociologists have not concerned themselves with whether adolescence is biologically or culturally determined. Instead, the primary contribution of sociologists (Davis, 1944; Havighurst, 1953) has been their description of social development during adolescence. Davis emphasized the emergence of "internalizing socialized anxiety" during adolescence. He postulated that adolescents control their behavior because of their anticipation and fear of punishment. Havighurst emphasized developmental tasks of adolescents, such as achieving a masculine or feminine social role and achieving socially responsible behavior. Both Davis and Havighurst emphasized how social class differences affect expectations of social development.

Sociological theories of adolescent development account for contrasts in adolescents' behavior by social class differences, but how social class differences warrant different educational and clinical approaches has not been investigated.

Psychological Theories

Neither the sociologists nor the psychologists listed in Table 1.1 have debated whether adolescence is primarily determined by biological or cultural factors. Instead, psychologists have attempted to document theories of psychological development, both in personality and cognition, during adolescence.

Psychological theories of adolescent development can be grouped according to Central European theories, psychoanalytic theory, field theory, social learning theory, and stage theories (Larson and McKinley, 1995; Muuss, 1975). Each of these theoretical groups is discussed in the sections that follow, except Central European theories (Kretschmer, 1951; Kroh, 1944; Remplein, 1956; Spranger, 1955; Zeller, 1952), which have had minimal influence on American psychologists and educators.

Psychoanalytic Theory

Sigmund Freud (1953) catalyzed American inquiry into psychoanalytic theory by documenting universal psychosexual stages that he believed to be genetically, not environmentally, determined. Freud believed that character formation during adolescence results from a struggle between two forces: the id (i.e., the biological-instinctual force) and the superego (i.e., the socially oriented force). Anna Freud (1948) placed greater emphasis on adolescent development and the role of puberty in character formation than did her father. Rank (1936), unlike Sigmund and Anna Freud, placed more emphasis on positive human dimensions of creativity and productivity, the conscious ego, and the present than he did on human repression and neurosis, the unconscious ego, and the past.

Field Theory

An alternative explanation of psychological development during adolescence has been offered by field theory (Lewin, 1939). In this theory, adolescence is viewed as a period of transition during which the individual changes group membership. The adolescent belongs partly to the child group and partly to the adult group, without belonging completely to either. Lewin believed that various cultures differ regarding their requirements for changing from the child to the adult group. Muuss (1975), who offered an interpretation of Lewin, noted that the greater the differentiation between the adult group and the child group in a given culture or social class, the more difficult the transition.

Social Learning Theory

A third theory to explain psychological development during adolescence has been offered by social learning theorists (Bandura and Walters, 1963; N. Miller and Dollard, 1941). These theorists attempted to integrate psychoanalytic and behavioristic theories by stressing reliance on environmental events (e.g., imitation of parents, teachers, and peers), rather than biological factors, to explain development. They seem to agree with the anthropologists in that they view adolescence as part of the continuous development from childhood to adulthood, not as a separate stage of development.

Stage Theories

Finally, stage theories attempt to explain psychological development during adolescence (Elkind, 1974, 1978, 2000; Erikson, 1968; Feuerstein, 1979, 1980; Gesell, Ilg, and Ames, 1956; Inhelder and Piaget, 1958; Kohlberg, 1975; Mitchell, 1979; Piaget 1952, 1970). Some theories concentrated attention on general development (Gesell et al., 1956; Mitchell, 1979), while others focused on specific aspects of development, notably identity development (Erikson, 1968), cognitive development (Elkind, 1974, 1978, 2000; Reuven Feuerstein, 1979, 1980; Inhelder and Piaget, 1958; Piaget, 1952, 1970), information processing (Case, 1984, 1985; Fischer, 1980; Sternberg, 1985), and moral development (Kohlberg, 1975). From these stage theories in particular, speech-language pathologists have extrapolated information on adolescents. For this reason, these theories are discussed in greater depth than the preceding theories.

General Development Theory

According to Muuss (1975), Gesell et al.'s (1956) theory of adolescence drew heavily from their general theory of recapitulation. That is, their theory of adolescence incorporated the concept that developmental trends and behavioral traits are biologically determined. Hence, the environment can only stimulate, modify, and support growth; it cannot sequence it.

Gesell et al. (1956) were mainly interested in studying overt behaviors as they are manifested in gradual stages or cycles of development. Their sequential patterns of development oscillate along a spiral course toward maturity: The child begins to master a skill, then reverts to earlier forms of behavior, and then may plateau before completely mastering the new skill and moving forward. Gesell et al. considered adolescence to be a transitional period from childhood to adulthood, with the most important changes occurring within the first five years. They believed that girls go through this period more rapidly than boys.

Mitchell (1979), not a theorist per se, advocated that adolescence covers too many years and too much growth to be considered one developmental period. Instead, Mitchell subdivided adolescence into three stages:

- **Stage I**—the early or child-adolescence stage
- **Stage II**—the middle or adolescence stage
- **Stage III**—the late or adult-adolescence stage

He emphasized the overlap between the upper limits of one age group and the lower limits of the next to indicate that general age clusters are more important than rigid chronological years. The major characteristics in each of his three stages of adolescence are discussed in detail in the context of developmental milestones in Chapter 2.

Identity Development Theory

Erikson (1968) studied with Sigmund and Anna Freud and was influenced by their psychoanalytic training. His theory of identity development, however, goes beyond their theories by encompassing socialization. The main concept in Erikson's theory is the acquisition of an ego-identity, and the most important characteristic of adolescence is identity crisis. Erikson maintained that the adolescent must search out an identity by asking, "Who am I?" Identity, then, is not given by society, nor is it a maturational phenomenon. Identity can be found only through interaction with, and feedback from, other people. Under this theory, peer group conformity is a means of testing roles.

Erikson (1968) also noted that pubescence is a time of rapid bodily changes; hence the identity crisis is partly the result of psychophysiological factors. Erikson believed that personal identity is achieved during adolescence through acceptance of the past, integration of the present, and orientation toward the future in terms of a decision about a career.

Another phenomenon occurring during adolescence is that of a psychosocial moratorium, or an "as if" period, when the adolescent can try on different roles as if not fully committed and accountable. Experimentation with various roles in life can occur without penalty. The moratorium is an essential prerequisite for identity achievement (Erikson, 1968).

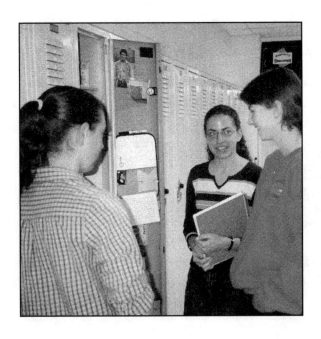

Cognitive Development Theory

Preadolescents and adolescents experience significant cognitive and metacognitive changes. To describe these changes, developmental theorists have taken two general approaches: the Piagetian theory (Elkind, 1974, 1978, 2000; Reuven Feuerstein, 1979, 1980; Inhelder and Piaget 1958; Piaget, 1952, 1970) and the information-processing theory (Case, 1984, 1985; Fischer, 1980; Sternberg, 1985). Both approaches describe cognitive development marked by quantitative and qualitative changes.

Piagetian Theory

Piaget's theory of cognitive development (Piaget and Inhelder, 1958; Piaget, 1952, 1970) has two interrelated aspects: a description of the four periods of development (sensorimotor, preoperational, concrete operational, and formal operational) and an explanation of concepts such as assimilation, accommodation, and equilibrium, which are as applicable to the formal operational period as to the sensorimotor period.

The formal operational period is the most relevant to adolescence. According to Inhelder and Piaget (1958), this period has two stages:

- **Stage IIIA** (approximately ages 11 or 12 to 14 or 15 years)
- **Stage IIIB** (approximately ages 14 or 15 years and upward)

Stage IIIA appears to be a preparatory stage in which the adolescent can handle some formal operations, but in a cumbersome way, and with systematic, rigorous proof. In Stage IIIB, however, the adolescent is capable of performing formal operational tasks in a spontaneous, systematic, rigorous way. In general, in the formal period, adolescents can reason on the basis of verbal propositions, leave the world of reality behind and enter the world of ideas, and think about their thinking.

David Elkind (1974, 1978, 2000) has written extensively on children and adolescents and has done much to popularize Inhelder and Piaget's (1958) theory in the United States. He described two developmental phenomena that emerge at adolescence as a result of higher levels of thinking (summarized in the sidebar on page 20). Elkind's ideas supplement, rather than supplant, Inhelder and Piaget's theory of cognitive development.

The Imaginary Audience

Adolescents, with their newly acquired skill of thinking about what others are thinking of them, act as though they are constantly on stage performing for everyone. The imaginary audience phenomenon is a new form of egocentrism through which adolescents must pass and which was not present earlier in childhood. This phenomenon is more prominent during the early years of adolescence.

The Personal Fable

Adolescents think that they are not like other people. Others might die in a car accident, but they could not; nothing bad could happen to them. The personal fable phenomenon contributes to the risks that adolescents will take—risks not typically taken by children or adults.

Sources: Elkind (1974, 1978, 2000)

Reuven Feuerstein (1979, 1980), who worked with Piaget and expanded his theory, has also made a significant contribution to adolescents with learning problems. His theory of cognitive modifiability holds that the human organism, even one judged to be severely impaired, is capable of change at any age—even if adolescents had inadequate development earlier in life or were exposed to conditions typically considered as barriers to change. Some of these barriers are exogenic (i.e., outside the person, such as poverty or lack of stimulation at early ages), and others are endogenic (i.e., inside the person, such as genetic defects or sensory impairments).

Cognitive modifiability results from direct exposure to stimuli and mediated learning experiences. However, while direct exposure to stimuli may explain some learning, it does not explain the diversity of learning that occurs within different individuals given the same situation. People who have the same biological parents and similar environmental stimuli can turn out to be very different individuals. According to Reuven Feuerstein (1980), differences in mediated learning experiences are the primary way to explain this phenomenon.

In a mediated learning experience, an adult selects and organizes stimuli for the youth (e.g., the adult might select and organize a list of words with specific prefixes and suffixes so that certain word comprehension strategies can be taught). An experience becomes mediated when there is an intention on the part of the adult to focus on an experience and to transmit the meaning of the experience (e.g., the adult explains to the student when understanding prefixes and suffixes is critical, such as in a social situation when distinguishing between judgmental and nonjudgmental behavior). An attempt to generalize the learning should occur. The adult needs to think continually,

"How can I make the adolescent acquire alone what I now need to facilitate?" The cognitive structure of the individual is affected through this process of mediation, and as learning sets are acquired, the capacity to become modified through direct exposure to stimuli increases in efficiency.

According to Reuven Feuerstein (1979, 1980), the more and the earlier that children are subjected to mediated learning experiences, the greater their capacity to be affected by and to learn from direct exposure to stimuli. Adolescents with typical development have had consistent mediated learning experiences, according to Feuerstein, and have benefited from direct exposure to stimuli. In essence, they have learned how to continue learning on their own. Feuerstein's theory maintains that when barriers obstruct learning, they can be overcome or bypassed, thus making it possible to restore a normal pattern of cognitive growth during adolescence. Chapter 12 has an extensive discussion of mediation that elaborates on Feuerstein's theory.

Information-Processing Theory

Developmental theorists who embrace information-processing theories are concerned with how information is taken into the organism, interpreted, represented, transformed, and acted upon (T. Gross, 1985). Three of the more fully developed views are:

- **Neo-Piagetian theory** (Case, 1984, 1985)

- **Skill theory** (Fischer, 1980)

- **Triarchic theory** (Sternberg, 1985)

Neo-Piagetian theory postulates that an executive system governs the way humans process and use information (Case, 1984, 1985; Pascual-Leone, 1980). As children grow, they assemble executive control structures (i.e., a mental plan) for solving various problems. Similar to Piagetian theory (Inhelder and Piaget, 1958; Piaget 1952, 1970), neo-Piagetian theory specifies age-related restrictions on processing capacity (e.g., Case's [1985] stages are 0 to 18 months, 18 months to 5 years, 5 to 11 years, and 11 to 18 years). Four substages of cognitive development during the preadolescent and adolescent years have been proposed by Case (1985): ages 9 to 11 years, 11 to 13 years, 13 to 15 years, and 15 to 18 years. According to neo-Piagetian theory, preadolescents use increasingly complex dimensional operations, and adolescents use increasingly complex and abstract operations.

Skill theory postulates 10 developmental levels that occur in three tiers; sensorimotor, representational, and abstract (Fischer, 1980; Fischer and Corrigan, 1981; Fischer, Hand, and Russell, 1984; Fischer and Pipp, 1984). Levels 1 through 6 occur prior to preadolescence. Preadolescents (i.e., children around the ages of 9 to 11 years) begin to demonstrate Level 7 single abstractions, which is the most primitive form of abstractions. Not until approximately 14 or 15 years of age, according to Fischer et al. (1984), can adolescents coordinate two or more abstractions in a single skill (i.e., Level 8 abstract mapping). Level 9 abstract systems emerge at about age 18 or 19 years, which means the adolescent now understands the complexities of relations between abstractions. Integrating abstract systems to form Level 10 general principles occurs around age 25; individuals at this level are now capable of fully mature organization of such areas as identity, morality, and political ideology.

What sets skill theory apart from Piagetian and neo-Piagetian stage theories is its emphasis on the different paths children and adolescents follow in acquiring skills. Stage theories assume that when a particular stage is reached, most of the skills exist at that level. Skill theories, however, assume that behavior may vary widely across levels below the optimal level, which sets the upper limit on skills. According to skill theory, environmental differences also contribute to the varied paths adolescents follow in acquiring skills. Different experiences

among adolescents lead to unevenness in development (e.g., there is more diversity among high school courses than during elementary years, so a student taking a literature course might show advanced performance in critical reading skills and average performance in chemistry).

Triarchic theory (Sternberg, 1985) does not specify developmental stages or levels. Rather, it describes mechanisms that underlie developmental changes, as well as the three kinds of components involved in intelligent thinking: metacomponents, performance components, and knowledge-acquisition components. Metacomponents (i.e., higher-order executive processes) are used in planning, monitoring, and decision-making and are crucial mechanisms in cognitive development (see the sidebar).

According to Sternberg (1985), a crucial aspect of adolescent thought is the ability to

Metacomponents for Intelligent Thought

- Recognition of the problem to be solved

- Selection of the components that execute the task

- Selection of the mental representations on which the components or strategy can operate

- Selection of a strategy for combining lower order components into a working algorithm for problem solving

- Decision of how to allocate attentional resources

- Awareness of what one has done, what one is doing, and what one still needs to do in problem solving

- Sensitivity to external feedback

Source: Sternberg (1985)

monitor and evaluate the effectiveness of problem-solving strategies. Improved monitoring of the function of the metacomponents also underlies cognitive development during adolescence.

Moral Development Theory

Kohlberg's (1975) theory of moral development was greatly influenced by Piaget's (Inhelder and Piaget, 1958; Piaget, 1952, 1970) cognitive development theory. Kohlberg advanced three levels of moral development: the preconventional or premoral level, the

conventional or moral level, and the post-conventional or autonomous level. Each level is divided into two stages. The conventional level is where most adolescents and many adults function. At this level, the person conforms to authority and obeys laws and social rules. The sidebar summarizes Kohlberg's six stages.

Kohlberg's (1975) theory of moral development incorporates the following principles: Moral stages form an invariant sequence of development, and moral development can terminate at any stage. According to

Stages of Moral Development

The Preconventional Level involves a punishment/reward system.

> **Stage 1**—Punishment-Obedience is defined by the person's judgments based on avoiding punishment or obtaining rewards.

> **Stage 2**—Instrumental Relativist Orientation is determined by the person's judgments based upon reciprocal favors or fulfillment of needs.

The Conventional Level involves social conformity.

> **Stage 3**—Interpersonal Concordance is based on judgments determined by conformity to persons in authority.

> **Stage 4**—Law and Order Orientation is based on judging or obeying laws and social rules.

The Postconventional Level involves humanistic concerns.

> **Stage 5**—Social Contract Orientation is defined as judgments made on the basis of individual rights and standards that have been agreed upon by the whole society.

> **Stage 6**—Universal Ethical Principle Orientation is defined as judgments made on the basis of consequence in accord with ethical principles such as justice and respect for human dignity.

Source: Kohlberg (1975)

Kohlberg, the advancement through the stages of moral reasoning depends on the interplay of three factors: cognitive developmental level, ability to empathize, and cognitive disequilibrium. He also maintains that these stages are universal and cut across cultures and socioeconomic levels.

Kohlberg's (1975) theory has been criticized by several of his colleagues. Siegal (1980) questioned the invariant sequence of the early stages and the methodology that posed moral dilemmas. Gilligan (1982) criticized Kohlberg's theory for failing to consider differences in stages of moral development between boys and girls during early adolescence. In Gilligan's research, young girls have not adhered to the stages postulated by Kohlberg.

Professionals need to be aware of the interaction between thinking skills and moral development and choices. The adolescent is creating a value system from which to operate on a daily basis.

Summary of Psychological Theories

The psychological theories are extremely diverse. Therefore we discuss them with regard to their educational/clinical implications in the following categories: psychoanalytic theory, field theory, social learning theory, and stage theories.

A psychoanalytical theory takes the position that:

(E)ducators can help by not making rules or expectations more frustrating than necessary and by discouraging heavy reliance on defense mechanisms. Educators also can look beyond a problem behavior to the underlying psychological conflict and encourage teenagers to talk about and try to understand their feelings. (P. Miller, 1989, pp. 20–21)

According to field theory, educators should be concerned about environmental factors that affect students' behavior. These factors can include high school class size and number of school clubs available.

Social learning theory maintains that educators must recognize that children learn behaviors by watching others or by having their behavior reinforced by others. Thus, educators are important role models, who can influence and shape adolescents' behavior.

According to stage theories, educators need to be aware of the developmental level of the adolescent. Educators must not skip over stages, but realize that each stage serves as the foundation for the next level of development. Curriculum and other school activities should be designed and implemented in a developmental hierarchy. One of the major thrusts of cognitive stage theorists, in particular, is that educators should look at events and situations from the adolescent's point of view and assess whether the adolescent is cognitively ready to learn a new concept. Adolescents need to be actively involved in the learning process, manipulating developmentally appropriate materials and ideas. As adolescents develop more advanced thinking skills, they are ready to develop a more advanced moral philosophy (P. Miller, 1989).

Summary of Theories of Adolescence

Muuss (1975) compared and contrasted the various theoretical positions, noting disagreements in definitions, characteristics, and general patterns of adolescent development. However, once the older and more extreme theoretical positions (e.g., Hall's (1904) biological theory and the Central European Theories) are eliminated, agreement does exist.

In our review of the literature, we found that all theorists agree on the existence of endocrinological changes during early adolescence and on behavioral changes due to an increase in sexual interests, awarenesses, and tensions. They disagree on the amount of importance placed on the endocrine changes, and on the extent to which the behavioral changes are caused by physiological or sociological events.

Most theorists discuss physiological changes that result in the individual's need to adjust to a new body image, and they view adolescence as a transitional period. The exceptions are those social learning theorists who view human development as a continuous process. A few theorists agree that adolescence is a multistage period of development, but they disagree as to the number, characteristics, and psychological meaning of each of the stages. All theories of adolescence emphasize physical growth, sexual maturation, increased autonomy, and cognitive sophistication (Lipsitz, 1980). The various theoretical positions collectively postulate that adolescence is a time of rapid physiological and psychological changes influenced by sociocultural determinants.

Coping with Different Theories of Adolescence

When confronted with varying theoretical perspectives, a professional is faced with choosing one of the following options. We would urge the last choice because it takes the best from various theories and then creates a comprehensive and synthesized perspective of adolescence.

Ignore all theories—This option has been advocated by professionals who believe theories are too impractical, abstract, and obtuse to be of any clinical value. Perhaps this attitude is responsible for the lack of a theoretical framework in many tests and educational materials. For example, when critiquing standardized tests and commercial intervention programs used with adolescents, we discovered how frequently professionals either do not state, or do not have, a theoretical model on which they base their test or program. However, stating the theory or theories upon which a test or program is based is essential for providing a rationale as to why it was developed and why it should be used. Knowles (1973) supports this view with the following statement:

> There is a cliché in the applied social sciences, often attributed to Kurt Lewin, that nothing is as practical as a good theory to enable you to make choices confidently and consistently, and to explain or defend why you are making the choices you make. (p. 93)

Select one theory—Another option is to conclude that one theory is the most appropriate, regardless of any conflicting evidence. Picking one theory may be initially advantageous in that it might minimize confusion. The disadvantage is that this option reflects a rigid position and may be erroneous, thus resulting in negative consequences. The state of the art is such that concepts, assumptions, and hypotheses about adolescents are constantly changing; therefore, a single theoretical position may result in a narrow perspective of the problem and the assessment and intervention procedures.

Select one theory for research and another for clinical application—This option is selected by professionals who view research and clinical application as opposing or mutually exclusive entities. Individuals are seen not as whole people, but as fragments to be either investigated or treated. Selecting one theory for research and another for clinical application creates false dichotomies

within a discipline. This results in researchers and clinicians failing to communicate and work cooperatively for the benefit of the person with a communication disorder.

Select precepts from a variety of theories and develop a more comprehensive, synthesized perspective—Currently, no one theory exists to account for the wide array of adolescent behaviors that require a speech-language pathologist's assessment and intervention. For example, cognitive functions of adolescents may be accounted for by one theory, while syntactic and semantic features may be accounted for by other theories.

Although selecting precepts from a variety of theories may be time consuming, this alternative may ultimately prove to be the most effective. The selection of precepts, when thought through carefully, avoids a superficial eclecticism. If professionals select this option of incorporating features from a variety of prevailing theories into a unified whole, they must do so in a systematic fashion to guarantee compatibility and consistency among the various theoretical constructs. For example, according to Lipsitz (1980), one of the problems of categorizing adolescence into a biological, anthropological, sociological, or psychological camp is that there is little dialogue among these disciplines. Each theoretical position is insufficient by itself, but each may be necessary when developing a comprehensive theoretical perspective of adolescence.

In conclusion, nothing is as practical as a good theory to provide a rationale as to why professionals are doing what they are doing. If professionals do not spend the necessary time building a theoretical perspective into research and clinical services, the result will be a confusing, invalid, and unreliable foundation from which to derive assessment and intervention strategies.

The Theoretical Tenets Underlying This Text

As authors who have focused for many years on the topic of adolescents with language disorders, we chose the last option presented above (i.e., to select precepts from a variety of theories and develop a more comprehensive, synthesized perspective) when developing the theoretical base for this text. No one theoretical position adequately explains what we believe about adolescents.

Our theory of adolescence holds that both biological and environmental factors influence adolescent development, although environmental factors may be stronger. This viewpoint has been influenced by Reuven Feuerstein (1979, 1980), who has documented bringing some individuals to near normal levels of functioning, despite negatively loaded genetics or disadvantaged socioeconomic backgrounds, by bombarding them with mediated learning experiences.

Adolescence involves unique and genetically predetermined bodily changes (e.g., puberty) to which the American culture has had different responses across racial and socioeconomic strata. For example, in some lower and middle socioeconomic strata, adolescence marks the time when children are expected to contribute significantly to family finances by getting a job or working in the family business; in some middle or higher socioeconomic strata, adolescents are not expected to work, but rather are sent away to private high schools to better prepare themselves for future careers. These responses constantly change as new generations of adults seek to improve their communication with adolescents. We believe that adolescence is a major developmental period within the life cycle, filled with its own unique challenges and stressful moments, but no more than other developmental periods have. Nor is adolescence any more "transitional" than are the periods from infancy to toddlerhood to childhood. It can be said that any period of time in human development is transitional (Sheehy, 1981, 1995).

[A]dolescence is a major developmental period within the life cycle, filled with its own unique challenges and stressful moments, but no more than other developmental periods have.

27

Communication Solutions
for Older Students

We concur with Muuss (1975), who argued that adolescence manifests both continuous and stagelike patterns. Adolescence is continuous (i.e., part of a continuum from infancy to adulthood), but there are stages within the adolescent period (i.e., early, middle, and late; see Chapter 2, pages 33–35, for more information on stages according to Mitchell (1979)). Furthermore, professionals should be guided in their assessment and intervention decisions by a student's stage of adolescence.

We extrapolate from the psychological theories of Inhelder and Piaget (1958) and Reuven Feuerstein (1979, 1980) when making decisions about cognitive functioning of adolescents. This cognitive functioning, in turn, influences intervention procedures.

Adolescents at lower cognitive levels will probably need more concrete, hands-on activities; adolescents at higher levels may participate in communication activities requiring abstract reasoning.

Finally, we have observed that the physical development of adolescents influences their psychosocial development and, in turn, these two domains affect communication development. It would be artificial to assume that only biological or only environmental factors affect the adolescent's overall development. Rather, a combination of developmental factors, both biological and environmental, occurs simultaneously. These developmental milestones during adolescence are presented in the next chapter.

Points of Discussion

1. How does your own comprehensive theory of adolescence interact with your theory(ies) of cognition, language, and communication development?

2. Why are well-developed theoretical tenets important to the assessment and intervention of older students with language disorders?

Suggested Readings

Muuss, R. (1975). *Theories of adolescence.* New York: Random House.

Sheehy, G. (1995). *New passages: Mapping your life across time.* New York: Random House.

Chapter 2

Developmental Milestones during Adolescence

Goals

- Provide an overview of typical physical and psychological development
- Summarize information on typical cognitive development and its relationship to language and communication development
- Describe conceptual development during adolescence
- Define critical thinking and intellectual standards that apply across all curricula

Physical Development

Adolescence is a time when children experience physical changes (Gullotta, Adams, and Markstrom, 2000; Hamburg, 1992). Early adolescence involves a more rapid period of physical growth than any other period in life, including infancy and early childhood (Lipsitz, 1979).

Professionals working with adolescents need to be cognizant of how preoccupied adolescents can be with their own bodily changes. For example, the adolescent who is late in making bodily changes may feel uncomfortable being grouped with peers who have already begun those changes. Adolescents, desiring peer conformity, do not easily tolerate noticeable developmental differences in others. Thus, adolescents with an obvious physical disability, delayed development, or accelerated development are often at a disadvantage when it comes to peer acceptance and peer popularity. Recall from Chapter 1 the developmental phenomenon of the imaginary audience that Elkind (1974, 1978, 2000) describes as prominent during adolescence (see the sidebar on page 20).

Failure by professionals to recognize the impact of physical development can undermine attempts to communicate with adolescents. Professionals need to empathize with the growing pains present during adolescence.

Failure by professionals

to recognize the impact of

physical development

can undermine attempts

to communicate with

adolescents.

During adolescence, pronounced bodily changes take place because of the presence of testosterone in males and estrogen in females. This time of rapid biological growth, which gives way to the first indications of sexual maturity, is known as *puberty* (Turner and Helms, 1979). Other factors of puberty can be seen in the sidebar. Puberty now begins earlier than it used to, probably because of better nutrition and fewer serious infections (Hamburg, 1992).

Part of the bodily changes that take place during adolescence includes brain growth. H. Epstein (1974, 1978) studied brain growth stages and concluded that five stages exist (i.e., 3 to 10 months, 2 to 4 years, 6 to 8 years, 10 to 12 years, and 14 to 16-plus years). Epstein recognized the first four stages as coinciding with mental growth described by Inhelder and Piaget's (1958) periods of cognitive development.

Puberty Factors

- An adolescent growth spurt (which can occur in the individual with variations in onset, intensity, magnitude, and duration, resulting in an increase in the skeleton, muscles, and viscera); usually lasts 2–3 years, with gains in height of up to 4 inches a year

- Changes in body composition, such as bone, fat, and muscles

- A sex-specific growth rate, varying between the sexes and leading to differences in body dimensions

- Development of the adult reproductive system and secondary sex characteristics

- Emotional changes brought about by hormone changes, resulting in strong emotions or extra sensitivities that have not existed before

Sources: Health Strategies (2002); Tanner (1974)

H. Epstein (1974, 1978) further hypothesized a fifth stage of brain growth (i.e., 14 to 16-plus years) that has no identifiable counterpart in Inhelder and Piaget's (1958) periods of cognitive development. However, Arlin (1975) reported that such a cognitive period does exist, having its onset between 14 and 16 years of age. Why is this important? H. Epstein and Toepfer (1978) have speculated that the adjustment problems and the social and educational difficulties of middle school students may be tied to a brain-related growth plateau. (These difficulties have been commonly blamed on sexual maturation.) During brain growth spurts, however, older students may be more capable of learning behaviors that previously eluded them.

Adolescents appear to be self-conscious about their bodily changes whether they physically mature early or late. Generally, those who mature early are found to be more adept in overall social adjustments than those who mature late (Turner and Helms, 1979). And boys appear to be more affected by the timing of maturation than girls (Papalia and Olds, 1975). A discussion of adolescent physical development is incomplete without acknowledging its interaction with psychological development.

Psychological Development

Psychological development can be considered from various perspectives. Psychological development can be viewed by examining developmental tasks, developmental stages, and self-concept and self-esteem.

Developmental Tasks

Preadolescents and adolescents face a specific set of developmental tasks as they approach maturity. Some of these tasks begin during childhood and continue into adolescence, whereas others are primarily a concern of adolescence (P. Miller, 1989). Each developmental task involves some degree of problem solving and personal decision making.

Developmental tasks are interrelated and not mutually exclusive. Progress in one task results in progress in another. For example, cognitive development assists in moral development and thus begins the building of a value system that will be applied to various aspects of one's life. Failure to acquire the developmental tasks of adolescence will result in arrested psychological development. P. Miller (1989) presents a broad perspective of adolescent developmental tasks in the sidebar on page 34, and Adams, Montemayor, and Gullotta (1989) add more specificity to the tasks in Table 2.1, on page 36.

Developmental Stages

Mitchell (1979) suggested (and we concur) that adolescence be viewed in stages. Recall from Chapter 1 that according to Mitchell, adolescence spans too many years and too much growth to be considered one developmental period. Thus, he subdivides adolescence into three stages:

Developmental Tasks of Adolescence

- Develop a sense of self-identity that is a unique combination of values, attitudes, beliefs, and behaviors

- Adapt to a physically changing body, as well as make psychological adjustments, including gender identity

- Develop a more abstract thought process about the physical world, as well as the social world of people, events, and social structures

- Acquire interpersonal skills that will allow building strong relationships with people of the same and opposite sex

- Establish a new relationship with family members that is the result of needing autonomy and having less emotional dependence, while still needing psychological and financial support

- Formulate a personal value system that guides decision making and interpersonal interactions

- Set goals for future achievement in terms of education, career, marriage, and so on

---

Source: P. Miller (1989)

- **Stage I**—the early or child-adolescence stage

- **Stage II**—the middle or adolescence stage

- **Stage III**—the late or adult-adolescence stage

Mitchell uses chronological age clusters for each stage, but recognizes the overlap between the upper limits of one age group and the lower limits of the next. This was done intentionally, to indicate that general age clusters are more important than rigid chronological years. Note that Mitchell extends adolescence to age 20 (in contrast to the World Health Organization's (WHO's, n.d.) definition of *adolescence* as ranging from 10 to 19 years). The following describes each stage in more detail.

Stage I—Early (or Child) Adolescence

Chronological ages for Stage I are 10 through 13 years for girls and 12 through 14 years for boys. This developmental stage is dominated by body growth spurts in height and weight and in primary and secondary sex characteristics. As a result of rapid bodily growth, the psychological response of the adolescent is one of concern about how the body looks and feels. These individuals are childlike and limited in their emotional range. Of the three stages, this is the time the adolescent is the most egocentric.

Socially, the peer group exerts influence, but the home and family remain the most important social and emotional factors in the adolescent's life. Moral outlook is at the conventional level (i.e., social conformity; Kohlberg, 1975). The future carries less importance during this stage than it does during the next two stages.

Stage II—Middle Adolescence (or Adolescence)

Characteristics exhibited during this developmental stage most closely reflect the typical image of adolescents. The individual in this stage is neither a child nor an adult (Mitchell, 1979). Chronological ages for both boys and girls in this stage include 13, 14, 15, and 16 years. Physical growth continues, but not at as rapid a pace as during early adolescence. Mental growth increases dramatically: It is now more abstract, theoretical, and idealistic. Because of the mental growth factor, the person shows more awareness of the outside world, engages in introspection, and experiences an increase in self-doubt. Along with introspection, idealism is tested. The adolescent is more interested in the opposite sex, and dating is more common than during early adolescence. The individual's social life is primarily with peers. This is the time in which Erikson's (1968) psychosocial moratorium (i.e., the "as if" period, when the adolescent can try on different roles as if not fully committed and accountable) is most likely to take place.

Stage III—Late (or Adult) Adolescence

The ages for both boys and girls in this developmental stage are 16 through 20 years (Mitchell, 1979). Physically and mentally, these individuals are adults and have achieved most of their adult growth. However, in terms of their social roles, they remain primarily adolescents. In Western society, Stage III is more a social phenomenon than a biological fact (Mitchell). During this stage, sexual intimacy increases and the person is more capable of dealing with interpersonal complexities. In addition, the individual becomes increasingly concerned about the future.

Mitchell (1979) suggests that the differences between early and late adolescence are profound, and that professionals should treat these differences with more respect. This is a critical concept to keep in mind when planning assessment and intervention. Table 2.1 summarizes the developmental tasks described by Adams, Montemayor, and Gullotta (1989) and the developmental stages described by Mitchell.

Self-Concept and Self-Esteem

Self-concept refers to the attributes that the individual believes characterize himself or herself (i.e., "Who am I?"). *Self-esteem* refers to the evaluative notions that one holds about oneself (i.e., "How do I feel about myself?"; Suls, 1989).

Characteristics of Tasks and Stages
of Typical Adolescence

Table 2.1

Developmental Task	Stage of Typical Adolescence		
	Early (10–13F; 12–14M)	**Middle (13–16)**	**Late (16–20)**
Acceptance of the Physical Changes of Puberty	• Physical changes occur rapidly but with wide range of person-to-person variability • Self-consciousness, insecurity, and worry about being different from peers	• Pubertal changes almost complete for girls; boys still undergoing physical changes • Girls more confident; boys more awkward	• Adult appearance, comfortable with physical changes • Physical strength continues to increase, especially for males
Attainment of Independence	• Changes of puberty distinguish early adolescents from children, but do not provide independence • Ambivalence (childhood dependency unattractive, but unprepared for the independence of adulthood) leads to vacillation between parents and peers for support	• Ability to work, drive, date; appearance of more maturity; dependency lessens and peer bonds increase • Conflict with authority, limit testing, experimental and risk-taking behaviors at a maximum	• Independence a realistic social expectation • Continuing education, becoming employed, getting married—all possibilities that often lead to ambivalence about independence
Emergence of a Stable Identity	• Am I OK? Am I normal? • How do I fit into my peer group? • Paradoxical loss of identity in becoming a member of a peer group	• Who am I? • How am I different from other people? • What makes me special or unique?	• Who am I in relation to other people? • What is my role with respect to education, work, sexuality, community, religion, and family?
Development of Cognitive Patterns	• Concrete operational thought: present more real than future; concrete more real than abstract • Egocentrism • Personal fable • Imaginary audience	• Emerging formal operations: abstractions, hypotheses, and thinking about future; personal interests and identity emerging	• Formal operations: thinking about the future, things as they should be, and options; consequences can be considered

Sources: Adams, Montemayor, and Gullotta (1989); Elkind (1974); Inhelder and Piaget (1958); Mitchell (1979)

Self-concept in older students shifts from an emphasis on the social exterior to psychological elements (Rosenberg, 1986). To illustrate, when Montemayor and Eisen (1977) asked youth in grades 4, 6, 8, 10, and 12 to answer "Who am I?" in 20 words or less, the younger subjects (those in grades 4, 6, and 8) described themselves in these categories: possessions; physical, self-body image; and territoriality (where they lived). In contrast, older subjects (like those in grades 10 and 12) described themselves in terms of internal beliefs and standards and stable personality traits. These changes in self-concept are gradual (Suls, 1989).

Self-esteem can be treated as a global concept (i.e., the overall evaluation of oneself either in positive or negative terms), as a domain-specific concept (i.e., one's perceived worth academically, socially, athletically, etc.), or both. Children show relative stability in global self-esteem between ages 8 and 11 years, lower scores between 12 and 14 years, and a rise again from ages 15 to 18 years (Harter and Connell, 1984; Rosenberg, 1979). Self-esteem continues to rise during the five years after high school (ages 18 to 23 years) as well (O'Malley and Bachman, 1983).

In discussing the dip in self-esteem during early adolescence, Suls (1989) concluded that the transition from elementary to middle school is a time of uncertainty, particularly for girls, as they "sort out" their position in a new school. As an aside, Simmons, Blyth, Van Cleave, and Bush (1979), when studying children in a K–8 school, found no decrease in self-esteem when the shift from sixth to seventh grade did not involve a change in schools. This finding has major implications for how schools are structured for preadolescents and adolescents and for how transitions are orchestrated. (We address these transitions further in Chapter 14.) Beyond physical and psychological development, a discussion of cognitive development is also important.

Cognitive Development

Cognition is the mental organization of experience. Cognition subsumes thinking, which is the application of cognition for a purpose (e.g., reasoning, judging, analyzing, recalling, inferring, imagining, and problem solving).

In general, the cognitive developmental changes that occur from childhood to adolescence can be summarized as follows:

- A growing ability to think about one's own thinking (metacognition)

- The ability to consider events removed in time or space, real or imagined

- The ability to consider all possible alternatives to a problem or situation

- The ability to formulate hypotheses and test them

- The ability to engage in deductive and inductive reasoning

- The ability to talk about their talking (metalinguistics)

Metacognition involves knowing what one knows, and what needs to be known, to achieve a goal (Wallach and L. Miller, 1988); it refers to a collection of means by which individuals assess the successes and failures of their problem-solving strategies (Flavell, 1976, 1977). Use of "meta-" abilities is optional (i.e., people choose whether or not to use their metacognitive and metalinguistic abilities). When they are needed, they are invoked (James, 1990). Metalinguistic awareness depends on linguistic knowledge.

The development of metacognitive and metalinguistic abilities is marked by increases in children's ability to engage in deliberate, controlled mental activities (Hakes, 1980). Metalinguistic abilities show their greatest development during middle childhood (i.e., 4 to 8 years of age; Hakes). However, development continues through adolescence.

The connection between cognition and language is open to debate. Rice (1983) provided a summary of the range of hypotheses about the relationship between cognition and language to which professionals might ascribe (see the sidebar).

Theorists, such as Piaget (1952, 1970) and Vygotsky (1962), supporting the different hypotheses summarized in the sidebar have cited varying levels of linguistic competence and varying kinds of linguistic phenomena. The hypotheses that emphasize the strength of cognition focus on the earlier stages of language acquisition. Those hypotheses that emphasize linguistic influence tend to be based on later stages. In essence, the cognition and language relationship may vary as a function of age, type of cognitive task, and linguistic ability (Rice, 1983; Schlesinger, 1977).

Potential Relationships between Cognition and Language

- **Strong cognition hypothesis**–Cognition precedes and accounts for language acquisition.

- **Local homologies hypothesis**–Simultaneous emergence of parallel cognitive and linguistic knowledge.

- **Interaction hypothesis**–Language and cognition mutually influence each other's development.

- **Cognition-anchored-in-language hypothesis**–Concepts are unstable until anchored with linguistic forms.

- **Weak cognition hypothesis**–Cognition does not account for all language development.

- **Mental-processes-not-rooted-in-meanings hypothesis**–Language disorders are associated with perceptual processing, memory problems, or both.

Source: Rice (1983)

Of the six primary possible relationships, our stance centers around the interaction hypothesis. For older students, we maintain that cognition influences language but that language—both oral and written—influences the development of cognitive skills. This position is also supported by such professionals as Lahey (1990); Cromer (1994); K. Cole, Mills, and Kelley, 1994; and Bellugi, Marks, Bihrle, and Sabo (1993).

For older students,

we maintain that cognition

influences language but

that language—both oral

and written—influences

the development of

cognitive skills.

Rhea Paul (2001) presents Rice's (1983) potential relationships between cognition and language as part of a discussion on discrepancy-based criteria for caseload selection. That is, do you serve students if their cognitive level is at or below their language level? Some would say no. We, however, would say yes because we believe that language can influence cognition, just as cognition can influence language.

Piagetian View

An abundance of research studies, journal articles, and book chapters have debated the existence of Piaget's (Inhelder and Piaget, 1958) formal operational thought during adolescence, as well as who engages in such thinking, when, and under what experimental conditions (Berzonsky, 1978; Elkind, 1975; Ellsworth and Sindt, 1991; Hains and D. Miller, 1980; Kamhi and Lee, 1988; Lawson and Wollman, 1976; Leadbeater and Dionne, 1981; Martorano, 1977; Neimark, 1979; Overton and Meehan, 1982). Formal operational thought includes the ability to reason systematically and logically about abstract ideas, which may have no basis in reality.

Formal operational thinking begins to emerge between 12 and 15 years. Several studies found that adolescents apply formal operational thought in some contexts, but not in others (Bart, 1971; Martorano, 1977). Adolescents of average intellectual ability probably attain formal operations, but do not apply them equally to all aspects of reality (Elkind, 1975). For example, formal operational thought may be applied in English literature but not in chemistry. Some researchers found that the transition from concrete to formal operational thought may never be complete across all content areas and that as many as half of the adults in the United States either do not engage in formal operational thought, or do so only in their field of expertise (Ellsworth and Sindt, 1991; Labinowicz, 1980; Lawson and Wollman, 1976).

Elkind (1975) found that adolescent boys consistently outperform girls in traditional Piagetian tasks requiring application of formal operational thought. However, he found that adolescent girls are more likely to apply their formal operational thinking to interpersonal matters, perhaps for social role reasons. Martorano (1977) found that mean scores on formal operational tasks completed by girls increased consistently during grades 6 through 12.

Other researchers found no gender differences when formal operational tasks were attempted (Jackson, 1965; Killian, 1979; Kishta, 1979). Overton and Meehan (1982) found that learned helplessness,

the perception of a lack of control over response outcomes, combined with feminine gender roles, resulted in inconsistent formal operational deficits. However, with most tasks presented during their research, no gender differences were found. Table 2.2 summarizes the percentage of students at each cognitive level found by H. Epstein (1979) at each age level.

Thus, while research on attaining formal operational thought would indicate that most adolescents achieve hypothetic-deductive reasoning in some situations, in a few individuals and in some settings, abstract thinking does not occur. Empirical research indicates that to expect formal

Table 2.2

Percentage of Students at Each Cognitive Level

Age (in years)	Preoperational	Concrete Onset	Concrete Mature	Formal Onset	Formal Mature
5	85	15			
6	60	35	5		
7	35	55	10		
8	25	55	20		
9	15	55	30		
10	12	52	35	1	
11	6	49	40	5	
12	5	32	51	12	
13	2	34	44	14	6
14	1	32	43	15	9
15	1	14	53	19	13
16	1	15	54	17	13
17	3	19	47	19	12
18	1	15	50	15	19

From "Cognitive Growth and Development," by H.J. Epstein, 1979, *Colorado Journal of Educational Research, 19*,(1), pp. 4–5. © 1979 by Herbert J. Epstein. Reprinted with permission.

operational thought to occur consistently within the adolescent population, across a variety of contexts, is unrealistic. In consideration of H. Epstein's (1979) findings, teachers of secondary curricula in American schools should not expect formal operational thought across all content areas. Yet, secondary-level curricula tend to demand formal operational thought.

Empirical research indicates that to expect formal operational thought to occur consistently within the adolescent population, across a variety of contexts, is unrealistic.

Ellsworth and Sindt (1991) addressed this mismatch between school curricula and cognitive levels of preadolescents and adolescents, which indicate that the majority of students fail to perform the abstract thinking tasks required in the curricula. Ellsworth and Sindt reason that students still graduate from high school, despite their lack of abstract reasoning, because teachers sense that the majority of their students do not have the reasoning abilities to succeed in the established curriculum and accommodate these students by providing lower level tasks (e.g., testing memory for facts rather than application of ideas).

Higher level language behaviors have had an uncertain relationship with formal operational thought. Piaget's (1952, 1959) view that the level of cognitive development is not dependent on concurrent language development has been supported by empirical research (Davelaar, 1977; P. Jones, 1972). Performance on formal operational reasoning tasks, for example, has not been found to be related significantly to subordinate clause use or to tentative statement use such as "it looks like" (Davelaar). D. Rosenthal (1979), however, found a relationship between formal operational thought and use of dimensional language. Concrete operational thinkers describe events by using comparatives and superlatives (e.g. "it's longer" or "it's the longest"), while formal operational thinkers cite the most general statement possible (e.g., "The most important thing is the length of the string"). Kamhi and Lee (1988) summarized the debate: "It is generally agreed that language plays a more important role in thinking as children get older" (p. 155).

Inductive Reasoning/Analogies

According to Nippold (1998) "analogical (inductive) reasoning occurs when an individual perceives similarities and differences between objects or events and uses that information to solve problems or to learn about the world" (p. 59). Performance on verbal analogies (e.g., *A* is to *B* as *C* is to <u>what</u>?) improves during adolescence. The improvements are in such areas as "increased speed and accuracy in reaching solutions, greater use of systematic problem-solving strategies, enhanced comprehension of semantically and structurally complex problems, becoming more adept at explaining and defending their solutions to analogy problems" (Nippold, pp. 59–60).

Piaget, Montangero, and Billeter (1977) noted that it was not until the formal operational period that students successfully completed most of the analogies without a trail-and-error strategy. Reuven Feuerstein (1979) investigated the relationship of chronological age and cognitive level to verbal analogical reasoning and found the following mean accuracy scores at each age level:

8-year-olds had 23 % correct responses
9-year-olds had 60% correct responses
10-year-olds had 72% correct responses
11-year-olds had 75% correct responses
12-year-olds had 87% correct responses
13-year-olds had 89% correct responses
14-year-olds had 91% correct responses

For adolescents with cognitive disabilities, a mean score of 57% was obtained compared to a mean score for the older (ages 12 to 14 years) adolescents with typical development of 89%.

Armour-Thomas and Allen (1990) researched the relationship between verbal analogical reasoning and high and low academic achievers in ninth grade (ages 14 and 15 years). In all types of analogies, the high achievers (mean score = 84%) outperformed the low achievers (mean score = 63%). This discrepancy is predictable and explains some of the academic challenges of students with low achievement.

Sternberg and Nigro (1980) studied the influence of semantics on verbal analogical reasoning and found that functional (*time* is to *clock* as *weight* is to *scale*) and antonymous (*clear* is to *cloudy* as *shallow* is to *deep*) analogies were easier than synonymous (*weep* is to *cry* as *smile* is to *grin*), sequential (*Tuesday* is to *Sunday* as *Friday* is to *Wednesday*) and categorical (*shirt* is to *clothing* as *hammer* is to *tools*) analogies. The students' performance improved with age with mean accuracy scores as follows:

9-year-olds had 72% correct responses
12-year-olds had 78% correct responses
15-year-olds had 83% correct responses
18-year-olds had 92% correct responses

Students continue to be challenged well into adolescence by classic four-part analogies when the problems contain more difficult words (Cashen, 1989). Using low-moderate-, and high-level problems (based on the difficulty of the words used), Cashen reported a mean accuracy score for each grade for each of these three problem sets respectively as follows:

Grade 5   = 90%, 73%, 42%
Grade 8   = 95%, 85%, 59%
Grade 11 = 95%, 93%, 66%

Nippold (1994) studied third-order analogies—that is, [(A : B :: C : D) :: (A : B :: C : D)]—in students who were 10, 12, 14, and 16 years of age and found that performance steadily improved through age 14 and then plateaued. The mean accuracy score for each age group was as follows:

> 10-year-olds had 59% correct responses
> 12-year-olds had 73% correct responses
> 14-year-olds had 88% correct responses
> 16-year-olds had 86% correct responses

Given the semantic difficulty of these analogies, the order of increasing difficulty was functional, categorical, antonymous, synonymous, then sequential.

In summary, analogical reasoning improves with age through adolescence, but there is a wide range of competence within age groups. The most successful students are those who have higher cognitive levels, greater academic achievement, and a more reflective problem-solving style, as well as increased word and world knowledge (Nippold, 1998).

(A)nalogical reasoning

improves with age through

adolescence, but

there is a wide range

of competence within

age groups.

Deductive Reasoning/Syllogisms

According to Nippold (1998), "a syllogism is a form of argument that contains two premises and a conclusion that follows logically from those premises" (p. 73). She noted that developmental studies reveal improvement in syllogisms throughout the school-age and adolescent years. For example, Sternberg (1980) investigated changes in accuracy as a function of age. Mean accuracy scores improved with age as follows:

> 8-year-olds had 60% correct responses
> 10-year-olds had 75% correct responses
> 13-year-olds had 77% correct responses
> 15-year-olds had 82% correct responses
> 16-year-olds had 84% correct responses

Nippold (1998) also cited a study by Taplin, Staudenmayer, and Taddonio (1974) that revealed that valid (i.e., logical connections between premises) and invalid (illogical connections between premises) syllogisms are difficult to understand, even by late adolescents. Performance does improve some by age, as indicated by the following mean accuracy scores:

> 9-year-olds had 39% correct responses
> 11-year-olds had 44% correct responses
> 13-year-olds had 45% correct responses
> 15-year-olds had 54% correct responses
> 17-year-olds had 63% correct responses

Roberge and Paulus (1971) examined how older students responded to categorical vs. *if-then* conditional syllogisms. The results were mean accuracy scores for 9, 11, 13, and 15 years, respectively, of 43%, 45%,

54%, and 63% for categorical syllogisms and 42%, 41%, 56%, and 59% for *if-then* conditional syllogisms.

Using subjects aged 7, 9, 11, 13, 17, and 19 years, Sternberg (1979) researched performance on five types of syllogisms. Combining all subjects, mean accuracy scores indicated this performance for the five syllogism types: conjunctive syllogisms (69%) were easiest, followed by exclusive disjunctive syllogisms (35%), *only-if* conditional (21%), biconditional (20%), inclusive disjunctive (6%), and *if-then* conditional (6%). The mean accuracy scores organized by age were as follows:

7-year-olds had 8% correct responses
9-year-olds had 17% correct responses
11-year-olds had 24% correct responses
13-year-olds had 31% correct responses
17-year-olds had 44% correct responses
19-year-olds had 57% correct responses

Similar to analogical reasoning, deductive reasoning improves with age. However, even at the upper age ranges, accuracy scores are much lower than for inductive reasoning.

Taxonomy of Educational Objectives

Any discussion of cognition would be incomplete without mention of the taxonomy of educational objectives, which began as a seminal work by Bloom, Engelhart, Furst, Hill, and Krathwohl (1956). As relevant today as when it was first created, the taxonomy serves as a classification device for educational objectives related to the cognitive domain. It was intended to facilitate communication among educators to aid in defining such vague terms as *thinking* and *problem solving*. Bloom stated, "What we are classifying is the intended behavior of students—the ways in which individuals are to act, think, or feel as the result of participating in some unit of instruction" (p. 12).

Bloom et al.'s (1956) taxonomy is organized into six major levels within the cognitive domain:

- **Knowledge**—Remembering (through either recall or recognition) ideas, material, or phenomena

- **Comprehension**—Knowing what has been communicated and making use of the material or ideas contained within the communication

- **Application**—Selecting the appropriate abstraction (theory, principle, idea, rule, or method) suitable to a problem that is new, but similar to, past problems presented

- **Analysis**—Breaking material into its constituent parts, determining the relationships among the elements, and recognizing the organizational principles

- **Synthesis**—Combining parts and elements from various sources to make a whole (creatively but within limits set by particular problems or materials)

- **Evaluation**—Making judgments about the value (for some purpose) of ideas, works, solutions, methods, and so on

The taxonomy is hierarchical (i.e., the objectives in one level are built on the behaviors found in the preceding levels). Table 2.3 illustrates the six levels along with the types of questions that can be used to ascertain students' levels of understanding. These levels can be helpful as professionals determine curricula relative to students' cognitive performance. In examining textbooks for adolescents, one can quickly recognize that all six of Bloom et al.'s (1956) levels within the cognitive domain are part of the expectations within middle and high school curricula.

Conceptual Development

The adolescent's conceptual ability is more flexible than that of the child's, as conceptual orientation in adolescents can shift back and forth between abstract-categorical

Table 2.3 **Overview of Bloom et al.'s (1956) Taxonomy**

Level	Definition	Questions/Tasks
Given Information		
Knowledge	Remember given information	Who? Which? What? When? How many?
Comprehension	Grasp meaning and abstract patterns to explain meaning	How? Why? Explain. Describe. Give an example.
Beyond Given Information		
Application	Apply information to new, related situations by analogy	What if? Tell what. Name some other.
Analysis	Take information apart for similarities and differences	What's wrong with? Why? What are some of the causes?
Synthesis	Create, invent, bring concepts and ideas together in problem solving	How are...alike or different? Suppose. How else? How can you improve? Predict. Design. What if?
Evaluation	Judge and evaluate according to social, academic, or other criteria	What's best or worst? What do you feel? Think about. Why?

From *The Learning Ladder* (p. 10), by E.H. Wiig and C.C. Wilson, 2002, Eau Claire, WI: Thinking Publications. © 2002 by Elisabeth H. Wiig and Carolyn C. Wilson. Reprinted with permission.

Communication Solutions for Older Students

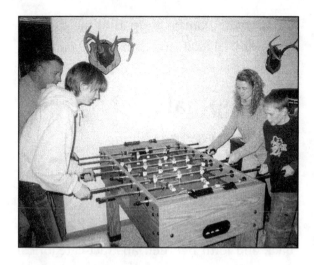

and perceptual orientations (Crager and Spriggs, 1969; Elkind, Barocas, and Johnsen, 1969; Kagan, Rosman, Day, Albert, and Phillips, 1964). Adolescents' thinking becomes increasingly freed from perception (Olver and Hornsby, 1966). There remains however, the flexibility to classify perceptual characteristics at an analytic level (e.g., both a ruler and a watch have numbers; Elkind et al., 1969; Kagan et al., 1964). Adolescents have a greater ability than children to classify by homogeneous functions (e.g., a lighter and a match go together because they can both start fires) and abstract functions (e.g., a camera and a pencil go together because they can both make a record of events; Crager and Spriggs, 1969).

The adolescent has an increasing ability to use words as a means of conceptualizing. Vygotsky (1962) suggested that the ability of the adolescent to use language as a vehicle for the acquisition of new concepts is the major intellectual advancement during this period. He also observed that while the young child thinks by remembering, the adolescent remembers by thinking. Acquisition of concepts becomes increasingly important for the adolescent as the secondary-school curriculum focuses almost exclusively on the acquisition of conceptual knowledge in the content areas (Wiig and Semel, 1980).

(W)hile the young child thinks by remembering, the adolescent remembers by thinking.

Wiig and Secord (1992a) note that older children and adolescents translate their word knowledge into world knowledge. This is in contrast to early (i.e., up to age 7) concept development, when the child's world knowledge translates into word knowledge (Crais, 1990).

"On graduating from high school, the average adolescent has learned the meaning of at least 80,000 different words" (Miller and Gildea, 1987, as cited in Nippold, 1988e, p. 29). From ages 9 to 19 years, new words and concepts are added to the lexicon, old words take on new and subtle meanings, and it becomes easier to organize the lexicon's content (Nippold, 1988b). For example, double-function terms such as *cold* and *bright* are understood by 6-year-olds when physical meanings are intended, but their psychological meanings may not be understood until preadolescence

(Asch and Nerlove, 1960). McGhee-Bidlack (1991) investigated concrete versus abstract noun definitions in 10-, 14-, and 18-year-olds. The results indicated that for all three age groups, concrete nouns were easier to define than abstract nouns.

Nippold (1998) cautioned that learning new words is not an all or none process, but rather learning of the full meaning of a word is a gradual process. The learning process is enhanced through direct instruction (i.e., in school and home), contextual abstraction (i.e., contextual cues in books, newspapers, and so on), and morphological analysis (i.e., understanding compound and root words, suffixes and prefixes, and so forth). According to Nippold, older students take on a more formal style to define words, demonstrating a qualitatively different style as they get older (e.g., the student will specify a category for a word rather than a description). She also pointed out that the developmental studies and standardized subtests on word definition focus primarily on the students' ability to define words in isolation, rather than in more natural contexts.

Nippold (1998) and Rhea Paul (2001) noted that vocabulary acquisition for adolescents involves:

- Advanced adverbial conjuncts (e.g., *moreover, nonetheless*)

- Adverbs of likelihood (e.g., *possibly, definitely*) and magnitude (e.g., *extremely, considerably*)

- Precise and technical terms related to curricular content (e.g., *bacteria, democracy*)

- Verbs with presuppositional (e.g., *regret, promise*), metalinguistic (e.g., *predict, infer*), and metacognitive (e.g., *hypothesize, observe*) components

- Words with multiple meanings (Adolescents don't just quantitatively increase their vocabulary, they also experience qualitative differences in vocabulary, (e.g., the word *run* has multiple meanings))

- Meanings of known words (e.g., *warm* in regard to temperature and *warm* meaning to affect one's emotions)

- Derivational connections among words (e.g., *clinic* and *clinician*)

- Meanings by antonyms (e.g., *reluctant* and *enthusiastic*)

- Synonyms (e.g., *huge* and *enormous*)

- Homonyms (e.g., *pair* and *pear*)

Critical Thinking

The National Council for Excellence in Critical Thinking Instruction's working definition of *critical thinking* is "the intellectually disciplined process of actively and skillfully conceptualizing, applying, analyzing, synthesizing, or evaluating information gathered from, or generated by, observation, experience, reflection, reasoning, or communication, as a guide to belief and action" (as cited in Richard Paul and Nosich, 1993, p. 110).

According to Richard Paul and Willsen (1993), critical thinking is:

- Forming and shaping one's thinking in a systematic way, which results in thinking about how to evaluate one's thinking

- Functioning in a purposeful and exact way

- Thinking that is disciplined and comprehensive

- Evaluating one's thinking based on intellectual standards of relevance, accuracy, precision, clarity, depth, and breadth

Overall, Richard Paul (1993) believes that critical thinking is excellence of thought based on intellectual standards and that "we attain genuine knowledge only when the information we possess is not only correct but, additionally, we know that it is and why it is" (p. 57). He claims that all definitions of critical thinking are, at best, scaffolding for the mind:

> (C)ritical thinking is thinking about your thinking while you're thinking in order to make your thinking better. Two things are critical: (1) critical thinking is not just thinking, but thinking which entails self-improvement, and (2) this improvement comes from skill in using standards by which one appropriately assesses thinking. To put it briefly, it is self-improvement (in thinking) through standards (that assess thinking). (p. 91)

The intellectual standards that students are to apply to their thinking across all academic classes are noted in the sidebar that follows. If students apply these intellectual standards and objectively critique their own thinking, they can be deemed critical thinkers (Richard Paul, 1993).

Speech-language pathologists often note that good critical thinkers possess the ability to engage in metacognitive tasks that emphasize (1) thinking about their thinking, (2) knowing when their thinking has gone astray, and (3) how to fix, repair, or revise their thinking strategies. Metacognitive ability and critical thinking capacity rely heavily on students' ability to assess their own thinking and to know what is accurate or inaccurate about their thinking process or application of thinking strategies. These types of abilities, not observed until early adolescence, develops more completely during middle adolescence, but is not fully developed across a variety of subject areas until late adolescence.

Intellectual Standards that Apply to Thinking in Every Subject

Thinking that is:		**Thinking that is:**
clear	vs.	unclear
precise	vs.	imprecise
specific	vs.	vague
accurate	vs.	inaccurate
relevant	vs.	irrelevant
plausible	vs.	implausible
consistent	vs.	inconsistent
logical	vs.	illogical
deep	vs.	superficial
broad	vs.	narrow
complete	vs.	incomplete
significant	vs.	trivial
adequate (for purpose)	vs.	inadequate
fair	vs.	biased or one-sided

Source: Richard Paul (1993)

Points of Discussion

1. Think back to your own adolescence. What are some instances when your preoccupation with physical changes or self-esteem affected your communication with others?

2. How would you use knowledge of characteristics of developmental tasks and stages of cognitive development to determine if a student is functioning at an early, middle, or late stage of development?

Suggested Readings

Mitchell, J. (1979). *Adolescent psychology.* Toronto, Canada: Holt, Rinehart, and Winston.

Elkind, D. (2000). *All grown up and no place to go.* Boulder, CO: Perseus.

Chapter 3

Oral and Nonverbal Communication Development

Goals

- Compare and contrast early and later language learning
- Describe typical oral communication development during preadolescence and adolescence
- Summarize the development of nonverbal communication skills

Professionals skilled in language assessment and intervention with adolescents are often called upon to sort out what's typical and what's not with regard to the communication skills of older students. As illustrated by the example in the sidebar on page 52, typical adolescent language may, at first, appear disordered. Astute professionals need to observe large numbers of adolescents in a variety of situations to develop awareness and knowledge of what's typical in the fluctuating language world of older students. They also must amass information on later language development. As cited throughout this chapter, a considerable amount of research has documented semantic, syntactic, and pragmatic aspects of typical language within older students.

The linguistic development that occurs during preadolescence and adolescence is much more subtle than the rapid language acquisition during early childhood (Nippold, 1988b). From ages 9 to 19 years, language development unfolds in a slow and protracted manner. Changes become obvious only when nonadjacent age groups are compared and sophisticated linguistic phenomena, such as examining the use of low frequency

Is This Typical Language, or Is It Disordered?

And we...like we found this really like awesome CD and we...um...we decided to play it and um...Jeremy's mom came in and she was SO mad, like she was yelling and screaming at us. And all we did was play her CD!

For the particular adolescent quoted, the language was determined to be typical. Knowledge of language development is crucial to making this determination.

Source: Larson and McKinley (1995)

syntactic structures and intersentential linguistic phenomena in spoken and written context, are studied further (Nippold, 1988b, 1998). Also, increasing individualism in language development (as a result of variability in coursework, extracurricular activities, and social contacts) makes it difficult for researchers to establish guidelines for typical linguistic performance in preadolescents and adolescents (Kamhi and Lee, 1988; Nippold, 1988c, 1998). Major contrasts between early language learning and later language development are summarized in the sidebar that follows. Also, general and specific trends during later language development are listed.

Linguistic Features

Definitions

Comprehension of linguistic features refers to the understanding of morphologic, syntactic, and semantic components of language. We often use the term *listening* (instead of *comprehension)* in our discussion because of its predominance in textbooks used for

adolescents and in much of the professional literature involving adolescents. The literature distinguishes between comprehension of a message and monitoring comprehension of a message. The latter task "is a metacognitive skill that allows listeners to notice and respond when they encounter messages that are difficult to comprehend" (Dollaghan, 1987, p. 46).

Listening is difficult to define because of the complexity of the behavior. What's more, just about as many definitions of listening exist as persons who have written about the topic (Barker, 1971; Nichols and Lewis, 1954; H. Weaver, 1972; Wolff, Marsnik, Tacey, and Nichols, 1983). Listening must be considered an integral part of the total communication process: The function of the listener is to derive meaning from the speaker's intent.

Listening is the basic language skill that is used the highest percentage of the time. Markgraf (1966) determined that high school students are expected to spend 46% of their classroom time listening. Rankin (1926) was one of the first to study how adults spend their verbal communication time. The study

Contrasts, General Trends, and Specific Trends
Between Early and Later Language Learning

Contrasts

- The major language goal for young children is to acquire spoken language. The major language goal for school-age students is to acquire written communication skills.

- The primary source of language stimulation for young children is spoken communication. For preadolescents and adolescents, both spoken and written communication forms are significant sources of language stimulation.

- Young children learn language in nondirected, informal settings. Older children and adolescents learn a great amount of language through formal instruction.

- Language development in younger children does not require metalinguistic competency. Metalinguistic competency is required for language development in older children and adolescents, especially as they learn to read and write.

- Young children are literal in their interpretations of language. Older children demonstrate increasing ability to appreciate figurative meanings.

- Young children's language and reasoning are concrete. Preadolescents and adolescents are learning language and acquiring reasoning processes that are abstract.

- Young children do not always take the perspective of others when communicating. Preadolescents and adolescents are more aware of listeners' and readers' needs and adjust their spoken and written messages accordingly.

General Trends

- In adolescence, it is difficult to state in detail by age level the specific thinking, language, and communication developmental milestones because individuals become increasing individualistic in their thinking and language abilities.

- During early childhood (birth to age 5), language is acquired rapidly, and the changes that occur from year to year are highly visible. During preadolescence and adolescence, these changes are more subtle, which has probably reinforced the concept that not much happens in language development after age 5.

- Analyzing written communication is as critical as oral communication after about the fourth grade. Written communication may influence oral communication and vice versa during the preadolescent years and beyond.

Continued on next page

Continued

- During preadolescence and adolescence, the student develops a meta awareness (i.e., the ability to think about one's own thinking, listening, and speaking performance) and thus is capable of revising communication performance based on evaluative feedback.

Specific Trends

- The child's lexicon (word development), especially word usage, improves greatly during the adolescent years. Quantitatively, upon graduating from high school, the average adolescent has learned the meaning of at least 80,000 different words. Qualitatively, old words take on new and subtle meanings, and it becomes easier to organize and reflect on the content of the word meanings.

- Syntactic structure is greatly affected by the context in which the utterances occur (i.e., setting (school or home); channel (spoken or written); and discourse genre (narrative, persuasive, or expository)). The more structured the setting, channel (written), and discourse genre, the more formal, complex, and complete the syntactical utterance.

- At about the age of 9, an important transition occurs in the literacy acquisition process. Children who have thus far been exposed primarily to narrative structures (stories) must begin to comprehend textbooks that are written in expository prose. Around the third grade, the student must read to learn instead of learn to read.

- Thinking becomes more abstract around age 11 years and older. At this time, the adolescent can think about thinking and operate on ideas, not just tangible objects and events.

- Figurative language includes metaphors, similes, idioms, and proverbs. It has been suggested that growth in figurative language production follows a U-shaped curve (i.e., novel, imaginative expressions are frequently produced by preschoolers; then decrease during the elementary years; and then increase during the adolescent years).

- Linguistic ambiguity can be in various forms, such as in isolated sentences, humor, and advertisements. Humor continues to develop during adolescence, and ambiguity alone is viewed as too simplistic by most adolescents. They like humor that is cognitively challenging with abstract themes, such as irony or witty remarks and spontaneous anecdotes.

- Narratives or story-telling ability occurs around 7 years of age; at 7 to 11 years of age, students are producing stories with multiple, embedded narrative structures. Between 13 and 15 years of age, students are capable of analyzing stories. From 16 through adulthood, individuals are capable of more sophisticated analysis (i.e., can generalize about the story meaning, formulate abstract statements about the message or theme of the story, and focus on their reaction to the story).

Sources: Grunwell (1986); Larson and McKinley (1995); Nippold (1988c, 1998)

revealed that adults spend 42% of their time listening, 32% speaking, 15% reading, and 11% writing. In 1975, Werner conducted an update of the Rankin study with adult subjects. She found that 55% of verbal communication time is spent listening, 23% speaking, 13% reading, and 9% writing. Clearly, the need for listening spans a lifetime.

Production of linguistic features refers to the appropriate expression of morphologic, syntactic, and semantic components during speaking. (NOTE: We use the term *speaking*, instead of *production*, in the intervention section of this book because preadolescents and adolescents understand this term, and it is part of their curriculum.)

Typical Development

Comprehension of Linguistic Features

Until the 1980s, child language researchers focused most of their efforts on charting and analyzing linguistic developments that occur between birth and age 6. Since then, interest in aspects of later language development has begun to escalate, and researchers have posed questions concerning differences between early and later development (Nippold, 1998; Nippold, Schwarz, and Undlin, 1992).

Subtle changes occur in the adolescent's ability to understand oral communication. Professionals should not expect preadolescents and adolescents to comprehend everything that is spoken to them, since certain linguistic features may not be entirely understood even by adults. For example, in both children and adults, sentences with relative clauses in the middle are more difficult to comprehend than sentences with such clauses at the end (Sheldon, 1977). And sentences that violate the minimal distance principle (i.e., those in which the subject and verb are not in reasonably close proximity) are difficult to comprehend (Chomsky, 1969; N. Reed, 1977; Sanders, 1971). Also, comprehension of the ask/tell distinction is late developing and is never fully resolved by some individuals (Kramer, Koff, and Luria, 1972). To illustrate, using ninth graders as subjects in a pilot study, Thomas and Walmsley (1976) found that the students erred in sentences with *ask, tell, promise, persuade,* and *threaten.* These investigators reported that errors might have been caused by the students' linguistic deficiencies or by their current level of metalinguistic development.

Given that comprehension of morphology and syntax is expected to be intact in older students, most research has focused on semantics, especially figurative language.

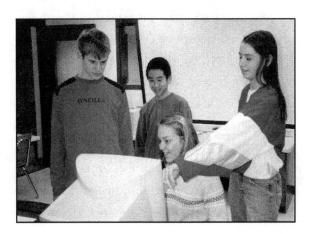

Communication Solutions
for Older Students

Comprehension of figurative language is particularly important to adolescents (V. Reed, 1994). They frequently encounter figurative language in textbooks and classroom discourse (Nippold, 1991, 1993) and in the slang and jargon of their peers. The ability to comprehend and use slang and jargon has been linked to peer acceptance and the ability to establish friendships during adolescence (Donahue and Bryan, 1984; Nippold, 1985, 1993). Nippold (1998) suggests that slang occurs most likely in spoken context, whereas idioms are produced in written and spoken language.

The ability to comprehend

and use slang and jargon

has been linked to peer

acceptance and the ability

to establish friendships

during adolescence.

Researchers have investigated the development of metaphor comprehension in students with typical development between the ages of 4 and 15 years (Galda, 1981). Results indicate that metaphoric understanding increases with age. Once students are in the concrete operational period, their metaphoric understanding and linguistic abilities increase, resulting in their ability to comprehend and explain abstract metaphors.

Studies cited in Nippold (1998) by Billow (1975); Kogan, Connor, A. Gross, and Fava (1980); Malgady (1977); and Siltanen (1981) have shown that comprehension of metaphors and similes steadily improves during adolescent years but that no specific cognitive prerequisites (either Piagetian or non-Piagetian) are found. Metaphor and simile comprehension depend on a number of factors: knowledge of semantic features and conceptual domains, the ability to manage syntactic complexities, the presence of linguistic contextual support, the type of response mode, and so on (Nippold).

Similarly, comprehension of idioms is acquired gradually during adolescence and remains incomplete even at the age 19 (Nippold, 1988a). Preadolescents tend to understand novel idioms at a literal level, although even 8-year-olds interpret sentences figuratively if familiar idioms and/or idiomatically biasing contexts are used (Ackerman, 1982). The degree of success in idiom comprehension depends on numerous factors, including the frequency of exposure to specific idioms, the manner in which understanding is to be indicated, and the degree of supporting contextual information (Abkarian, A. Jones, and West, 1992; Nippold and Martin, 1989). Nippold (1998) summarized idiom comprehension as being more difficult when students have to explain the figurative meanings of idioms than when choosing from multiple-choice tasks or pointing to a picture that illustrates the meaning.

Nippold and C. Taylor (2002) found that 11-year-old children were less familiar with idioms and had greater difficulty comprehending them than 16-year-old adolescents did. The adolescents rated all the idioms as highly familiar, but despite their high familiarity, certain idioms were difficult for them to comprehend. The two groups did not differ in their transparency judgments. An idiom is more transparent if the literal and nonliteral meanings closely compare, whereas it is more opaque if the idioms literal and nonliteral meanings are more unrelated. Transparent idioms are easier to understand.

Nippold (2000) noted that figurative language as an aspect of semantics grows during adolescence. Proverbs are one of the most difficult forms of figurative language. Nippold, Hegel, Uhden, and Bustamante (1998) reported that proverb comprehension increased with age level as follows:

Grade 6 = 51%
Grade 8 = 71%
Grade 10 = 73%
Grade 12 = 81%
University = 93%

Nippold, Uhden, and Schwarz (1997) investigated proverbs in eight age groups, ranging in age from 13 to 79 years of age. They used an explanation response mode. No age group reached a ceiling on the task, and performance appeared to decline in the 60-year age group. It should be noted that those with the most formal education performed the best. Proverbs containing abstract language are more difficult than those containing concrete language. This was true for every grade level. Nippold and Allen (1998) reported in their study that students' knowledge of words contained in proverbs was significantly correlated to their understanding of proverbs. However, word knowledge was not sufficient unto itself. Other factors, such as inferring meaning from larger linguistic context in which the proverb occurs, were also important.

Some researchers claim that students have little or no comprehension of proverbs before adolescence (Douglas and Peel, 1979; Lutzer, 1988). However, one study by Nippold, Martin, and Erskine (1988) found proverb comprehension among preadolescents to be markedly better than other studies have found. Their task did not demand explanation of proverbs, nor were proverbs presented out of context. Thus, when task demands are simplified, it appears preadolescents comprehend proverbs reasonably well, a finding consistent with the development of metaphors and idioms. In general, 9-year-olds have a basic understanding of the various figurative language types, but major improvements occur throughout adolescence (Nippold, 1988a).

According to Nippold (1998), developmental studies have examined the understanding of linguistic ambiguity in three domains—isolated sentences, humor, and advertisements. Shultz and Pilon (1973) examined 6-, 9-, 12-, and 15-year-olds' understanding of ambiguous sentences. They found that phonological ambiguities were easier than lexical, and that lexical were easier to understand than surface and deep structure ambiguities. Humor development in adolescence is unclear, and it is unknown as to what degree performance improves beyond age 15 (Nippold, 1998). Nippold, Cuyler, and Braunbeck-Price (1988) studied ambiguous advertisements and found that the ability to understand them improved throughout adolescence and that it was not completely mastered by 18 years of age.

Production of Linguistic Features

One of the most extensive studies to date that explored language production of adolescents is that of Loban (1976). He completed a 13-year longitudinal study on 211 typical subjects from kindergarten through grade 12. He selected a group high in language ability (as reported by teachers), a group low in language ability, and a random group of subjects representative of the total group. The characteristics that teachers used to describe those in the high-ability group included the use of a varied vocabulary, the adjustments of speaking pace to listeners' needs, and the ability to remain in control of ideas expressed. Subjects in the high-ability group spoke freely, fluently, and effectively, and listened attentively. The characteristics that teachers used to describe those in the low-ability group included reduced awareness of listeners' needs and meagerness of vocabulary. Their language rambled without apparent purpose and projected a hesitant, faltering style.

Each year, Loban (1976) completed an oral interview with all subjects, and from grade 3 on, he collected one or more written compositions. The purpose of Loban's research was to determine what differences existed between pupils who ranked high in language proficiency compared with those who ranked low with regard to both oral and written language. He also wanted to know if growth in language followed a predictable year-by-year sequence.

Using communication units as his basic measurement, Loban (1976) measured the average number of words per communication unit during oral language. A *communication unit* was defined as an independent clause with its modifiers. Loban found that those students with a high average number of words per communication unit were the same students who were rated high-ability by teachers.

Loban's (1976) investigation of a random group of subjects (i.e., a mixture of students rated high or low on language skills by teachers) revealed that a plateau typically followed a year of language growth. See Table 3.1 for a comparison of the average number of words per communication unit, the relative growth, and the year-to-year velocity of the three groups during grades 1 through 12.

Average Number of Words Used per
Communication Unit (by Grade)—Oral Language

Table 3.1

Grade	Average Number of Words per Communication Unit (mean)			Relative Growth[a] (in percent)			Year-to-Year Velocity[b] (in percent)		
	High Group	Random Group	Low Group	High Group	Random Group	Low Group	High Group	Random Group	Low Group
1	7.91	6.88	5.91	67.61	58.80	50.51	—	—	—
2	8.10	7.56	6.65	69.23	64.62	56.84	+1.62	+5.82	+6.33
3	8.38	7.62	7.08	71.62	65.13	60.51	+2.39	+0.51	+3.67
4	9.28	9.00	7.55	79.32	76.92	64.53	+7.70	+11.79	+4.02
5	9.59	8.82	7.90	81.97	75.38	67.52	+2.65	-1.54	+2.99
6	10.32	9.82	8.57	88.21	83.93	73.25	+6.24	+8.55	+5.73
7	11.14	9.75	9.01	95.21	83.33	77.01	+7.00	-0.60	+3.76
8	11.59	10.71	9.52	99.06	91.54	81.37	+3.85	+8.21	+4.36
9	11.73	10.96	9.26	100.26	93.68	79.15	+1.20	+2.14	+2.22
10	12.34	10.68	9.41	105.47	91.28	80.43	+5.21	-2.40	+1.28
11	13.00	11.17	10.18	111.11	95.47	87.01	+5.64	+4.19	+6.58
12	12.84	11.70	10.65	109.74	100.00	91.03	-1.37	+4.53	+4.02

From Language Development: Kindergarten through Grade Twelve (p. 27), by W. Loban, 1976, Urbana, IL: National Council of Teachers of English. © 1976 by the National Council of Teachers of English. Reprinted with permission.

[a] Relative Growth uses the scores of the Random Group at grade 12 to equal 100 percent.

[b] Year-to-Year Velocity is the percentage change in any given group from one year to the following year.

In addition to examining the average number of words per communication unit during oral language, Loban (1976) analyzed the percentage of total words that were in mazes. *Mazes* are words or unattached fragments not necessary to the message. When a maze is removed from a communication unit, "the remaining material constitutes a straightforward, acceptable communication unit" (Loban, p. 102). As illustrated in Table 3.2, all groups ended grade 12 with virtually identical percentages of verbal mazes used in grade 1, with erratic fluctuation evidenced during the middle years of school.

Loban (1976) also analyzed the average number of words per maze and found relative stability throughout all 12 grades (his findings

Percentage of Total Words in Mazes Used (by Grade)—Oral Language

Table 3.2

Grade	High Group	Random Group	Low Group
1	7.61	7.46	9.04
2	6.21	8.03	8.31
3	4.71	6.39	7.98
4	6.39	8.38	11.06
5	6.41	7.53	9.04
6	6.98	8.29	10.33
7	5.82	7.76	11.08
8	6.08	8.12	9.30
9	5.31	7.29	10.18
10	7.45	7.40	7.51
11	7.32	7.04	9.01
12	7.25	7.04	9.19

From *Language Development: Kindergarten through Grade Twelve* (p. 29), by W. Loban, 1976, Urbana, IL: National Council of Teachers of English. © 1976 by the National Council of Teachers of English. Reprinted with permission.

are displayed in Table 3.3). The high-ability group consistently showed the smallest degree of maze behavior as a percentage of total words, and the lowest average number of words per maze. Although students in the low ability group used a lower average number of words, they simultaneously used a larger amount of verbal maze behavior.

Leadholm and J. Miller (1992) and J. Miller, Freiberg, Rolland, and Reeves (1992) urge us to use verbal maze data cautiously since mazes may be common in the speech of students when they are attempting to formulate long, complex utterances. These researchers observed students in a variety of communication situations and reviewed students' academic and social success, and they found maze behavior even though the students had typical development.

In comparing the average number of communication units in oral language with those in written language, Loban (1976) found that his subjects tended to speak and write in units that had similar average lengths. He found that those students who were superior in oral language skills in

Average Number of Words Produced per Maze (by Grade)—Oral Language

Table 3.3

Grade	High Group	Random Group	Low Group
1	1.94	2.09	1.81
2	1.89	1.89	1.90
3	1.88	1.85	1.98
4	1.97	2.06	1.99
5	1.93	2.09	2.07
6	2.15	2.21	2.16
7	1.90	2.06	2.17
8	1.96	2.01	2.11
9	1.78	1.98	2.18
10	1.85	1.92	1.92
11	1.94	1.97	1.97
12	1.77	1.99	2.24

From *Language Development: Kindergarten through Grade Twelve* (p. 31), by W. Loban, 1976, Urbana, IL: National Council of Teachers of English. © 1976 by the National Council of Teachers of English. Reprinted with permission.

kindergarten and first grade, before they learned to read and write, were the same students who excelled in reading and writing by the time they were in sixth grade. (Written language results are elaborated on in Chapter 4.) The inclusion of longer and more complex dependent clauses, especially adjectival clauses, was a primary mark of increasing language development, both oral and written. The growth of adjectival clauses was centered mainly in grades 7 through 9. Table 3.4 shows the grade-by-grade changes in dependent clause use in oral communication.

The inclusion of longer and more complex dependent clauses, especially adjectival clauses, was a primary mark of increasing language development, both oral and written.

Average Number of Dependent Clauses per Communication Unit—Oral Language

Table 3.4

Grade	Average Number of Dependent Clauses per Unit (mean)			Relative Growth[a] (in percent)			Year-to-Year Velocity[b] (in percent)		
	High Group	Random Group	Low Group	High Group	Random Group	Low Group	High Group	Random Group	Low Group
1	0.24	0.16	0.12	41.38	27.59	20.69	—	—	—
2	0.25	0.21	0.17	43.10	36.21	29.,31	+1.72	+8.62	+8.62
3	0.27	0.22	0.18	46.55	37.93	31.03	+3.45	+1.72	+1.72
4	0.37	0.30	0.20	63.79	51.72	34.48	+17.24	+13.79	+3.45
5	0.37	0.29	0.25	63.79	50.00	43.10	0.00	+1.72	+8.62
6	0.41	0.37	0.30	70.69	63.79	51.72	+6.90	+13.79	+8.62
7	0.44	0.35	0.31	75.86	60.34	53.45	+5.17	-3.45	+1.73
8	0.45	0.39	0.30	77.59	67.24	51.72	+1.73	+6.90	-1.73
9	0.52	0.43	0.31	89.66	74.14	53.45	+12.07	+6.90	+1.73
10	0.61	0.48	0.33	105.17	82.76	56.90	+15.51	+8.62	+3.45
11	0.63	0.52	0.36	108.62	89.66	62.07	+3.45	+6.90	+5.17
12	0.67	0.58	0.46	115.52	100.00	79.31	+6.90	+10.34	+17.24

From *Language Development: Kindergarten through Grade Twelve* (p. 37), by W. Loban, 1976, Urbana, IL: National Council of Teachers of English. ©1976 by the National Council of Teachers of English. Reprinted with permission.

[a] Relative Growth uses the scores of the Random Group at grade 12 to equal 100 percent.

[b] Year-to-Year Velocity is the percentage change in any given group from one year to the following year.

One of the most ambitious components to Loban's (1976) research was to determine the use of all strategies by which students expanded communication units beyond simple one-word subjects and predicates (e.g., dependent clauses, adverbs, infinitives, propositonal phases, and adjectives). He called this the elaboration index. Table 3.5 shows the number of elaboration index points across all grade levels. Of note are the following observations:

• The low-ability group is consistently about four years behind the high language-ability group. For example, their elaboration index at grade 5 (early adolescence) matches the index of high-ability users at grade 1.

• The random group (a mixture of high and low language users) is about two years behind the high-ability group.

Average Number of Elaboration Index Points per Communication Unit—Oral Language

Table 3.5

Grade	Elaboration Points per Unit			Relative Growth[a]			Year-to-Year Velocity[b]		
	High Group	Random Group	Low Group	High Group	Random Group	Low Group	High Group	Random Group	Low Group
1	3.18	2.47	2.05	52.56	40.83	33.88	—	—	—
2	3.05	2.73	2.43	50.41	45.12	40.17	-2.15	+4.29	+6.29
3	3.33	2.78	2.57	55.04	45.95	42.48	+4.63	+0.83	+2.31
4	3.96	3.63	2.98	65.45	60.00	49.26	+10.41	+14.05	+6.78
5	4.14	3.67	3.12	68.43	60.66	51.57	+2.98	+0.66	+2.31
6	4.77	4.33	3.46	78.84	71.57	57.19	+10.41	+10.91	+5.62
7	5.36	4.38	3.94	88.60	72.40	65.12	+9.76	+0.83	+7.93
8	5.48	4.95	4.24	90.58	81.82	70.08	+1.98	+9.42	+4.96
9	5.70	5.16	4.16	94.21	85.29	68.76	+3.63	+3.47	-1.32
10	5.93	5.11	4.22	98.02	84.46	69.75	+3.81	-0.83	+0.99
11	6.80	5.75	4.92	112.40	95.04	81.32	+14.38	+10.58	+11.57
12	6.92	6.05	5.41	114.38	100.00	89.42	+1.98	+4.96	+8.10

From *Language Development: Kindergarten through Grade Twelve* (p. 59), by W. Loban, 1976, Urbana, IL: National Council of Teachers of English. © 1976 by the National Council of Teachers of English. Reprinted with permission.

[a] Relative Growth uses the scores of the Random Group at grade 12 to equal 100 percent.

[b] Year-to-Year Velocity is the percentage change in any given group from one year to the following year.

- The elaboration index results show the same essential growth patterns as the average number of words per communication unit (shown in Table 3.1). Thus, Loban concluded that one could use the easier word count measurement with students and trust the elaboration index would mirror the same results.

In most oral language measurements taken by Loban (1976), the subjects in the high-ability group were approximately four to five years advanced in comparison with subjects in the low-ability group. There was a strong correlation between high socioeconomic status and entry into the high-ability group. A similar correlation existed between the low-ability group and low socioeconomic status. While subjects from minority ethnic groups (i.e., Asian, Mexican, and African Americans) comprised a disproportionately high percentage of the low-ability group and a low percentage of the high-ability group, social inequity—not ethnic background—

affected language proficiency. As Loban (1976) stated, "Minority students who came from securely affluent home backgrounds did *not* show up in the low proficiency group. The problem is poverty, not ethnic affiliation" (p. 23).

Language production during preadolescence and adolescence has also been discussed extensively by others (Nippold 1988c, 1998; Rhea Paul, 2001; Scott, 1988). Syntactic growth during adolescence is subtle (Scott). Between the ages of 8 and 12 years, the frequency of phrases like *and everything, and stuff,* and *or something* increases threefold. Connectives are gradually mastered, with these being more difficult than others: *although, which, yet* (intrasentential), and *thus* and *however* (intersentential). During adolescence, new syntactic structures develop—such as growth within sentences (intrasentential), resulting in longer, more complex sentences and growth between sentences (intersentential), resulting in increased use of subordinate and coordinate clauses (Nippold, 1998; Rhea Paul, 2001).

Production of figurative language also shows gradual improvement throughout preadolescence and adolescence. Nippold (1988c) summarized the work of Gardner, Kircher, Wonner, Bechhofer, Wolf, and Perkins, "It has been suggested that growth in production follows a U-shaped curve such that novel, imaginative expressions are frequently produced by preschoolers, decrease during the elementary school years, but increase during adolescence" (p. 180).

The ability to explain sentential ambiguity also improves steadily during the preadolescent and adolescent years (Nippold, 1988d). Nelsen and Rosenbaum (1972), as cited in Nippold (1998), studied boys and girls in grades 7 through 12 and found that boys generated more slang than girls on topics of money, autos, and motorbikes, but girls outperformed boys on topics of clothing and appearance, boys, and popular and unpopular people. The use of slang appears to be contingent upon both topic and gender.

Discourse

Discourse encompasses conversations, narations, expository language, persuasion, and negotiation. Discourse is composed not of words or sentences, but of speech acts (Austin, 1962). Austin maintained that speech acts can be analyzed in three parts:

- Locutions (propositions or idea units composed of a predicate and its related arguments)

- Illocutions (the speaker's intentions)

- Perlocutions (the listener's interpretations)

Discourse is a broader term than *pragmatics*, which involves "the ways in which normally developing children link consecutive utterances within discourse to maintain coherency and to clarify messages" (Craig, 1983, p. 106). Craig's definition considers the integrated nature of structural and conversational rules. Writing in 1971, before the popularity of the term *pragmatics*, Hymes discussed the importance of sentence acceptability, or "who can say what, in what way, where, and when, by what means and to whom?" (p. 15). His insight into sentence acceptability in the 1970s paved the way to pragmatics in the 1980s and to social skills in the 1990s and beyond. As Gallagher (1991) so astutely noted, "Social cognition, social skills, and the attainment of age-appropriate friendship skills provide the foundation on which peer relationships are built. Central to each of these is language skill" (p. 13).

Conversations

Definition

The term *conversation* frequently "is used loosely and nontechnically to refer to any interactional stretch of talk involving at least two participants, and taking place in a non-formalized setting" (Edmondson, 1981, p. 6). Hoskins (1996) explained how conversation can be seen as a series of moves:

- Introducing a topic
- Maintaining a topic
- Introducing a topic in an elaborated form
- Extending a topic
- Changing a topic
- Requesting clarification
- Responding to requests for clarification

Typical Development

Grice's (1975) classic work proposed four fundamental rules of conversations (see the sidebar that follows) that summarize expectations held by speakers and listeners, and they have held true over time. These rules are intact by late adolescence and frequently emerge by the middle grades.

Various researchers have investigated communicative maturity during conversations. For example, Wiig (1982) found communicative maturity to be developed by age 13. At this time, youth can make the transition between an informal language code (i.e., peer register) and a more formal language code (i.e., adult register). Moreover, Wiig found that by age 15, teenagers use the more formal register not only with adults, but also with their own peer group, unless the peers are their closest friends. Different surface structures of the speech act are appropriate for different situations, depending on the listener, setting, topic, and objectives (Wiig, 1983). Modification of the verb phrase is the most important aspect in making the surface structure changes from an informal code to a formal one (e.g., "Close the door" vs. "Would you mind closing the door?"). A mature communicator will have many different structural forms to express the same intent.

Four Fundamental Rules of Conversation

Quantity: Informativeness

"1. Make your contribution as informative as is required (for the current purposes of the exchange).

2. Do not make your contribution more informative than is required" (p. 45).

Quality: Sincerity

"1. Do not say what you believe to be false.

2. Do not say that for which you lack adequate evidence" (p. 46).

Relationship: Topic Management

"1. Be relevant" (p. 46).

Manner: How to Be Clear

"1. Avoid obscurity of expression.

2. Avoid ambiguity.

3. Be brief (avoid unnecessary prolixity).

4. Be orderly" (p. 46).

Source: Grice (1975)

A mature communicator will have many different structural forms to express the same intent.

As communicative maturity increases, inept communication acts decrease. By third grade, students are able to recognize an inept communication act, but they cannot yet correct it (R. Johnson, Greenspan, and G. Brown, 1980). By sixth grade, students improve inept communication acts if those acts attempt to influence others' actions (e.g., Listen to this situation: "You're studying for a test at school. Lou calls you up and wants to come over to visit. You say, 'You picked a fine time to visit.' How would you correct your statement?"). Not until ninth grade can students correct inept attempts to have others feel better (e.g., "Tom is sad because his dog died. You say, 'Cheer up, it's nothing to be upset about. Pretty soon you'll forget all about it.' How would you correct your statement?").

A possible explanation as to why inept communication acts decrease in late adolescence is that the person is capable of using more sophisticated communication strategies—for example, taking the perspective of the listener. Also, older adolescents have a greater range of interpersonal constructs (e.g., adjusting their communication to the emotional state of the communication partner) that they apply to communication situations (Ritter, 1979).

We have completed a six-year longitudinal study in which we analyzed the spontaneous conversational speech of eight typical adolescents (four boys and four girls), while they were in the seventh through twelfth grades, under two experimental conditions (Larson and McKinley, 1998; McKinley and Larson, 1991, 1996). In one condition, adolescents talked with a familiar peer of their choice (e.g., a close friend); in the other condition, they talked with an unfamiliar adult of the opposite sex. These two conditions were selected to represent bipolar situations.

The study revealed that adolescents conversing with a peer were more likely to use a variety of question types, more frequent figurative language expressions, and new and abrupt topic shifts, as well as the communication functions of entertaining, getting information, and getting the listener to feel/believe/do something. Table 3.6 summarizes the data on conversational partner differences.

Only a few gender-related differences were revealed. Males used returns to topic and the functions of getting the listener to feel/believe/do something and entertaining more frequently than females. Table 3.7 summarizes the gender-related differences across conversational samples.

The grade-level differences indicated three dominant patterns for the communication behaviors: (1) a trend upward (e.g., negative interruptions increased with advanced grades) or a trend downward (e.g., abrupt topic shifts decreased with grade level); (2) a more or less equal frequency of occurrence at seventh and twelfth grades, with significant differences in one or more middle grades (e.g., nonspecific language and verbal mazes); (3) a relatively flat pattern with similar frequencies of occurrence at all grades (e.g., one-appearance negation and giving information). Table 3.8 summarizes the grade-level differences across conversational samples.

In summary, the findings of our study indicated a noticeable pattern of fluctuation and a relative lack of gender-related differences in characteristics of normal adolescents' conversations from grades 7 through 12. There was notable evidence that characteristics of the adolescents' conversations were adjusted depending on their partners (i.e., a more formal register with the adult and a more informal one with the peer).

Topic maintenance patterns have been studied by Dorval (1980), who found significant differences between children and

Frequency of Communication Behaviors in 10-Minute Conversations:
Table 3.6 **Conversational Partner Differences (Reported as Means)**

Communication Behavior	Conversational Partner	
Number of Conversational Turns	Adult	Peer
	80.02	74.72
Linguistic Features		
Negation		
One appearance	26.13	22.15
Double	0.44	0.34
Questions		
Interrogative reversal	1.44	4.72
Tag	0.63	1.38
Rising intonation	3.46	8.04
Wh	1.63	6.11
Total	7.16	20.25
Figurative language	3.23	8.38
Nonspecific language	8.02	7.45
Pragmatics		
Interruptions: Verbal-positive	8.56	5.38
Interruptions: Verbal-negative	5.48	6.19
Topic shift—Direction		
Return	0.19	0.70
New	1.52	3.62
Topic shift—Manner		
Abrupt	0.58	3.04
Gradual	1.13	1.40
Verbal mazes	10.21	9.96
Paralinguistics		
Vocalized pauses	6.38	4.21
Functions		
Giving information	50.46	31.36
Getting information	4.50	13.60
Describing ongoing event	0.13	0.60
Getting listener to feel/believe/do	0.29	1.47
Describing beliefs, feelings	13.08	15.26
Indicating readiness	10.63	8.04
Problem solving	0.19	0.36
Entertaining	0.77	4.04

From "Characteristics of Adolescents' Conversations: A Longitudinal Study," by V. Lord Larson and N.L. McKinley, 1998, *Clinical Linguistics and Phonetics, 12*(3), p. 189. © 1998 by Taylor and Francis. Reprinted with permission.

Frequency of Communication Behaviors in 10-Minute Conversations:
Table 3.7 **Gender Differences (Reported as Means)**

Communication Behavior	Gender	
	Male	Female
Number of Conversational Turns	81.40	73.44
Linguistic Features		
Negation		
One appearance	22.21	26.06
Double	0.17	0.60
Questions		
Interrogative reversal	3.28	2.85
Tag	1.04	0.96
Rising intonation	6.19	5.27
Wh	4.23	3.46
Total	14.74	12.54
Figurative language	7.34	4.25
Nonspecific language	7.68	7.79
Pragmatics		
Interruptions: Verbal-positive	6.89	7.08
Interruptions: Verbal-negative	6.21	5.46
Topic shift—Direction		
Return	0.60	0.29
New	2.32	2.79
Topic shift—Manner		
Abrupt	1.72	1.88
Gradual	1.19	1.33
Verbal mazes	9.51	10.65
Paralinguistics		
Vocalized pauses	5.11	5.50
Functions		
Giving information	44.74	37.35
Getting information	9.64	8.38
Describing ongoing event	0.34	0.38
Getting listener to feel/believe/do	1.21	0.54
Describing beliefs, feelings	14.38	13.94
Indicating readiness	7.40	11.25
Problem solving	0.28	0.27
Entertaining	3.47	1.33

From "Characteristics of Adolescents' Conversations: A Longitudinal Study," by V. Lord Larson and N.L. McKinley, 1998, *Clinical Linguistics and Phonetics, 12*(3), p. 190. © 1998 by Taylor and Francis. Reprinted with permission.

Frequency of Communication Behaviors in 10-Minute Conversations: Grade-Level Differences (Reported as Means)

Table 3.8

Communication Behavior	Grade					
Number of Conversational Turns	7th	8th	9th	10th	11th	12th
	70.00	82.87	82.63	70.88	70.25	88.00
Linguistic Features						
Negation						
One appearance	23.75	25.53	23.63	22.50	24.69	24.94
Double	0.63	0.47	0.38	0.19	0.38	0.31
Questions						
Interrogative reversal	2.81	2.93	3.25	2.06	4.13	3.19
Tag	0.56	0.73	0.69	1.31	1.63	1.06
Rising intonation	4.06	4.93	6.44	4.81	6.31	7.75
Wh	4.19	4.00	3.56	3.38	3.56	4.38
Total	11.62	12.66	13.94	11.68	15.55	16.38
Figurative language	5.56	4.93	3.69	5.81	7.94	6.69
Nonspecific language	5.50	7.73	4.44	10.31	13.19	5.25
Pragmatics						
Interruptions: Verbal-positive	3.63	5.67	7.94	6.25	5.31	13.06
Interruptions: Verbal-negative	2.38	4.00	4.56	8.31	6.19	9.44
Topic shift—Direction						
Return	0.94	0.20	0.44	0.56	0.38	0.13
New	4.19	2.80	1.75	2.44	1.69	2.50
Topic shift—Manner						
Abrupt	3.19	1.47	1.13	1.88	1.69	1.44
Gradual	1.94	1.53	1.06	1.13	0.75	1.19
Verbal mazes	12.06	10.67	4.56	8.75	13.69	10.81
Paralinguistics						
Vocalized pauses	8.44	4.93	3.38	5.38	5.06	4.63
Functions						
Giving information	37.88	42.80	43.94	34.69	36.81	50.06
Getting information	8.63	7.93	8.75	8.19	9.81	10.63
Describing ongoing event	0.06	0.13	0.19	0.38	0.56	0.81
Getting listener to feel/believe/do	0.63	1.93	1.06	0.31	0.50	0.88
Describing beliefs, feelings	16.19	17.33	13.25	15.31	12.38	10.88
Indicating readiness	2.88	9.67	13.69	9.88	7.44	12.56
Problem solving	0.38	0.67	0.56	0.00	0.06	0.00
Entertaining	3.56	2.40	1.19	2.31	2.69	2.19

adolescents. The results of the study revealed the following:

- Nonelaborated topic-related remarks increased in frequency during the elementary years, but started to decrease during high school as more complex topic-related remarks increased.

- More complex remarks such as factual and perspective-oriented evaluations/ elaborations/questions were made during ninth grade and increased in frequency thereafter.

- In ninth grade, but declining thereafter, a high proportion of evaluation comments were made relative to elaboration comments and evaluations, elaborations, and questions that focused on people's perspectives or feelings.

Thus, conversational quality (i.e., coordination associated with topic management) changes with age.

Topics of conversation have been indexed and classified by Rutherford, Freeth, and Mercer (1969) using taped transcripts of 15-year-old adolescents. While analyzing younger children, two broad topics surfaced: domestic and educational. Rutherford et al. (1969) found these to be insufficient when classifying topics of adolescents, so they added a third general topic, "philosophical." This added category absorbed topics that did not relate to the individual's immediate environment of school and home. Philosophical topics were discussed without immediate personal experience or knowledge and often reflected facts or opinions derived from television. Although these data were obtained from England, it is probable that the classification of the conversational topics of American youth would also require a philosophical category.

Rutherford (1976) made the astute observation that it is the way in which adolescents talk about certain topics, such as popular music groups, that causes adults to complain that adolescents "speak another language." The current system of beliefs and attitudes of adolescents can be seen through the medium of their conversations. Adolescents make remarks that allow peer group members to share the feeling expressed, but which intentionally prevent adult onlookers from understanding (e.g., "Well, just...(laugh) him" and "Well, not just his voice...but himself" (Rutherford, p. 113)). Such utterances are not analyzable, according to Rutherford. They are part of normal adolescent secretiveness, a necessary mechanism that allows children to grow up and grow away from parents. Much of the secret nature of their lives is reflected through their language (Rutherford).

Raffaelli and Duckett (1989) investigated conversational development from grades 5 through 9. They found the following: (1) as grade level increased, students (especially girls) spent more time socializing with friends (i.e., girls in grade 5 spent 9% and in grade 9 spent 18%, whereas boys spent 7% at grade 5 and 9% at grade 9); (2) topics of conversation differed depending on who the conversational partner was (e.g., personal issues, such as being kissed or planning a dance party were more likely discussed with peers than with family); and (3) higher levels of affect (e.g., cheerfulness) were displayed with peers than family. It is evident that well-developed conversational skills serve a highly social function and thus increase one's possibility of being accepted by peers and of developing friendships, which in turn minimizes loneliness and asocial behaviors (Asher and Gazelle, 1999).

Narrations

Definition

Structurally, narrations are midway between oral and literate language (Westby, 1984, 1991a). They form a transition from the language style of the home to the language style of the school. Personal narratives (on the oral end of Westby's (1984, 1991a) continuum) are either reports of "what happened," called *personal experience narratives*, or reports of the imagination, called *stories* (Lahey, 1988). Narrations can be viewed as extended monologues, in contrast with conversations, which are interactive dialogues.

> Narrations may be viewed as suprasentential discourse units with underlying organizational rules, or *story grammars*; as conceptual units that reveal the speaker's expectations about event sequences, or scripts; as lin-

guistic expressions requiring specific formal devices to bind them into coherent texts; and as *communication events* that demand thoughtful assessment of the listener's needs. (Johnston, 1982, p. 144)

Other differences between the two include these (Roth and Spekman, 1986):

- Narrations have more extended or elaborated units of text than conversations.

- Narrations are expected to have story markers (e.g., an introduction and a closing) and an orderly presentation of events leading to a logical resolution.

- Narrations carry the expectation that the speaker will engage in an oral monologue and that the listener's role can be more passive. More responsibility is placed on the speaker to be organized, coherent, and interesting.

Typical Development

A study done by Leadholm and J. Miller (1992) found that children produced a longer mean length of utterance (MLU) when talking in a narrative mode, than in a conversational mode. See Table 3.9 for a summary of their results presented by Nippold (1998). The organization of those longer utterances has been the focus of study for other researchers (Applebee, 1978; Stein and Glenn, 1979).

Applebee's (1978) typical developmental information has become a standard for

MLUs Obtained by Leadholm and J. Miller (1992) for Children in Two Speaking Modes (*N* = 167)

Table 3.9

Age (in years)	Conversation	Narration
5.4	5.71	6.06
7.1	5.92	7.32
9.1	6.50	8.80
11.1	7.62	9.83
13.0	6.99	9.32

From *Later Language Development: The School-Age and Adolescent Years* (2nd ed.; p. 159), by M.A Nippold, 1998, Austin, TX: Pro-Ed. © 1998 by Pro-Ed. Reprinted with permission.

explaining the sequence that children go through when learning narrative structure (see the sidebar on page 74). Typically, children reach the true narrative stage by approximately 8 years of age, and complex stories with multiple embedded narrative structures emerge at approximately 11 to 12 years of age (Westby, 1984). In fact, even as early as age 5 or 6 years, children can begin to produce structurally complete fantasy narratives during oral storytelling (Botvin and Sutton-Smith, 1977). Thus, professionals would expect that by adolescence, Applebee's sequence has been mastered and complex stories have emerged. This is often not the case, however, with adolescents who have language disorders (see Chapter 6).

Another way that narrations have been studied is through the use of story-reformulation tasks. Several researchers have proposed that story schemata are used by listeners to guide comprehension and recall (Mandler and N. Johnson, 1977; Rumelhart, 1975; Stein and Glenn, 1979). P. Weaver and Dickinson (1982) summarized

the way that efficient listeners maximize verbatim recall by using these processes:

- Recognition of verbal formulae (e.g., "Once upon a time there was...")

- Prediction of sentence structures based on the constraining power of preceding sentences

- Recognition and use of conjunctions and prepositions to mark relationships (i.e., temporal, causal, spatial) among propositions during encoding

- Integration of information gathered from these multiple sources

Chappell (1980) found that early adolescents were pragmatically aware of what information needed to be retold, and they used appropriate syntactic structures. By adulthood, a story being retold is "filled in" if the original story does not follow a predictable story sequence (Johnston, 1985).

The amount of information recalled during story-reformulation tasks showed developmental changes as age increased; however,

---

Summary of the Development of Narrative Structure

- Initially, children use prenarrative structures starting with "heap stories." They talk about whatever attracts their attention, without regard for a relationship among the elements or a macrostructure.

- A second preparative stage is "sequence stories," which have macrostructure, but the storyteller does not actually have a temporal sequence in mind. Rather, characters, objects, or events are put together because they are perceptually associated with each other.

- The next stage is "primitive narratives," in which characters, objects, or events are put together because they complement each other in some logical way. These narratives are the students' first use of inference in stories. However, their inferences go in only one direction and they do not perceive the reciprocal causality between thoughts and events.

- Another developmental stage is the chained narrative, which is first "unfocused," then "focused." In unfocused chain stories, the elements are logically related to each other but not related to any macrostructure. Thus, the story has no theme or plot. In the "focused chain," all the elements or events sequenced and related to the story's macrostructure. However, the story still lacks reciprocal relationships between characters' attributes and events, and among main events. Thus, the story does not have a strong plot.

- The last stage of development is the "true narrative" that integrates logical cause-and-effect chaining of the macrostructure elements, which are linked to the macrostructure of the story. This results in the story having a strong, well-developed plot.

Source: Applebee (1978)

---

basic organizational structure did not vary across ages (Mandler and N. Johnson, 1977). Young children tended to emphasize action sequence outcomes, but older children and adults emphasized the actions themselves or the internal events motivating them (Mandler and N. Johnson). Across all age levels, the most important units of a story were recalled most frequently (A. Brown and Smiley, 1977).

Thus, while some aspects of story reformulation differed with age (e.g., the amount of information recalled or emphasis placed during recall), other aspects did not (e.g., organizational structure or judgment of the importance of units). As P. Weaver and Dickinson (1982) pointed out, story grammar taxonomies such as Stein and Glenn's (1979) are relatively insensitive to developmental changes.

Expository Language

Definition

Expository language—on the literate end of Westby's (1984, 1991a) continuum—is used for the planning and transmission of logic-based knowledge and involves comparisons, explanations, and opinions (McFadden, 1991). The major purpose of expository language—often called *expository text,* whether oral or written—is to instruct (Hughes, McGillivray, and Schmidek, 1997). The discourse of instruction is closely tied to metalinguistic skills and the onset of formal operations in Piaget's (1952, 1970) view of cognition. The major distinctions between narrative and expository text are outlined in Table 3.10.

Table 3.10

Text Differences

Narrative	Expository
Purpose to entertain	Purpose to inform
Familiar schema content	Unfamiliar schema content
Consistent text structure; all narratives have same basic organization	Variable text structures; difference *(sic)* genres have different structure
Focus on character motivations, intentions, goals	Focus on factual information and abstract ideas
Often require multiple perspective taking—understanding points of view of different characters	Expected to take the perspective of the writer of the text
Can use pragmatic inferences, i.e., inference from similar experiences	Must use logical-deductive inferences based on information in texts
Connective words not critical—primarily *and, then, so*	Connective words critical—wide variety of connectives, e.g., *because, before, after, when, if-then, therefore*
Each text can stand alone	Expected to integrate information across texts
Comprehension is generally assessed informally in discussion	Comprehension often assessed in formal, structured tests
Can use top-down processing	Relies on bottom-up processing

From *Language and Reading Disabilities* (p. 159), by H. Catts and A. Kamhi, 1999, Boston: Allyn and Bacon. © 1999 by Pearson Education. Reprinted with permission.

Typical Development

From third grade on, students are expected to spend a significant amount of academic time describing, defining, discussing, and explaining information in small and large groups and as individuals (N. Nelson, 1993). Expository text encompasses the oral/ listening tasks of the classroom as well as a rather sudden change to expository text in their reading, away from story narratives. As Spor and Schneider (1999) observed, the emphasis of reading changes from learning to read to learning from text at about age 9. Street (2002) observed:

> This gives students approximately two years to master the skills required to learn from texts before facing the challenging reading demands of middle school. No longer are they in elementary school where they likely spent a great deal of time reading short novels and chapter books. Now they are in middle school, where they are often shocked by the reading expectations of their content area teachers. (p. 35)

Hughes, McGillivray, and Schmidek (1997), citing McCabe's (1995) work, summarized expository development as follows:

> Developmentally, narrative discourse seems to be the earlier and more common way that preschool and early school-age children make sense of experience, while informational, non-story discourse develops later (McCabe, 1985). However, some studies indicate that even kindergarten-age children can produce good informational discourse, and that by adolescence, expository performance may exceed narrative performance. (p. 5)

An important aspect of expository language is the requirement of explicitness (Wallach and L. Miller, 1988). In written exposition, explicitness is taken to an extreme, since punctuation must be used to map the meanings carried by gesture, facial expression, intonation, and prosody (McFadden, 1991). Furthermore, if a teacher is familiar with the information (e.g., the correct answers to a written essay test), then the student will be judged on the breadth and depth of his or her knowledge (Hughes, McGillivray, and Schmidek, 1997).

Persuasion and Negotiation

Definitions

Both persuasion and negotiation are reasoned forms of discourse, and therefore we included them in this section (see Table 3.11).

Areas of Gradual Improvement in
Persuasion and Negotiation as School-Age Children
and Adolescents Mature*

Table 3.11

Persuasion	Negotiation
• Adjusts to listener characteristics (e.g., age, authority, familiarity) • States advantages to the listener as a reason to comply • Anticipates and replies to counterarguments • Uses positive strategies such as politeness and bargaining • Gives up negative strategies such as whining and begging • Generates a large number and variety of different arguments • Controls the discourse assertively	• Takes the social perspective of another • Shows awareness of the needs, thoughts, and feelings of others • Reasons with words (verbal reasoning) • Uses cooperative and collaborative strategies • Shows concern for group welfare • Shows concern for long-term implications of conflict • Shows willingness to compromise

From *Later Language Development* (p. 190), by M.A. Nippold, 1998, Austin, TX: Pro-Ed. © 1998 by Pro-Ed. Adapted with permission.

*Ages 5–18+ years

Persuasion involves the use of argumentation to convince another person to perform an act or to accept a point of view desired by the persuader...(and negotiation) involves communication to resolve conflicts and to achieve goals in mutually acceptable ways.

(Nippold, 1998, p. 189)

Typical Development

Persuasion

Spoken persuasion is a distinct type of discourse in which the speaker must adjust the style of communication to relevant interpersonal and situational factors (Nippold, 1998). Nippold goes on to state that developmental studies have shown improvement in students' ability to engage in persuasive speech after the third grade. Older groups of students, such as those in the seventh and eleventh grades, are able to generate a greater number of different arguments than those in the third grade. Likewise, older students:

- Use politeness and bargaining more

- Take the perspective of the listener and modify their strategies based on listener characteristics such as age, authority, and familiarity in relation to themselves

- Are capable of refusing the persuasive strategies of others

Nippold (2000) showed that persuasive contexts result in the most advanced syntactic forms in adolescents' writings. She went on to state that a growing "body of research on syntactic development suggests that persuasive writing develops gradually over time and that it is more difficult to perform than other types of writing such as narrative or descriptive" (p. 22).

Negotiation

Selman, Beardslee, Schultz, Krupa, and Podorefsky (1986) investigated the development of interpersonal negotiation abilities in three age groups of students: younger (11 through 13 years), middle (14 through 16 years), and older (17 through 19 years). The results revealed that a negotiation is, indeed, a challenging task and that not even the oldest group had developed all the necessary strategies, such as those shown in Table

3.11. The older students were, however, more aware of the participants' wants and feelings, showed concern for long-term consequences of the conflict, and were most interested in resolving the conflict through compromise and mutual agreement. Also, it was found that girls demonstrated more advanced negotiation skills than boys. Eckert's (1990) study of conversational patterns revealed that girls used more interpersonal negotiation strategies than did boys in more natural conversational contexts.

In summary, Nippold (1998) so ably stated that, collectively, studies have shown that as students mature:

> they show an increasing tendency to resolve conflicts in ways that reflect greater social perspective-taking, verbal reasoning, cooperation and collaboration with others, and concern for group welfare. They also show increasing concern for the long-term implications of a conflict and a willingness to compromise if necessary. Growth in conflict resolution is especially active during adolescence, a time when the peer group becomes more important and opportunities for social interaction expand. (p. 201)

Nonverbal Communication

Definition

Nonverbal communication refers to communication that transcends spoken words. It includes six components (see the sidebar). While the discipline of communication sciences and disorders typically has not included paralanguage within nonverbal communication, we have selected to use Knapp's (1978) comprehensive definition of nonverbal communication. Paralanguage features include purposeful, directed, and controllable behaviors that may accompany or substitute for language and thus contribute to the development of a conversation (Edmondson, 1981).

Nonverbal factors are major determinants of meaning in the interpersonal context. Birdwhistell (1970) asserted that only 30 to 35% of the social meaning of a conversation is carried by words, while Mehrabian (1968) estimated that nonverbal factors are even more important. According to Knapp (1978), nonverbal communication serves these purposes:

- Repetition
- Contradiction
- Substitution
- Complementation
- Accentuation
- Regulation

Typical Development

The power of nonverbal communication cannot be overlooked. In studying undergraduate university students (i.e., primarily late adolescents), Rashotte (2002) summarized her primary findings as follows:

> (S)ingle nonverbal elements each have distinct meanings and create distinct impressions in those who view them; nonverbal behaviors work in combination with

Nonverbal Communication Components

- Kinesic behaviors
- Physical characteristics
- Touching behavior
- Paralanguage (including voice quality and vocalizations)
- Proxemics
- Artifacts (e.g., perfume, clothes)

Source: Knapp (1978)

overt behaviors to create modified impressions of actions; and nonverbal behaviors play as important a role as overt behaviors in those combinations. (p. 99)

French (1978) has described several nonverbal behaviors considered typical for adolescents that in the past would have been signs of hostility and rebellion. One such behavior is the blank stare, or focusing the eyes beyond the listener when engaging in a conversation. Another is the eye roll, once used as an expression of impudence. Now, the eye roll is used so extensively that the message it once conveyed has been weakened (French). Another behavior is the back turn, or shifting the body slightly, to expose the back to the receiver during the conversation. French believes the back turn has been influenced by Black culture, which views it as a sign of trust and of understanding what was said. He also described the "Black Walk," which is slower than the "White Walk." It is more of a stroll, with the head slightly elevated and casually tipped to one side. French suggests that the nonverbal message conveyed by the Black Walk is, "I am strong. I am 'cool.' I can't be bothered by anything in this world" (p. 544) and that the nonverbal message conveyed by the White Walk is, "I am a strong (person), and I'm in a hurry to get somewhere" (p. 544). French has observed that both White and Black youth have adopted nonverbal communication patterns of Black culture.

Some of the research in nonverbal communication during adolescence has analyzed recognition of facial expressions. In the 1920s, Gates (1923) conducted a facial expression recognition study and found that laughter was identified by age 3, pain by ages 5 to 6, anger by age 7, fear by ages 9 to 10, and surprise by age 11. None of the individuals studied had recognized scorn by age 14. The findings of this study have not been seriously challenged (Knapp, 1978). According to a report by Blanck and R. Rosenthal (1982), older children develop some degree of distrust toward facial expressions when accompanied by discrepant vocal cues. They summarized the data on older children as evidence that these children put more weight on facial expressions under normal conditions of communication and less under conditions of discrepancy.

Age changes in deceiving and detecting deceit have been reported by DePaulo and Jordan (1982). Before adolescence, children's distinction of deception from truth by reading only facial expressions is by chance. When given both verbal and nonverbal cues, adolescents perceive feigned expressions of liking as less positive than sincere expressions of liking, and feigned expressions of disliking as less negative than honest expressions of disliking. Girls between 5 and 12 years of age are increasingly adept at masking their deceptions facially; the reverse tends to occur for boys. The strategy that seventh graders use to deceive a person is to convey the feigned affect with the same degree of intensity as when it occurs naturally when telling the truth, while college students deceive by exaggerating the dissimulated affect. DePaulo and Jordan (1982) speculated that students learn and practice deception by playing card games, board games, party games, and sports.

Two studies examining the development of eye contact, or gazing, up to adolescence disagree on whether there is a gradually increasing or decreasing trend in looking behavior (Ashear and Snortum, 1971; Levine and Sutton-Smith, 1973). Knapp (1978) reported that adolescence represents a low point for eye gazing. Such lack of eye contact noted in adolescents with typical development is important data for professionals to keep in mind when they are assessing gazing behavior during conversational speech.

Listening feedback, such as head nods and vocalizing "mm-hmm," has been found to be nearly absent through fifth grade (Dittman, 1972). Before middle school, adults probably cannot expect much overt feedback, such as head nods, to indicate that children are listening to them. Our findings (McKinley and Larson, 1983, 1991) support Dittman's results. We found eighth-grade students provided considerable nonverbal listener feedback during conversations, even more than they did while in seventh grade.

> *Before middle school, adults probably cannot expect much overt feedback, such as head nods, to indicate that children are listening to them.*

The decoding of nonverbal cues is a gradually increasing skill from kindergarten through ages 20 to 30, after which a leveling off occurs (Dimitrovsky, 1964). On tests of nonverbal sensitivity, females consistently outperformed males from grade school through the middle 20s (Knapp, 1978). Nonverbal ability was not found to be significantly related to intelligence quotients, class rank, Scholastic Aptitude Test (SAT) scores, or vocabulary test scores (Knapp). The findings show that, in general, if persons were good senders of nonverbal communication, they were also good receivers (Knapp).

The empirical research reported in this section underlines the continuing development of nonverbal communication during adolescence. Developmental changes in both encoding and decoding nonverbal cues occur in preadolescents and adolescents with typical development.

Points of Discussion

1. Critique the oral and nonverbal communication development data presented in this chapter.

2. Describe several research topics that would significantly add to our database on typical language development in older students.

Suggested Readings

Street, C. (2002). Expository text and middle school students: Some lessons learned. *Voices from the Middle, 9*(4), 33–38.

Nippold, M. (1998). *Later language development: The school-age and adolescent years.* Austin, TX: Pro-Ed.

Chapter 4

Literacy Development

Goals

- Summarize milestones in written language development (i.e., in reading, writing, and spelling)

- Explain the primary differences between oral and written language skills

Before discussing the various aspects of written language (reading, writing, and spelling), we believe it is important to consider the concept of literacy. According to a report by the American Speech-Language-Hearing Association (2001b), *literacy* is defined by the National Literacy Act of 1991 as "an individual's ability to read, write, and speak in English and compute and solve problems at levels of proficiency necessary to function on the job and in society, to achieve one's goals, and to develop one's knowledge and potential" (p. 6).

According to N. Nelson (1998), it is in the later stages of language development that literacy activities gain importance. Language development in the later stages involves the integration of listening, speaking, reading, writing, and thinking. These modalities should be viewed as interactive processes and should not be examined in isolation (Nelson). For the purpose of organizing this book, however, we talk about each modality separately.

Whether language is oral or written, two people are needed for communication to occur—speakers need listeners and writers need readers. Also needed are a reason to communicate (pragmatics), meaning (semantics), and structure (syntax), which is coded phonetically or graphically (Westby, 1990).

However, two differences between oral and written language should be noted: contextualization and immediacy of the audience (N. Nelson, 1988). "Although it is not altogether clear how knowledge of specific differences between spoken and written language emerges, it is clear that children apply their realizations about modality differences relatively late in the language development process" (Gillam and Johnston, 1992, p. 1304).

Reading
Definition

The American Speech-Language-Hearing Association (2001b) stated, "reading can be defined as the processes by which one constructs meaning from printed symbols" (p. 7). Reading has two general components: decoding and comprehension. *Decoding* is the process of word recognition that transforms print to words. *Comprehension* is a process by which language is understood and interpreted and thus meaning is constructed at the word, sentence, and discourse levels. According to Catts and Kamhi (1999), readers use word knowledge acquired in spoken language to construct meaning in reading. These researchers also noted that some of the higher order comprehension processes employed in reading are different from those used in spoken-language comprehension.

Typical Development

Chall (1983) outlined the stages of reading development. Five stages are included during the developmental process, preceded by prereading, which occurs during preschool and kindergarten. Literacy socialization is the main achievement during prereading (e.g., knowing which way to hold a book, learning how to turn pages, recognizing that print moves from left to right in the English language). Following prereading skills, the following stages occur:

- **Stage 1 (decoding) in grades 1–2—** The main achievement is phonological analysis and segmentation.

- **Stage 2 (automaticity) in grades 2–4—**The main achievement is fluent reading with greater comprehension than stage 1.

- **Stage 3 (reading to learn) in grades 4–8—**Children gain more complete comprehension and have an increased rate of reading.

- **Stage 4 (reading for ideas) in grades 8–12—**The main achievement is the use of inferences and recognizing different points of view.

- **Stage 5 (critical reading) in college/ post–high school—**Critical reading requires critical thinking and synthesis of new knowledge.

Reading initially requires bringing to conscious awareness the various categories and relations in language (Menyuk and Chesnick, 1997). Therefore, initial word reading brings to consciousness phonological awareness and lexical meaning; reading sentences brings to consciousness awareness of semantic and syntactic relations (such as subject-verb relationships); and reading passages brings to consciousness awareness of discourse relations (such as pronominal substitution) and text structure (such as narratives).

Moats (2000) summarized reading development yet another way. According to her, and supported by the work of Ehri (1994), children progress through four stages:

- Logographic
- Novice alphabetic
- Mature alphabetic
- Orthographic

At the logographic level, children are context dependent and rely on incidental visual cues to derive any meaning from print. At the novice alphabetic level, they acquire letter-name knowledge and partial phoneme awareness. At the mature alphabetic level, they recognize "chunks" (e.g., a stem such as "ing" or "and"). They also master grapheme-phoneme connections and, at this stage, have more elaborated phoneme awareness. Finally, at the orthographic level, students have both phoneme and morpheme awareness, sequentially decode print, and readily see connections between speech and print.

Good readers are skilled in the phonological processing system before the middle grades (Moats, 2000). Whereas comprehension at the first grade level is accounted for by how well students sound out words and recognize words out of context, by the middle grades, knowledge of word meanings becomes more of a factor (Foorman, Francis, Shaywitz, Shaywitz, and Fletcher, 1997; Moats).

By third grade, students are capable of automatically recognizing words and have been helped by their phonological awareness and knowledge of the alphabetic principles. By then, students have been exposed to comprehending oral and written narrative and expository discourse and have had world experiences that allow them to more readily comprehend what they are reading.

As students move into the upper elementary and secondary levels, they expand their knowledge of narrative, expository, and persuasive discourse. Older students learn how to adjust their reading depending on the varied demands of the text and the purpose

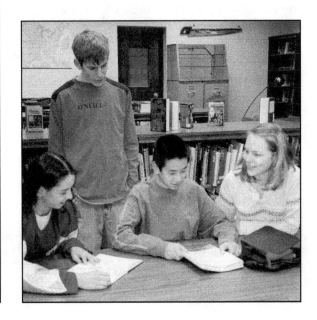

for reading. They are also capable of recognizing when they are having difficulty and can use metacognitive strategies, such as re-reading and asking questions, to facilitate comprehension. From upper elementary grades through college, students must read textbooks, reports, lab books and other lengthy materials across a variety of disciplines (American Speech-Language-Hearing Association, 2001b). Older students must be at the orthographic level, or they are severely disadvantaged within the general education curriculum.

Adolescent literacy, particularly reading skills, has become a national priority for the U.S. Department of Education and the National Institute of Child Health and Human Development (NICHD; National Institutes of Health, 2002). The NICHD provided major funding for two workshops in 2002 that helped set the agenda for research on the reading skills of older students. Curtis (2002) presented a synthesis of past research, encompassing 155 studies since 1990, on this topic. Much of the research has focused on struggling readers. Curtis observed:

> Such a focus is understandable, particularly given that as many as 40 percent of 13-year-olds seem to have difficulty interrelating ideas and making generalizations, while as many as 60 percent of 17-year-olds are unable to understand complicated literacy and informational passages. (p. 10)

In their grant announcement "Research in Adolescent Literacy" (2002), the National Institutes of Health emphasized the study of how reading develops in competent readers during middle grades and high school, rather than focusing in the deficits in struggling readers. This research will be applied to determine what is needed to raise literacy levels overall. As a nation, when considering all student levels, achievement in reading declines between grades 4–8, and again between grades 8–12. While this pattern currently represents "typical" development in the United States, other industrial countries do not have the extent of reading decline by older students that the United States does. For this reason and many others, the study of how to develop more competent older student readers is an encouraging national priority in the early part of this new century.

Ratner and L. Harris (1994) listed the skills needed to be a successful reader. They are presented in Table 4.1. Given the expectation that after third grade, students read to learn (rather than learn to read, as they did prior to grade three), adolescents should have the skills listed in Table 4.1. If they fail to have these skills, their reading deficits compound their difficulties in learning the academic content of school.

Writing
Definition

Written language requires that the meaning of the message be independent of an immediate reference (i.e., decontextualized), whereas spoken language is thought to be context dependent since it usually relies on the

Table 4.1   # Task Analysis of Reading Skills

Skills Required to Decode Unknown Printed Words	
Phonological Skills	• Awareness of differences and similarities between phonemes • Knowledge of phonological rules of the language • Ability to blend individual phonemes into a meaningful word • Knowledge of sound-letter association
Synthesis	• Ability to combine sounds into larger units
Attentional Skills	• Ability to focus attention on a specific sound or task • Ability to sustain attention for the length of time it requires to complete a specific task • Enough attentional capacity to simultaneously decode and comprehend the text
Auditory Perceptual Skills	• Ability to isolate a sound within a word in initial, medial, and final position • Ability to perceive relationships between words that rhyme (i.e., to perceive the sounds of parts of two or more words that sound the same) • Ability to perceive the double sound of consonant blends in words, such as *play* and *blue* (e.g., *bl, br, cl, cr, dr, dw, fl, tr, gr, pl, gl, pr, sc, sk, sl, sm, sn, sp, st, ng*) • Ability to perceive the consonant combinations that represent one sound (e.g., *sh, th, wh, ch, ph, ng, gh*) • Ability to perceive differences between the sounds of short vowels in words (e.g., *fan, fin, fun* and *tan, tin, ten*) • Ability to perceive the sounds of vowel combinations (e.g., *ie, ea, oo, oi, ou, oa, ai*)
Knowledge of Morphological Rules	• Ability to divide perceived words into their smallest grammatical units, or morphemes (e.g., *unanswerable* contains *un, answer,* and *able*)
Sequential Memory	• Ability to rapidly recognize and retrieve letters and words • Ability to remember the order of phonemes that when combined comprise a word • Ability to recall the sounds within a word and words within a phrase or sentence • Ability to recall from memory the syntactical, phonological, and morphological rules that govern the arrangement of words in a phrase or sentence

Continued on next page

Table 4.1–Continued

Visual Perceptual Ability	• Ability to distinguish different letter shapes • Ability to discriminate letters of varying size • Ability to perceive the differences between the amount of space separating letters within words and that which separates words in a phrase or sentence • Ability to distinguish the direction and orientation of different letters • Ability to perceive any angle, slant, or other deviation from the horizontal or vertical • Ability to understand that the letters have permanent shapes despite the fact that we view them vertically on a chalkboard, horizontally on a desk, and from a variety of orientations, and that we often move while we are viewing them (shape constancy) • Ability to separate the letters from the lined paper on which they are written and/or separate the printed letters from illustrations on the same page (figure-ground discrimination) • Ability to recognize or identify the letters despite distortion, illegibility, partial erasure, or overlap (closure)
Skills Required to Read with Comprehension	
Attention	• Ability to attend to and to simultaneously decode and comprehend the text • Ability to focus attention on the relevant and most important aspects of written text • Ability to withhold attention from irrelevant and incidental information in the text to be read
Syntax	• Ability to understand complex spoken sentences with embedded clauses • Ability to understand relationships between sentences and across sentence boundaries (paragraph)
Semantics	• Ability to understand the multiple meanings and subtle nuances of spoken language • Ability to use appropriate and adequate vocabulary • Ability to associate and generalize concepts • Ability to interpret idiomatic, figurative, and colloquial speech

Table 4.1—Continued

Memory	• Ability to access stored lexical knowledge • Ability to hold the sentences in working memory long enough to establish relationships among the concepts expressed by the sentences being read and related concepts stored in memory • Ability to hold the words of a relatively long and complex sentence in short-term memory long enough to extract the most pertinent and important components • Ability to tap past experiences and previously stored information that relate to the topic, the problem, and the meaning of the material to be read • Ability to draw from long-term memory lexical information pertaining to words and word meanings • Ability to appropriately and adequately use general information stored in long-term memory, based on past personal experiences with objects, situations, and events • Ability to draw from long-term memory information that enhances and supplements what is read (i.e., analogous reasoning ability) • Ability to hold in working memory the correct sequence of events in a story
Imagery	• Ability to envision the scene described by the author, not only the visual details, but also the smells, the sounds, and the entire physical and emotional environment
Pragmatics	• Ability to quickly identify the topic of the paragraph or chapter to be read • Ability to perceive the relationships between experiences of a character in the story and one's own • Ability to appropriately and adequately use social skills with peers and adults in real life • Ability to understand affect denoting emotions when communicating with another person • Ability to understand motivation that causes individuals to react and respond to another person, event, or situation in a particular way • Ability to recognize cause-effect relationships and to identify consequences of fictional characters' actions • Ability to predict what will happen in a story or how the character will react • Ability to role play • Ability to empathize with people who are unhappy, embarrassed, or frightened in real life

Continued on next page

Table 4.1–Continued

Pragmatics *(Continued)*	• Ability to understand the emotional reactions of a character in a story • Ability to predict the character's response in a given situation, and also to envision the character's affect indicating the emotions that are felt • Ability to determine just from the description of the dialogue the tone of voice, the stress of words, the sarcasm, and the inflection in the voices of the characters as they speak
Higher Level Cognitive Skills	• Ability to find evidence in a passage to support logical generalizations and conclusions • Ability to differentiate between the main idea of the story and supporting details • Ability to infer concepts that are not explicitly stated • Ability to perceive the author's purpose or intention • Ability to distinguish among facts, opinions, hypotheses, and assumptions • Ability to differentiate conclusions from supporting statements, facts from opinions, and explicit from implied statements • Ability to determine how details relate to main ideas, whether sufficient information is provided by the author, and whether the author's ideas are coherent • Ability to apply criteria or standards with which to make judgments on content, ideas, methods, products, and people that are presented by the author • Ability to combine components of information into a coherent and connected whole • Ability to apply ideas learned in one situation to new or related situations

From *Understanding Language Disorders: The Impact on Learning* (pp. 197–201), by V. Ratner and L. Harris, 1994, Eau Claire, WI: Thinking Publications. © 1994 by Thinking Publications. Adapted with permission.

immediate context to convey the communication message. Consider the following:

• In oral communication, the audience is generally physically present or on the phone and the communication is a shared turn-taking dialogue in which speaker and listener may share common information.

• In written communication, the audience may be unknown or must be imagined by the writer. The writer does not get immediate feedback as does the speaker, and thus the writer must anticipate the degree to which the written message must be made explicit (N. Nelson, 1988).

One of the major demands on high school students is the increasing requirement to produce longer, more elaborate complex written forms across a variety of discourse genre (N. Nelson, 1998). The types of writing required of adolescents in school are shown in the sidebar. Typical adolescents take years to master basic writing skills. For example, N. Nelson's (1988) and N. Nelson and Friedman's (1988) research on written personal narratives found that 63% of seventh graders with typical development still produced primitive narratives (see the sidebar in Chapter 3 on page 74 for Applebee's (1978) narrative development sequence). Of the tenth graders, 46% produced focused chains and only 39% produced true narratives. Of college freshmen, 25% produced focused chains and

75% produced true narratives. Data such as these need to be taken into account when judging the written language skills of those referred for suspected language disorders.

Typical adolescents

take years to master basic

writing skills.

Typical Development

Some professionals adhere to the idea that all areas of language are important and that each area assists the others. They maintain that listening, speaking, reading, and writing

---

Types of Writing Required of Adolescents in School

- Personal experience narratives (Describe your best experience.)
- Story retelling (Write a book report.)
- Factual retelling (Summarize a passage from your history book.)
- Fictional stories or guided stories (Write your own fantasy short story.)
- Expositions on how to do something (Explain how to plant a rose bush.)
- Descriptions (Describe the tourist trades in Wisconsin.)
- Reporting (Write a report of a sporting event.)
- Persuasive (Write an essay on why students should be allowed to listen to music during study hall.)
- Business letters (Write a letter applying for a job interview.)
- Friendly letter (Write to your friends inviting them to a party.)

Source: Scott and Erwin (1992)

abilities develop concurrently and interrelatedly, rather than sequentially (Schory, 1990; Teale and Sulzby, 1986; Westby, 1990). Perera (1986), while discussing later language development, suggested that complex linguistic structures are encountered first in reading and then are practiced in writing. She called writing "a potent agent in the process of language development" (p. 518). Writing is also an ideal medium for the acquisition of complex structures, "because it allows the language user to deliberate, to review and to correct, without pressure from conversational partners" (Perera, p. 518). Rubin (1987) identified several skills used by students who have developed adequate writing (see the sidebar).

Competent writers use three major processes while writing: planning, generating sentences, and revising (Hayes and Flower, 1987). Planning involves information retrieval and the shaping of that knowledge to match the audience. Generating sentences translates the plan into formal prose. Even the most extensive outline is expanded on average by a factor of eight in the final essay (Kaufer, Hayes, and Flower, 1986). Revising involves rewriting the generated sentences with the goal of improving the text.

Unfortunately, revisions are not always beneficial. One study found that fourth graders hardly revise at all, eight graders' revisions hurt more than they help, and twelfth graders' revisions that are helpful narrowly outnumber the harmful ones (Bracewell, Scardamalia, and Bereiter, 1982). One possible explanation for this is provided by Applebee (1981):

> However detailed and constructive a teacher's comments may be, their effectiveness depends upon the extent to which the students read the comments and upon whether simply reading them is enough to teach a student how to correct the errors. Since students rarely are asked to write another draft, they have few chances to learn how to use an editor's suggestions and revisions to produce a better manuscript. (p. 103)

Abilities of Students Who Have Developed Adequate Writing Skills

- Create subject matter, without the benefit of shared understandings with their communication partners
- Address unknown audiences
- Engage in writing to contribute to an ongoing knowledge base
- Revise their messages constantly

Source: Rubin (1987)

One of the most ambitious longitudinal studies ever undertaken on written language development is that of Walter Loban (1976). He collected a written language sample from the same subjects (in grades 3–12) from whom he collected an oral language sample (described in Chapter 3). One composition of a typical writing sample was obtained from each subject during grades 3–9, and two or more compositions per year from students in grades 10–12.

Loban (1976) analyzed the written samples along the same parameters as the oral samples. Table 4.2 shows the average number of words per communication unit (Loban defined a *communication unit* as an independent clause with its modifiers) for written language. That same table also shows the relative growth of length of communication unit across the grade span, as well as the velocity of that growth. The spurt in writing skills at grade 12 is particularly striking when comparing the low-ability group to the other two. Unlike the smooth developmental patterns for oral language, the pattern for written language was more erratic. In written language, large upward changes in the number

Average Number of Words per Communication Unit—Written Language

Table 4.2

Grade	Average Number of Words per Communication Unit (mean)			Relative Growth[a] (in percent)			Year-to-Year Velocity[b] (in percent)		
	High Group	Random Group	Low Group	High Group	Random Group	Low Group	High Group	Random Group	Low Group
3	7.68	7.60	5.65	58	57	43	—	—	—
4	8.83	8.02	6.01	67	60	45	+9	+3	+2
5	9.52	8.76	6.29	72	66	47	+5	+6	+2
6	10.23	9.04	6.91	77	68	52	+5	+2	+5
7	10.83	8.94	7.52	82	67	57	+5	-1	+5
8	11.24	10.37	9.49	85	78	72	+3	+11	+15
9	11.09	10.05	8.78	84	76	66	-1	-2	-6
10	12.59	11.79	11.03	95	89	83	+11	+13	+17
11	11.82	10.69	11.21	89	81	84	-6	-8	+1
12	14.06	13.27	11.24	109	100	85	+17	+19	+1

From *Language Development: Kindergarten through Grade Twelve* (p. 33), by W. Loban, 1976, Urbana, IL: National Council of Teachers of English. © 1976 by the National Council of Teachers of English. Reprinted with permission.

[a] Relative Growth uses the scores of the Random Group at grade 12 to equal 100 percent.

[b] Year-to-Year Velocity is the percentage change in any given group from one year to the following year. The impact of anticipating or not anticipating college apparently accounts for the velocities that emerge at grade 12.

of communication units were sometimes followed by downward shifts during the middle and high school years (as opposed to the plateaus he observed following growth in oral language samples). As for oral language use, the high-ability group in Loban's study engaged in written language that was approximately four to five years ahead of subjects whom teachers rated as being in the low-ability group for language skills. For example, looking at the number of communication units used by the low-ability group at grade 12 (11.24), this is the same number used by the high-ability group at grade 8. Note from Table 4.2 that all groups showed particularly rapid growth in written language from grades 9 to 10. The high-ability and random groups showed another surge in the number of words per communication unit from grades 11 to 12, but the low-ability group did not. Loban attributed this growth to the anticipation of and preparation for college, an experience not present for those in the low-ability group.

When comparing the development in average number of words per communication unit for oral vs. written language, a distinct pattern emerged from grades 1 through 12 (this pattern is illustrated in Table 4.3). From grades 1 through 9, the average words

Average Number of Words per Communication Unit— Comparison of Oral and Written Language (Mean)

Table 4.3

Grade	High Group		Random Group		Low Group	
	Oral	Written	Oral	Written	Oral	Written
1	7.91	—	6.88	—	5.91	—
2	8.10	—	7.56	—	6.65	—
3	8.38	7.68	7.62	7.60	7.08	5.65
4	9.28	8.83	9.00	8.02	7.55	6.01
5	9.59	9.52	8.82	8.76	7.90	6.29
6	10.32	10.23	9.82	9.04	8.57	6.91
7	11.14	10.83	9.75	8.94	9.01	7.52
8	11.59	11.24	10.71	10.37	9.52	9.49
9	11.79	11.09	10.96	10.05	9.26	8.78
10	12.34	12.59	10.68	11.79	9.41	11.03
11	13.00	11.82	11.17	10.69	10.18	11.21
12	12.84	14.06	11.70	13.27	10.65	11.24

From *Language Development: Kindergarten through Grade Twelve* (p. 35), by W. Loban, 1976, Urbana, IL: National Council of Teachers of English. © 1976 by the National Council of Teachers of English. Reprinted with permission.

per oral communication unit was slightly higher than the average for written language, but from grades 10 through 12, longer communication units occurred in writing.

The growth in dependent clauses in written language based on Loban's (1976) data is shown in Table 4.4. The average number of dependent clauses per communication unit for all three groups is more alike after the elementary grades than for any other measure in his study. In studying the data, readers can see that by grade 10, there were few differences among the averages of the groups, and that in grade 11, the low-ability group actually used more dependent clauses per communication unit than did those students in the high-ability group. The explanation for this lies in the quality of the writing of those in the high-ability group. They ceased to use dependent clauses as often in their writing in favor of more succinct and sophisticated word choices, such as appositives, gerunds, and participles. In fact, Loban reminds readers that excessive use of dependent clauses can result in complicated sentences that obscure rather than clarify meaning. Thus, while the low-ability group looks like it has closed the developmental

Average Number of Dependent Clauses per Communication Unit—Written Language

Table 4.4

Grade	Average Number of Dependent Clauses per Communication Unit (mean)			Relative Growth[a] (in percent)			Year-to-Year Velocity[b] (in percent)		
	High Group	Random Group	Low Group	High Group	Random Group	Low Group	High Group	Random Group	Low Group
4	0.38	0.19	0.06	63.33	31.67	10.00	—	—	—
5	0.35	0.21	0.14	58.33	35.00	23.33	-5.00	+3.33	+13.33
6	0.40	0.29	0.18	66.67	48.33	30.00	+8.32	+13.33	+6.67
7	0.48	0.28	0.20	80.00	46.67	33.33	+13.33	-1.66	+3.33
8	0.54	0.50	0.40	90.00	83.33	66.67	+10.00	+36.66	+33.34
9	0.46	0.47	0.37	76.67	78.33	61.67	-13.33	-5.00	-5.00
10	0.53	0.52	0.51	88.33	86.67	85.00	+11.66	+8.34	+23.33
11	0.43	0.45	0.55	71.67	75.00	91.67	-16.66	-11.67	+6.67
12	0.66	0.60	0.52	110.00	100.00	86.67	+38.33	+25.00	-5.00

From *Language Development: Kindergarten through Grade Twelve* (p. 40), by W. Loban, 1976, Urbana, IL: National Council of Teachers of English. © 1976 by the National Council of Teachers of English. Reprinted with permission.

[a] Relative Growth uses the scores of the Random Group at grade 12 to equal 100 percent.

[b] Year-to-Year Velocity is the percentage change in any given group from one year to the following year.

gap by the senior high years with regard to this aspect of written language, the quality of their writing when compared to the high-ability group is considerably less cohesive and efficient (i.e., with regard to the number of words needed to express the same thought).

Table 4.5 compares the growth in dependent clause usage in both oral and written language across the grades and across groups. When looking at data for grades 8–12, the low-ability group clearly showed dependent clause usage in written language that did not manifest itself in oral language samples. (Before grade 8, their oral language was more advanced.) The reverse is true for the high-ability language group. From grades 9–12, they tended to use more dependent clauses in their speaking than in their writing; prior to grade 9, their writing had more dependent clause usage than their speaking. Again, the shift for those in the high-ability group is more likely related to the use of more sophisticated elaboration strategies beyond dependent clauses in their written language.

Average Number of Dependent Clauses per Communication Unit— Comparison of Oral and Written Language

Table 4.5

Grade	High Group		Random Group		Low Group	
	Oral	Written	Oral	Written	Oral	Written
1	0.24	—	0.16	—	0.12	—
2	0.25	—	0.21	—	0.17	—
3	0.27	—	0.22	—	0.18	—
4	0.37	0.38	0.30	0.19	0.20	0.06
5	0.37	0.35	0.29	0.21	0.25	0.14
6	0.41	0.40	0.37	0.29	0.30	0.18
7	0.44	0.48	0.35	0.28	0.31	0.20
8	0.45	0.54	0.39	0.50	0.30	0.40
9	0.52	0.46	0.43	0.47	0.31	0.37
10	0.61	0.53	0.48	0.52	0.33	0.51
11	0.63	0.43	0.52	0.45	0.36	0.55
12	0.67	0.66	0.58	0.60	0.46	0.52

From *Language Development: Kindergarten through Grade Twelve* (pp. 37, 40), by W. Loban, 1976, Urbana, IL: National Council of Teachers of English. © 1976 by the National Council of Teachers of English. Adapted with permission.

Given the shortcomings of dependent clause usage for clear, cohesive writing, Loban (1976) turned to an elaboration index to study more advanced language structures. This index accounted for all strategies used to expand communication units beyond one-word subjects and predicates. The elaboration indexes for the written language samples from grades 4–12 are shown in Table 4.6. The high-ability group showed clear developmental superiority when all elaboration structures, not just dependent clause usage, were considered. The greatest developmental changes with regard to elaboration happened in grade 8 for the random and the low-ability groups and at grade 12 for the high-ability group (see the Year-to-Year Velocity column in Table 4.6). Note that these surges in writing occurred one or two years after similar surges in oral language elaboration. (See Table 3.5, on page 63.)

Table 4.7 compares the relative growth in elaboration for oral vs. written language. Similar to the growth-regression pattern illustrated in Table 4.2, the development of elaboration did not follow a smooth, steady progression. For example, note that all three groups slowed up or fell backwards at grades 9 and 11. The random group, which is most representative of all populations in a school, showed notable advances in writing development at grades 5, 8, 10, and 12.

Average Number of Elaboration Index Points per Communication Unit—Written Language

Table 4.6

Grade	Elaboration Points per Unit			Relative Growth[a]			Year-to-Year Velocity[b]		
	High Group	Random Group	Low Group	High Group	Random Group	Low Group	High Group	Random Group	Low Group
4	4.12	3.29	2.73	52.55	41.96	34.82	—	—	—
5	4.51	4.08	2.64	57.53	52.04	33.67	+4.98	+10.08	-1.15
6	5.06	4.18	3.12	64.54	53.32	39.80	+7.01	+1.28	+6.13
7	5.62	4.07	3.36	71.68	51.91	42.86	+7.14	-1.41	+3.06
8	6.22	6.05	4.89	79.34	77.17	62.37	+7.66	+25.26	+19.51
9	6.41	5.25	4.33	81.76	66.96	55.23	+2.42	-10.21	-7.14
10	7.15	6.79	5.40	91.20	86.61	68.88	+9.44	+19.65	+13.65
11	6.38	5.97	5.72	81.38	76.15	72.96	-9.82	-10.46	+4.08
12	8.51	7.84	6.11	108.55	100.00	77.93	+27.17	+23.85	+4.97

From *Language Development: Kindergarten through Grade Twelve* (p. 61), by W. Loban, 1976, Urbana, IL: National Council of Teachers of English. © 1976 by the National Council of Teachers of English. Reprinted with permission.

[a] Relative Growth uses the scores of the Random Group at grade 12 to equal 100 percent.

[b] Year-to-Year Velocity is the percentage change in any given group from one year to the following year.

Average Number of Elaboration Index Points per Communication Unit

Table 4.7

Grade	High Group		Random Group		Low Group	
	Oral	Written	Oral	Written	Oral	Written
1	3.18	—	2.47	—	2.05	—
2	3.05	—	2.73	—	2.43	—
3	3.33	3.25	2.78	2.43	2.57	2.11
4	3.96	4.12	3.63	3.29	2.98	2.73
5	4.14	4.51	3.67	4.08	3.12	2.64
6	4.77	5.06	4.33	4.18	3.46	3.12
7	5.36	5.62	4.38	4.07	3.94	3.36
8	5.48	6.22	4.95	6.05	4.24	4.89
9	5.70	6.41	5.16	5.25	4.16	4.33
10	5.93	7.15	5.11	6.79	4.22	5.40
11	6.80	6.38	5.75	5.97	4.92	5.72
12	6.92	8.51	6.05	7.84	5.41	6.11

From *Language Development: Kindergarten through Grade Twelve* (p. 63), by W. Loban, 1976, Urbana, IL: National Council of Teachers of English. © 1976 by the National Council of Teachers of English. Reprinted with permission.

Returning to the comparison of oral and written elaboration (see Table 4.7), all groups used more elaboration in writing than in speaking by grade 12. That pattern was present from fourth grade on for the high-ability group (with the exception of grade 11). The shift in pattern was more gradual for the random group; not until grade 8 was written elaboration used consistently more than oral elaboration. Finally, the low-ability group used written elaboration less than oral elaboration until grade 8 and overall their usage was depressed compared to the other groups. Loban (1976) observed that:

(L)earning to write in a way that uses a large repertoire of syntactical strategies develops more slowly for those who lack proficiency in oral language. Very plausibly, they need to develop and practice syntactical complexities in speech before they can use them in writing. (p. 63)

Writing skills continue to develop throughout late adolescent and adult years. According to Nippold (1998), research has demonstrated that certain lexical cohesion devices (such as synonyms and collocation) are used with increased frequency in written sentences during the adolescent years. Polanski (1989) found that the type of formal writing: expressive (descriptive), explanatory (expository), and persuasive played a role in the production of metaphors in grades 4, 8, and 12, and college students. The results indicated that metaphoric production increased with age in all three modes, but most often in the expressive mode and least often in the persuasive mode. This illustrates that it is important to evaluate students' writing in a variety of written modes. According to a report by the American Speech-Language-Hearing Association (2001b), students find planning and revising difficult well into their secondary school years, and although they are capable of writing well-formed narrative and informational texts, persuasive writing remains difficult even in high school.

Ratner and L. Harris (1994) noted that one type of writing skill that is important at the secondary level is that of note taking. They delineated the skills needed to be a good note taker (see the sidebar on page 100).

Particularly for individuals whose vocations depend on writing talent, development of additional skills may become a lifelong pursuit. For other adults, research suggests that writing is the language art least used (Werner, 1975); the average adult spends only 9% of his or her communication time engaged in writing. However, the written word long outlasts the spoken word, and thus the importance of the quality of one's written language cannot be underestimated throughout the life span.

Spelling
Definition

Spelling is a complex language skill that requires the integration of phonological, morphological, semantic, and orthographic knowledge (Lombardino and Ahmed, 2000). To this knowledge set, Masterson, Apel, and Wasowicz (2002) add knowledge of learned mental images of words (i.e., mental orthographic images). All combined, this knowledge is needed to understand how the sounds and structure of oral language relate to the letters and structure of written language.

Typical Development

According to a report by the American Speech-Language-Hearing Association (2001b), to be a fluent writer, one should be a fluent speller. Masterson and Crede (1999) found that students progress through five developmental stages:

Stage 1—Preliterate (emergent)
Stage 2—Letter-name (alphabetic)
Stage 3—Within-word pattern
Stage 4—Syllable juncture
Stage 5—Derivational

These stages, ages of development, and characteristics of each stage are presented in Table 4.8. One can conclude from Table 4.8 that older students should be at the derivational stage by the mid-elementary grades and beyond. Of course, this is not always the case, as shown in Chapter 6, where we present spelling deficit information.

Skills Required to Take Adequate Notes

- Adequate attention span

- Ability to focus on material being discussed

- Adequate short-term sequential memory

- Ability to process complex verbal sentences that contain embedded clauses

- Adequate vocabulary

- Ability to perceive relationships among objects, events, and situations presented both visually and auditorily

- Ability to grasp inference and figurative language

- Ability to follow 3–4 step directions

- Ability to differentiate the main idea, relevant details, and information that illustrates that idea

- Ability to hold words in mind while writing them down, at the same time listening to additional words

- Ability to process simultaneous visual and auditory stimuli

- Ability to copy from a chalkboard or overhead transparency and simultaneously listen while the teacher explains notations

- Ability to switch between sensory tracts: auditory (listening), visual (seeing), and motor-kinesthetic (writing)

- Auditory discrimination ability

- Auditory closure ability to "fill in" when information spoken has not quite been distinguished

- Auditory figure-ground ability

From *Understanding Language Disorders: The Impact on Learning* (p. 195), by V. Ratner and L. Harris, 1994, Eau Claire, WI: Thinking Publications. © 1994 by Thinking Publications. Adapted with permission.

(T)o be a fluent writer,

one should be a

fluent speller.

In a more comprehensive fashion, Ehri (2000) discussed behaviors that support the development of spelling skills:

- Word familiarity, which assists individuals to retain in memory a specific spelling

- Knowledge about the general alphabetic system (i.e., spelling regularities

Table 4.8

Stages of Spelling Development

Stage	Age (in years)	Characteristics
Preliterate (Emergent)	1–5	• Scribbling • Writing letterlike forms • Not understanding that writing represents sounds
Letter-Name (Alphabetic)	5–7	• Having writing-to-speech correspondence at the syllable level (e.g., one syllable equals one letter) • Spelling only simple sight words correctly • Developing letter-sound matches for initial and final consonants
Within-Word Pattern	6–12	• Spelling most sight words correctly • Using letter patterns to spell single syllables • Using short vowels correctly in invented spellings • Using silent letters for long vowels (e.g., *rain, rake*)
Syllable Juncture	8+	• Appreciating the meaning-spelling connection • Having invented spelling errors at the syllable juncture points and schwa positions
Derivational Relations	8+	• Learning that some words with the same derivation share the same spelling pattern • Acquiring derivations throughout life

Sources: Masterson and Crede (1999); J. Wasowicz (personal communication, January 7, 2003)

that recur in different words, including grapheme-phoneme and phoneme-grapheme units and spelling patterns and morphographs that symbolize syllabic units, root words, and affixes)

• Knowledge about specific words, frequently acquired through memory

It should be noted that reading and spelling are not entirely correlated (grapheme-phoneme relations are used for reading whereas phoneme-grapheme relations are used for spelling). Also, there are about 40 distinctive phonemes in English, but 70 letters or letter combinations to symbolize these phonemes. Thus, pronouncing spellings is easier than writing spellings.

Memory is often taxed by words that have a schwa vowel (e.g., note the second syllable in *lettuce, terrace,* and *bargain).* The schwa might be spelled with any vowel letter or pair of letters. Thus, the difficulty is in remembering each spelling. Also, words are difficult to spell when they include nonconventional graphemes, doubled letters, silent letters, and uncommon spelling patterns, as in words like *lieutenant, unnecessary, conscientious, accommodate, noticeable, receipt,* and *aisle.*

In summary, word reading and word spelling are closely related in that both take advantage of prealphabetic level, partial alphabetic level, full alphabetic level, and consolidated alphabetic level (Ehri, 2000). Templeton (in the foreword to Masterson, Apel, and Wasowicz, 2002) aptly observed, "Simply put, looking closely at how students spell words offers powerful insight into the nature of their word knowledge and thus the types of information they use when they read and write words" (p. X).

Points of Discussion

1. Critique the written language development data presented in this chapter.

2. Describe several research topics that would significantly add to our database on literacy development in older students.

Suggested Readings

American Speech-Language-Hearing Association. (2001). *Roles and responsibilities of speech-language pathologists with respect to reading and writing in children and adolescents.* Rockville Pike, MD: Author.

Ehri, L.C. (2000). Learning to read and learning to spell: Two sides of a coin. *Topics in Language Disorders, 20*(3), 19–36.

Loban, W. (1976). *Language development: Kindergarten through grade twelve.* Urbana, IL: National Council of Teachers of English.

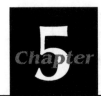

Communication in Culturally and Linguistically Diverse Populations

Goals

- Provide key statistics on cultural diversity within the United States, especially as they relate to older students

- Define and describe language differences vs. language disorders

- Illustrate how linguistic diversity and adolescence might intersect, thus creating implications for those who serve older students

The cultural composition of the United States is changing. This change consists of increased numbers of individuals from Africa, Central and South America, the Caribbean Islands, Asia, and the Pacific Rim (Rhea Paul, 2001). Also, within the United States there are changes in migration patterns, such as Native Americans moving away from reservations (i.e., 90% stayed in 1940 to 20% staying today). A second major change is that non-White, non-Western European citizens are having the majority of the children. In fact, by 2030, more than 40% of school children will be from non-White, non-European backgrounds (Rhea Paul).

These estimates are conservative. Already, almost 40% of students are from non-White, non-European backgrounds

(National Center for Educational Statistics, 2000a). The U.S. Department of Education (2000), as reported by Meece and Kurtz-Costes (2001), projects that by the year 2020, more than two-thirds of the school population will be African American, Asian, Hispanic, or Native American, with Hispanic youths representing over 20% of the 5- to 17-year-old population. By this same year, minorities will actually represent the majority of children under 18 in a number of states, such as Texas, California, Hawaii, and Florida.

According to Rhea Paul (2001), already in some states (e.g., California and Texas) the majority of residents (i.e., averaging all ages) are of non-European heritage. Likewise, in some cities in the United States (e.g., Miami, Philadelphia, and Baltimore) the majority of the children are from culturally different populations and are non-White.

The Evolving Definition of *Race*

Based on the 2000 U.S. Census Bureau report: Of the respondents to the 2000 census in the United States, 75% identified themselves as White alone; 12% as Black or African American alone; 1% as American Indian and Alaska Native alone; 4% as Asian alone; 0.1% as Native Hawaiian and Other Pacific Islander alone; and 5.5% as some other race alone.

The question on race for Census 2000 was different from the one for the 1990 census in several ways. Most significantly, respondents were given the option of selecting one or more race categories to indicate their racial identities (rather than having a forced choice of only one race). Because of these changes, the Census 2000 data on race are not directly comparable with data from the 1990 census or earlier censuses. Caution must be used when interpreting changes in the racial composition of the U.S. population over time.... According to Census 2000, 281.4 million people resided in the United States, and 35.3 million, or about 13 percent, were Latino.... The remaining 246.1 million people, or 87 percent, were not Hispanic (U.S. Census Bureau, 2001, pp. 2–4).

Professionals should note that the U.S. Census Bureau does not define Hispanic as a race, but as an origin; those who label themselves as Latino may be a member of any race.

As with all changes in how demographics are tracked and reported, it will take some time for all systems to report data using the same definitions. The educational statistics and projections available at the writing of this book typically included those individuals of Hispanic origin within the minority information reported.

Linguistic Diversity

With the demographic changes in the United States, it is critical that speech-language pathologists and other professionals understand the difference between a language difference and a language disorder. A *language difference* is a rule-governed language code or system that is different from Standard American English (SAE), but one that meets the norms of the individual's primary linguistic community (Rhea Paul, 2001). If a culturally different student has a *language disorder*, communication problems in both English and the student's primary language will be noted (Roseberry-McKibbin, 2002).

A language difference is a rule-governed language code or system that is different from Standard American English (SAE), but one that meets the norms of the individual's primary linguistic community.

Understanding typical language development and differences between SAE and the primary linguistic system of the student is critical for appropriate assessment and diagnosis and ultimately for intervention or service delivery. Professionals who do not recognize the effect of cultural influences on communication may violate legal mandates that require all students be provided with culturally and linguistically appropriate assessment protocols and instructional methods or service delivery models (Roseberry-McKibbin, 2002).

Immigration is a major contributor to the diversity within our schools. Approximately 4% of school-age children were foreign-born in 1990, compared with only 1% in 1970 (Meece and Kurtz-Costes, 2001). A majority of foreign-born residents live in only six states—California, Florida, Illinois, New Jersey, New York, and Texas. Asia and Latin America are the major sources of U.S. immigration (National Research Council, 1997).

Professionals must recognize that each person in any cultural group is first an individual and second a member of a particular cultural group, and that there is a great deal of heterogeneity within cultural groups (Roseberry-McKibbin, 2002). Professionals also cannot assume that all minority youths are linguistically diverse. Many are assimilated into the mainstream American culture and are monolingual English-speaking individuals. Others are bilingual, multilingual, or semilingual (i.e., neither the original language nor the new language is acquired satisfactorily).

Approximately 5% of all school-age children in the United States speak a language other than English at home (National Center for Educational Statistics, 2000a). Anyone who speaks a language other than Standard American English is considered to be in the linguistic minority (Ratner and L. Harris, 1994). This does not mean the individual's language is disordered. D. Taylor (1988) noted that "normal" for a particular speaker is determined by one's culture. Language that meets the cultural constraints of the linguistic community is normal. The purpose of this chapter is not to provide an in-depth review of each culture, although professionals need to seek out this information in order to work successfully with populations who are culturally diverse. For more in-depth knowledge, readers might consult Roseberry-McKibbin (2002) or Langdon and Cheng (2002).

Second Language Learning

Speech-language pathologists must understand the normal processes of second language learning, which include but are not limited to the following (Roseberry-McKibbin, 2002):

- Interference, or the process wherein a language behavior (i.e., in syntax, morphology, phonology, pragmatics, and/or semantics) from the first language is carried over to the second language

- Fossilization, wherein a specific second language "error" is firmly entrenched in the second language even though the person is very proficient in the second language

- Code-switching, or the alternation between two languages within sentences or discourse units; although code-switching is a normal behavior among second language learners and adolescents, it can become extensive in cases in which the individual is not proficient in the second language

Langdon and Cheng (2002) also considered *language loss*, which is the normal losing of how to express something in one's first language as one assimilates the second language. Language loss is common and should be anticipated as professionals study the language behaviors of those whose first language is not English.

The level of proficiency a child has in his or her primary language when initially exposed to a second language will affect the child's future development of both languages (Cummins, 1989). Regression in the primary language may occur from exposure to the second language at an unsuitable time. A threshold of competence in the primary language should be reached before a second language can be mastered; otherwise, semilingualism results (Cummins). This threshold often does not occur until the mid-elementary years, and there are data to suggest that age 10 is the best time to introduce a second language (Skutnabb-Kangas and Toukomaa, 1976, as cited in Pacheco,

1983). Even so, D. Duncan (1989) suggested that school-age children take 18 to 36 months to function linguistically in a new language. Cummins cautioned that academic language competence may take up to seven years to develop for children with typical development who are learning English after the age of 6. Roseberry-McKibbin (2002) stated that a culturally fair, dialectically non-biased method of assessment is that of obtaining language samples and in turn using the communication unit (C-Unit) rather than mean length of utterance (MLU), as the measurement of analysis. Recall from Chapter 3 that a C-Unit consists of an independent clause plus its modifiers.

Dialects

Standard American English (SAE) has many dialects. Competent language users can easily switch between SAE and their dialect in response to the communication situation. Dialects reflect only a difference in language use, not pathology of language (O. Taylor, 1988).

One of the most common dialects in the United States is African American English (AAE), previously called Black English (BE). O. Taylor and Peters (1982) presented a thorough description of AAE features by reviewing 29 linguistic rules. These 29 linguistic rules (e.g., invariant "be," negation, plurals, questions, and pronouns) have been analyzed to determine where there is overlap between AAE and several other dialects (i.e.,

Southern English, Southern White nonstandard English, and Appalachian English). They also briefly reviewed Spanish-influenced English in terms of phonological and syntactic features.

A more extensive study by Mendelberg (1984) investigated the language of Mexican-American adolescents of migrant origin. The analysis of the data revealed distinctive language patterns used in different settings. Initially, it would seem that the language patterns chosen are determined as a matter of the subject's personal choice. However, upon further investigation, it appears that underlying the choice is the role language plays as a symbol of the group and the position the group occupies in the social system. There is a relationship between language use and the development of a group identity. These findings concur with O. Taylor and Peters (1982), who concluded that major social and cultural factors influence language acquisition and behavior.

Significant dialect differences are delineated in Tables 5.1 through 5.6. The tables contrast the most salient features of Standard American English (SAE) with African American English (AAE), with Latino English (LE), and with Asian English (AE). These three dialects comprise the most common ones used by school-age students in the United States. In addition, pragmatic contrasts are summarized in Table 5.7. Competent professionals working with linguistically diverse cultures must recognize

Phonemic Contrasts between African American English (AAE) and Standard American English (SAE)

Table 5.1

SAE Phonemes	Position in Word		
	Initial	**Medial**	**Final***
/p/ /n/		Unaspirated /p/	Unaspirated /p/ Reliance on preceding nasalized vowel
/w/	Omitted in specific words *(I'as, too!)*		
/b/		Unreleased /b/	Unreleased /b/
/g/		Unreleased /g/	Unreleased /g/
/k/		Unaspirated /k/	Unaspirated /k/
/d/	Omitted in specific words *(I'on't know)*	Unreleased /d/	Unreleased /d/
/ŋ/		/n/	/n/
/t/		Unaspirated /t/	Unaspirated /t/
/l/		Omitted before labial consonants *(help-hep)*	"uh" following a vowel *(Bill-Biuh)*
/r/		Omitted or /ə/	Omitted or prolonged vowel or glide
/θ/	Unaspirated /t/ or /f/	Unaspirated /t/ or /f/ between vowels	Unaspirated /t/ or /f/ *(bath-baf)*
/v/	Sometimes /b/	/b/ before /m/ and /n/	Sometimes /b/
/ð/	/d/	/d/ or /v/ between vowels	/d/, /v/, /f/
/z/		Omitted or replaced by /d/ before nasal sound *wasn't-wud'n)*	

Blends

/str/ becomes /skr/   /ʃr/ becomes /str/
/θr/ becomes /θ/   /pr/ becomes /p/
/br/ becomes /b/   /kr/ becomes /k/
/gr/ becomes /g/

Final Consonant Clusters (second consonant omitted when these clusters occur at the end of a word)

/sk/   /nd/   /sp/
/ft/   /ld/   /ʤ d/
/st/   /rd/   /nt/

From *Language Development: An Introduction* (5th ed.; p. 418), by R.E. Owens, Jr., 2001, Boston, MA: Allyn and Bacon. © 2001 by Pearson Education. Reprinted with permission.

*Note weakening of final consonants.

Grammatical Contrasts between African American English (AAE) and Standard American English (SAE)

Table 5.2

	AAE Grammatical Structure	SAE Grammatical Structure
Possessive -'s	Nonobligatory where word position expresses possession Get *mother* coat. It *be* mother's.	Obligatory regardless of position Get *mother's* coat. It's *mother's*.
Plural -s	Nonobligatory with numerical quantifier He got ten *dollar*. Look at the *cats*.	Obligatory regardless of numerical quantifier He has ten *dollars*. Look at the *cats*.
Regular past -ed	Nonobligatory, reduced as consonant cluster Yesterday, I *walk* to school.	Obligatory Yesterday, I *walked* to school.
Irregular past	Case by case, some verbs inflected, others not I *see* him last week.	All irregular verbs inflected I *saw* him last week.
Regular present-tense third-person singular -s	Nonobligatory She *eat* too much.	Obligatory She *eats* too much.
Irregular present-tense third-person singular -s	Nonobligatory He *do* my job.	Obligatory He *does* my job.
Indefinite *an*	Use of indefinite *a* He ride in *a* airplane.	Use of *an* before nouns beginning with a vowel. He rode in *an* airplane.
Pronouns	Pronominal apposition: pronoun immediately follows noun Momma *she* mad. She…	Pronoun used elsewhere in sentence or in other sentence; not in apposition Momma *is* mad. She…

Continued on next page

Communication Solutions
for Older Students

Table 5.2—Continued

	AAE Grammatical Structure	**SAE Grammatical Structure**
Future tense	More frequent use of *be going to (gonna)* I *be going* to dance tonight. I *gonna* dance tonight. Omit *will* preceding *be* I *be* home later.	More frequent use of *will* I *will* dance tonight. I *am going* to dance tonight. Obligatory use of *will* I *will* (I'll) *be* home later.
Negation	Triple negative *Nobody don't never* like me. Use of *ain't* I *ain't* going.	Absence of triple negative *No one ever* likes me. *Ain't* is unacceptable form *I'm not* going.
Modals	Double modals for such forms as *might, could,* and *should* I *might could* go.	Single modal use I *might be able* to go.
Questions	Same form for direct and indirect What *it is?* Do you know what *it is?*	Different forms for direct and indirect What *is it?* Do you know what *it is?*
Relative pronouns	Nonobligatory in most cases He the one stole it. It the one you like.	Nonobligatory with *that* only He's the one *who* stole it. It's the one (*that*) you like.
Conditional *if*	Use of *do* for conditional *if* I ask *did* she go.	Use of *if* I asked *if* she went.
Perfect construction	*Been* used for action in the distant past He *been* gone.	*Been* not used He left a long time ago.
Copula	Nonobligatory when contractible He sick.	Obligatory in contractible and uncontractible forms He's sick.
Habitual or general state	Marked with uninflected *be* She *be* workin'.	Nonuse of *be*; verb inflected She's *working* now.

From *Language Development: An Introduction* (5th ed.; pp. 419–420), by R.E. Owens, Jr., 2001, Boston, MA: Allyn and Bacon. © 2001 by Pearson Education. Reprinted with permission.

Phonemic Contrasts between Latino English (LE)
Table 5.3 and Standard American English (SAE)

SAE Phonemes	Position in Word		
	Initial	**Medial**	**Final***
/p/	Unaspirated /p/		Omitted or weakened
/m/			Omitted
/w/	/hu/		Omitted
/b/			Omitted, distorted, or /p/
/g/			Omitted, distorted, or /k/
/k/	Unaspirated or /g/		Omitted, distorted, or /g/
/f/			Omitted
/d/		Dentalized	Omitted, distorted, or /t/
/ŋ/	/n/	/d/	/n/ *(sing–sin)*
/j/	/ʤ/		
/t/			Omitted
/ʃ/	/tʃ/	/s/, /tʃ/	/tʃ/ *(wish–which)*
/tʃ/	/ʃ/ *(chair–share)*	/ʃ/	/ʃ/ *(watch–wash)*
/ɪ/	Distorted	Distorted	Distorted
/ʤ/	/d/	/j/	/ʃ/
/θ/	/t/, /s/ *(thin–tin, sin)*	Omitted	/ʃ/, /t/, /s/
/v/	/b/ *(vat–bat)*	/b/	Distorted
/z/	/s/ *(zip–sip)*	/s/ *(razor–racer)*	/s/
/ð/	/d/ *(then–den)*	/d/, /θ/, /v/ *(lather–ladder)*	/d/

Blends

/skw/ becomes /eskw/*

/sl/ becomes /esl/*

/st/ becomes /est/*

Vowels

/ɪ/ becomes /i/ *(bit-beet)*

From *Language Development: An Introduction* (5th ed.; p. 424), by R.E. Owens, Jr., 2001, Boston, MA: Allyn and Bacon. © 2001 by Pearson Education. Reprinted with permission.

*Separates cluster into two syllables.

Grammatical Contrasts between Latino English (LE)
Table 5.4 **and Standard American English (SAE)**

	LE Grammatical Structure	**SAE Grammatical Structure**
Possessive -'s	Use postnoun modifier This is the homework of *my brother*. Article used with body parts I cut *the finger*.	Postnoun modifier used rarely This is *my brother's* homework. Possessive pronoun used with body parts I cut *my* finger.
Plural -s	Nonobligatory The *girl* are playing. The *sheep* are playing.	Obligatory, excluding exceptions The *girls* are playing. The *sheep* are playing.
Regular past -ed	Nonobligatory, especially when understood I *talk* to her yesterday.	Obligatory I *talked* to her yesterday.
Regular third-person singular present-tense -s	Nonobligatory She *eat* too much.	Obligatory She *eats* too much.
Articles	Often omitted I am going to store. I am going to school.	Usually obligatory I am going to *the* store. I am going to school.
Subject pronouns	Omitted when subject has been identified in the previous sentence Father is happy. Bought a new car.	Obligatory Father is happy. *He* bought a new car.
Future tense	Use *go + to* I *go to* dance.	Use *be + going to* I *am going* to the dance.
Negation	Use *no* before the verb She *no* eat candy.	Use *not* (preceded by auxiliary verb where appropriate) She does *not* eat candy.
Question	Intonation; no noun-verb inversion *Maria is* going?	Noun-verb inversion usually *Is Maria* going?

Table 5.4—Continued

	LE Grammatical Structure	SAE Grammatical Structure
Copula	Occasional use of *have* I *have* ten years.	Use of *be* I *am* ten years old.
Negative imperatives	*No* used for *don't* *No* throw stones.	*Don't* used *Don't* throw stones.
***Do* insertion**	Nonobligatory in questions You like ice cream?	Obligatory when no auxiliary verb *Do* you like ice cream?
Comparatives	More frequent use of longer form (*more*) He is *more* tall.	More frequent use of shorter *-er* He is tall*er*.

From *Language Development: An Introduction* (5th ed.; pp. 425–426), by R.E. Owens, Jr., 2001, Boston, MA: Allyn and Bacon. © 2001 by Pearson Education. Reprinted with permission.

these differences when conducting assessment procedures or providing intervention services to those individuals. Please note that Table 5.7 contains information on Native Americans, but the preceding six tables do not. The reason for this is the large number of Native American languages. While, culturally, Native American languages share some semantic and pragmatic features, the phonetic and syntactic variations among their indigenous languages are many. There are more than 200 American Indian languages spoken in the United States, and dialectal differences exist within them (Roseberry-McKibbin, 2002).

Cultural Diversity and Older Students

Attention to problems among adolescents must begin with knowing that this age group is not homogeneous. There are many subgroups, which, although they face common problems, have different degrees of risk depending on their social, ethnic, or racial backgrounds. "For example, black male adolescents are five to six times as likely to die as a result of homicide as white males, and black girls are two to three times as likely to become homicide victims as white girls" (Hechinger, 1992, p. 29). Thus, the degree

Phonemic Contrasts between Asian English (AE) and Standard American English (SAE)

Table 5.5

SAE Phonemes	Position in Word		
	Initial	**Medial**	**Final**
/p/	/b/§	/b/§	Omission
/s/	Distortion*	Distortion*	Omission
/z/	/s/†	/s/†	Omission
/t/	Distortion*	Distortion*	Omission
/tʃ/	/ʃ/§	/ʃ/§	Omission
/ʃ/	/s/†	/s/†	Omission
/r/, /l/	Confusion‡	Confusion‡	Omission
/θ/	/s/	/s/	Omission
/dz/	/d/ **or** /z/§	/d/ **or** /z/§	Omission
/v/	/f/‡	/f/‡	Omission
	/w/†	/w/†	Omission
/ð/	/z/*	/z/*	Omission
	/d/§	/d/§	Omission

Blends

Addition of /ə/ between consonants‡

Omission of final consonant clusters§

Vowels

Shortening or lengthening of vowels (*seat–sit, it–eat**)

Difficulty with /ɪ/, /ɔ/, and /æ/, and substitution of /ə/ for /æ/†

Difficulty with /ɪ/, /æ/, /U/, and /ə/§

From *Language Development: An Introduction* (5th ed.; p. 427), by R.E. Owens, Jr., 2001, Boston, MA: Allyn and Bacon. © 2001 by Pearson Education. Reprinted with permission.

*Mandarin Chinese only.

†Cantonese Chinese only.

‡Mandarin, Cantonese, and Japanese.

§Vietnamese only.

Grammatical Contrasts between Asian English (AE) and Standard American English (SAE)

Table 5.6

	AE Grammatical Structure	SAE Grammatical Structure
Plural -s	Not used with numerical adjective: *three cat* Used with irregular plural: *three sheeps*	Used regardless of numerical adjective: *three cats* Not used with irregular plural: *three sheep*
Auxiliaries *to be* and *to do*	Omission: I *going* home. *She not want eat.* Uninflected: I *is going.* *She do not want eat.*	Obligatory and inflected in the present progressive form: I *am going home.* *She does not want to eat.*
Verb *have*	Omission *You been here.* Uninflected *He have one.*	Obligatory and inflected: *You have been here.* *He has one.*
Past-tense -ed	Omission: *He talk yesterday.* Overgeneralization: *I eated yesterday.* Double marking: *She didn't ate.*	Obligatory, nonovergeneralization, and single marking: *He talked yesterday. I ate yesterday. She didn't eat.*
Interrogative	Nonreversal: *You are late?* Omitted auxiliary: *You like ice cream?*	Reversal and obligatory auxiliary: *Are you late? Do you like ice cream?.*
Perfect marker	Omission: *I have write letter.*	Obligatory: *I have written a letter.*
Verb-noun agreement	Nonagreement: *He go to school. You goes to school.*	Agreement: *He goes to school. You go to school.*
Article	Omission: *Please give gift.* Overgeneralization: *She go the school.*	Obligatory with certain nouns: *Please give the gift. She went to school.*
Preposition	Misuse: *I am in home.* Omission: *He go bus.*	Obligatory specific use: *I am at home. He goes by bus.*

Continued on next page

117

Communication Solutions for Older Students

Table 5.6—Continued

	AE Grammatical Structure	SAE Grammatical Structure
Pronoun	Subjective/objective confusion: *Him go quickly.* Possessive confusion: *It him book.*	Subjective/objective distinction: *He gave it to her.* Possessive distinction: *It's his book.*
Demonstrative	Confusion: *I like those horse.*	Singular/distinction: *I like that horse.*
Conjunction	Omission: *You I go together.*	Obligatory use between last two items (in) a series: *You and I are going together. Mary, John, and Carol went.*
Negation	Double marking: *I didn't see nobody.* Simplified form: *He no come.*	Single obligatory marking: *I didn't see anybody. He didn't come.*
Word order	Adjective following noun (Vietnamese): *clothes new.* Possessive following noun (Vietnamese): *dress her.* Omission of object with transitive verb: *I want.*	Most noun modifiers precede noun: *new clothes.* Possessive precedes noun: *her dress.* Use of direct object with most transitive verbs: *I want it.*

From *Language Development: An Introduction* (5th ed.; p. 428–429), by R.E. Owens, Jr., 2001, Boston, MA: Allyn and Bacon. © 2001 by Pearson Education. Reprinted with permission.

of risk to adolescents will depend on their ethnicity and how society responds.

Roseberry-McKibbin (2002) noted that "children entering their adolescence, must face the changes of adolescence as well as problems commonly encountered when adjusting to a new country" (p. 17). Certainly new immigrants who enter the United States as older students (i.e., past age 10) have major language challenges as they encounter U.S. school systems. Those with disorders in their primary language can be expected to have problems learning English as a foreign language. This can be determined through careful parental interview procedures (Langdon and Cheng, 2002).

There are significant racial and ethnic differences in students' levels of educational

Semantic and Pragmatic Contrasts between Standard American English (SAE) and Four Major Dialects

Table 5.7

	Semantics	Pragmatics
Native American English (NAE)	Many Native American students are "whole concept" rather than linear learners. They may understand explanations more easily when they progress from the whole to the parts, rather than from the parts to the whole. Many Indian languages have no word for time, contain no future tense verbs, and are based almost entirely on the present tense.	Bragging about oneself or one's abilities is considered rude; in SAE, bragging is usually tolerated. Giving advice or information only when asked honors their belief in not interfering in the affairs of others; in SAE, giving advice and information is commonplace. Avoiding eye contact signifies respect, and respect is highly valued; in SAE, it is disrespectful not to engage in eye contact. A lapse of time between the asking of a question and someone answering is required by etiquette; in SAE, such a lapse is uncomfortable.
African American English (AAE)	Many lexical items are used in AAE that are not used in SAE or that come into SAE from their use in AAE. Some examples include *funky* and *rap*. Other words are used to denote meanings in AAE that are not part of their meaning in SAE, although often these meanings migrate into mainstream use as well. Some examples are *hog* (expensive car), *all that* (excellent), and *dude* (man or person).	Preference for indirect eye contact during listening and direct eye contact during speaking; preferences are opposite in SAE. Use of direct questions is sometimes seen as harassment (e.g., "When will you be done?" is seen as rushing someone to finish something). Asking personal questions of a person someone has met for the first time is seen as improper and intrusive; such inquiry is considered "friendly" in SAE. Participating competitively in conversations is typical, with the most assertive participants doing most of the talking; this might be considered "rude" in SAE.

Continued on next page

Table 5.7–Continued

	Semantics	Pragmatics
Latino English (LE)	Number, color, and letter words often receive less emphasis in parent-child interactions in Hispanic households. Names and labels for objects, donors of objects, and particularly for relatives are emphasized in Hispanic parent-child interactions.	Hissing to gain attention is acceptable; in SAE, it is impolite. Direct eye contact may be interpreted as a challenge to authority; it is a sign of respect in SAE. Business conversations are preceded by lengthy exchanges unrelated to the main point; getting quickly to the point is valued in SAE.
Asian English (AE)	Literal translations from native language *(open-light* = turn on light). Difficulties with idioms and colloquialisms.	Interrupting a conversation is considered impolite; in SAE, interruptions are appropriate in certain circumstances. Kinship terms are very important in determining the relationship between two speakers and extend beyond the family; kinship terms have a less rigid effect on SAE. Expressing affection publicly, especially between men and women, "looks ridiculous"; kissing and hugging in public are acceptable in SAE.

Sources: Gilliland (1988); Rhea Paul (2001); Roseberry-McKibbin (2002)

attainment in the United States that professionals need to consider in their work with older students. For example, 17-year-old African American students score about the same as 13-year-old White students for reading and mathematics (National Center for Educational Statistics, 2000b). To what can professionals attribute this gap? Steele (1992) argued that mainstream society portrays African Americans as intellectually inferior and a fear of confirming this negative stereotype leads these students to "disidentify" with school, thus reducing their achievement efforts. Ogbu (1992) posited that African

American students may show poorer academic achievement lest they be seen as acting White. In contrast, Spencer, Noll, Stoltzfus, and Harpalani (2001) looked at adolescents' ethnic identity, self-beliefs, and achievement, and their findings were summarized by Meece and Kurtz-Costes (2001) as follows:

> As previously mentioned, the acting White assumption posits that African American adolescents who show academic success and *[sic]* have embraced a Eurocentric identity. Contrary to this hypothesis, Spencer et al. showed that in their large sample of African American adolescents, academic excellence was positively related to healthy self-esteem and to a strong Afrocentric identity. African American youth in their sample who had a stronger Eurocentric identity showed lower self-esteem and lower academic achievement. These research findings are invaluable in beginning to understand the processes at work in identity formation, motivation, and achievement striving in ethnic minority children and youth. (p. 4)

The lesson to be gained by speech-language pathologists and other professionals working with older students from non-White backgrounds is to view any deficit in a broader context than simply school performance as measured by tests. The adolescent's attitudes, motivation, and experiences must also be considered.

Meece and Kurtz-Costes (2001) cautioned that one of the most pervasive problems in research to date is the failure to untangle the confounding factors of ethnic background and socioeconomic status. Given the disproportionate percentage of ethnic minority families who live in poverty, to what extent does economic hardship affect educational disparities? Most studies have failed to control for the income of ethnic minorities and the income of the ethnic majority with whom they are compared. Statistics show that 19% of children under 18 are growing up below the poverty threshold of $16,500 for a family of 4; the poverty rate is roughly 35% each for African Americans and those with Hispanic origin compared with 14% for Whites (Forum on Child and Family Statistics, 1999). Professionals must be careful not to confuse ethnic diversity with language problems stemming from poverty (e.g., a lack of print materials in the home, inadequate food, and poor health service). Roseberry-McKibbin (2002) also cited the potential family issues that may surface as the student gets older, such as the conflict between laws in the United States (e.g., those mandating compulsory education) and the desires of a family who wants its teenage child to go to work to assist with the family's income level.

Communication Solutions
for Older Students

Statistics show that African American students and those from Hispanic origin have higher rates of school suspensions and expulsions than any other minority groups (National Center for Educational Statistics, 1999). Between 1971 and 1999, the percentage of students who completed high school increased from 82 to 92% for Whites, 59 to 89% for African Americans, and 48 to 62% for those of Hispanic origin (National Center for Educational Statistics, 2000a). This is encouraging progress. However, when these older students were followed beyond high school, a different pattern was revealed: 80% of White high school graduates, 14% of African American students, and 12% of students with Hispanic origin entered college. Studying those who were between 25 and 29 years of age, 36% of Whites had completed a bachelor's degree, compared with 17% of African Americans and 14% of Hispanics (National Center for Educational Statistics, 2000a). Clearly, minority students are much more at risk for not completing their degrees than their White counterparts. Professionals such as speech-language pathologists must ask themselves what they can do to assist those dropping out of high school or college to persevere, especially when language disorders are at the base of their academic challenges.

Slaughter-Defoe and Rubin (2001) conducted a longitudinal study of African American Head Start children and their matched peers to determine the factors that influence educational achievement during their adolescence. The findings of the study indicated that preschool and primary grade teachers were strong contributors to the later educational goal setting and academic achievement during adolescence. Parents were contributors, but were not solely responsible to the Head Start students' later educational success in adolescence. This study strongly encourages and supports Head Start programs that use a parent/teacher collaborative model to support early childhood educational achievement, which results in long-term educational benefits for these students into their adolescence.

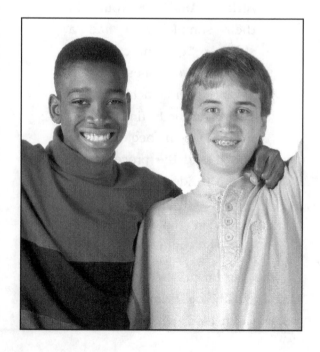

Asian Americans are a notable exception to the pattern of lower school achievement records by non-White populations. With the exception of Southeast Asians, this group shows higher graduation rates and graduate degree attainment than Whites (Barringer, Gardner, and Levin, 1993). The high academic performance and attainments of Asian American students is well documented (Fuligni, 1997; Kao, 1995). Kao noted that the parents of many Asian American groups place high premium on educational success and that educational achievement is a large part of the value system.

Roseberry-McKibbin (2002) observed that often young people from different cultures want to be Americanized, but their elders expect them to maintain traditional customs, resulting in conflict between the generations. These conflicts may escalate during adolescence when young people are developmentally wired to establish their independence from parents. Professionals need to be sensitive to both the needs of the older student and those of family members who may not share mainstream values and priorities.

The Role of Ethnography in Intervention

In 1974, Hymes described a new area of study called "the ethnography of speaking," which examines the role of speaking in the socialization of children. Anthropology and linguistics were brought together not in an attempt to establish communication universals, but to preserve the complexity of language use. Duranti (1988) explained:

> Ethnographers...like the people they study...struggle both to capture and maintain the whole of the interaction at hand. The elements of one level (e.g., phonological register, lexical choice, discourse strategies) must be related to elements at another level (e.g., social identities, values).... Ethnographers act as linking elements between different levels and systems of communication. (p. 220)

An ethnographic approach is different from a pragmatic analysis approach because there is stronger concern for the sociocultural context of language use.

Ethnography is critical when intervening with minority students. Speech-language pathologists from the majority culture will not typically share assumptions, values, or communication patterns with children from minority cultures. Thus, formulation of appropriate intervention strategies is prevented when professionals lack awareness of the importance of the cultural-socialization relationships within a given minority population.

Professionals should develop a database of typical development in children from culturally diverse backgrounds, rather than continuing to use Whites as the norm against which other groups are compared (McLoyd, 1998; Meece and Kurtz-Costes, 2001). Well-designed studies of a single group that are restricted in terms of ethnicity and social status may be more informative than comparative studies across groups that differ on a number of demographic variables (C. Wong and Rowley, 2001).

Crago and E. Cole (1991) described nine basic assumptions that characterize the ethnographic approach (see the sidebar that follows). These nine assumptions should become part of the foundation upon which solid, practical intervention goals and activities are created.

J. Damico and S. Damico (1993) echo the need to respect the complexity of the relationships between language and social skills when considered from a diversity perspective. As speech-language pathologists are called upon more and more to recommend intervention for students from culturally and linguistically diverse backgrounds, it is critical that the students' home languages are not seen as detriments and that their home cultures are not devalued in any way (J. Damico and S. Damico). Rather, professionals should assist students from diverse backgrounds to become more empowered in the educational system (J. Damico and Armstrong, 1991).

Basic Assumptions to the Ethnographic Approach

- "The everyday details of life can be made comprehensible" (p. 107). Study the details of people's everyday life experiences and build knowledge of what people say, what they do, and what people say they ought to say or do. Incorporate these details into intervention.

- "Accurate description requires extensive contact" (p. 108). Learn extensively about the culturally groups treated. Only then are appropriate speech-language services delivered.

- "Interpretation is an inherent part of observation" (p. 108). Seek and capture accurate interpretations of people's beliefs and actions to select appropriate times, forms, places, and people for intervention.

- "Analysis is an interactive spiral and not predetermined" (p. 108). Start with an initial set of questions during intervention and collect the response data. This should lead to more questions. Analysis during intervention is ongoing.

- "All descriptions are partial and subjective" (p. 109). Understand your influence on any findings and results. Describe and account for your own life situations that might contribute to partiality. Open, honest reckoning may lead to more productive clinical outcomes.

- "Descriptions have emic and etic dimensions" (p. 109). *(Emic* refers to the people being investigated (e.g., the culturally diverse students; *etic* refers to the outsider studying the people (e.g., a speech-language pathologist).) Shape etic frameworks to suit the client at hand, which may or may not fit into such a mold. Recognize how clients see your perspectives, actions, and interpretations.

- "More than one perspective is needed" (p. 110). Gain multiple perspectives on a student's functioning. Avoid misinterpretations, such as deficiency interpretations of cultural differences, by tapping into culturally informed points of view.

- "Both macro and micro levels of analysis are needed" (p. 110). Use language samples to pinpoint important gaps that are not culturally related (micro level). Document how language is integrated with cultural and socioeconomic dimensions (macro level).

- "Themes are generalizable from the careful study of a small number of people" (p. 111). Gather information on the communicative interactions of a few families within a particular cultural group, as it can be relevant to several students on your caseload.

Source: Crago and E. Cole (1991)

Points of Discussion

1. What resistance to assessment and intervention might you anticipate from an older student who has a language disorder and is also in the linguistic minority?

2. What would you ask teachers and family members about a student to determine if a language disorder or difference exists? If you did a classroom observation, what would you be looking for?

Suggested Readings

Meece, J.L., and Kurtz-Costes, B. (2001). Introduction: The schooling of ethnic minority children and youth. *Educational Psychologist, 36*(1), 1–7.

Roseberry-McKibbin, C. (2002). Multicultural students with special language needs (2nd ed.). Oceanside, CA: Academic Communication Associates.

Language Disorders
in Older Students

Goals

- Cite the prevalence of communication disorders in adolescents in schools and in juvenile detention facilities

- Discuss characteristic deficits in older students with language disorders

The theories of adolescence and the typical developmental milestones during preadolescence and adolescence presented in Chapters 1 through 4 frame the discussion that follows regarding the nature of language disorders in older students. This chapter reports the available statistics about this age group, discusses the expectations of typical adolescents, and highlights the myriad of problems that older students with language disorders often face.

Prevalence of Communication Disorders

Statistics for Adolescents in School

Statistics on the number of older students with disorders of speech and language are scattered because specific data on this age group have not often been gathered. Over a span of nearly 20 years, we have made three separate attempts to gather such data from state consultants for speech-language programs.

Statistics on the number of older students with disorders of speech, language, or hearing are scattered because specific data on this age group have not often been gathered.

Our first attempt was in late 1983. We conducted a national survey of state consultants for speech-language programs to determine the prevalence of communication disorders among adolescents. At the time of the initial survey, we defined the age range of older students as 12 to 20, in contrast to our present definition of 9–19 years. For purposes of comparative analysis, subsequent surveys have retained the original age range.

The return rate for the first survey was 26% (13 of 50 states). The majority of the surveys returned indicated that consultants had no means of retrieving statistics specifically for adolescents with communication disorders in their states. Thus, we could not compute a national prevalence figure. However, one reporting state, Florida, did compute prevalence figures and reported that 1.4% of students aged 13 to 21 years

were receiving services. Florida implemented Project Adolang (Task Force on Secondary Programs for the Speech-Language Impaired, 1983) to identify adolescent language problems and their implications for education.

In 1992, we conducted an update to our 1983 national survey. Only 8 of 50 states (16%) responded, and the majority of those reported that their states still had no way to retrieve statistics specifically for the 12- to 20-year-old age group. The few who were able to derive numbers showed a considerable difference between those receiving speech-language services in the 6- to 11-year-old range (5.3%) vs. the 12- to 20-year-old range (0.8%). Of those reported, 2.9% of the 6- to 11-year-old group had speech-language identified as their *only* disability, compared to 0.4% of the 12- to 20-year-old group.

Another state could report only the unduplicated count (i.e., students who have speech-language as their *primary* disability) and cited that 4.1% of their 6- to 11-year-olds received speech-language services, compared to 0.8% of their 12- to 20-year-olds. One state "translated" our age ranges to grades (i.e., grades 1–6 and grades 7–12) and reported that 4.7% of the younger group received speech-language services, compared to 1.5% of the older age group.

Particularly striking was the observation that only a fraction of students between 12 and 20 years of age were receiving speech-language services, compared to those between the ages of 6 and 11 years.

The implication was that relatively few students continued to receive speech-language services beyond the age 12. An unanswered question is whether the overwhelming decline in secondary students receiving speech-language services is due primarily to "curing" communication disorders by age 12 or to other factors.

In the spring of 2002, we repeated our survey for the third time. Eleven of the 50 states (22%) completed and returned it. Once again, not all states were able to break down their numbers of students receiving speech-language services among the 6- to 11- and 12- to 20-year age range. For example, one state reported their prevalence figure as 2.6% served through a resource room and .5% served through self-contained classrooms for those with communication disorders, across the age range of 6 to 20 years. Based on our past two surveys, we speculated that the number was artificially low when considering younger children, and high when considering older students.

Only two states cited both the total number of students between 12 and 20 years of age receiving speech-language services and the total number of students in their state in that age range. Both states reported the unduplicated count (i.e., students were identified as having only speech-language needs and no other disability). One state reported 1.4% and the other reported 0.5%. Translated into "real" people, in a group of 1,000 adolescents, the number served

ranged from 5 to 14 students, depending on the state analyzed. This is in contrast to those same states in which 3.7% and 4.8% of 6- to 11-year-olds were served (unduplicated count), or 37 to 48 children out of 1,000.

Translated into "real" people, in a group of 1,000 adolescents, the number served ranged from 5 to 14 students depending on the state analyzed.

We were able to derive duplicated counts (i.e., counts that include students classified as receiving speech-language services in conjunction with another special education program and those classified as speech-language services only) for four more states using the 2000 census data to determine the total number of 12- to 20-year-olds in those states. These additional numbers ranged from 1.32% to 0.4%. Translated into "real" people, in a group of 1,000 adolescents, the number served in these four states ranged from 4 to 13 students, depending on the state analyzed.

Communication Solutions
for Older Students

It is unclear why the duplicated counts are essentially the same as the unduplicated counts. States track enrollment data differently, so responders appeared to supply data in the form most readily available to them. We could sense our survey was a work overload to them, and several states returned surveys with the comment that no one had time to complete the data analysis required, or there was no longer a state-level speech-language supervisor. For example, two states reported the number of students receiving speech-language services relative to the total number of students enrolled for special education services, rather than as a percentage of the total number of students in their state within the 12- to 20-year age range.

In sum, for our 2002 survey, the prevalence figures for older students ranged from 0.5 to 1.4% based on those receiving services. This percentage was up considerably from our 1992 survey, and amazingly consistent with the Fein (1983) report from the American Speech-Language-Hearing Association, which documented 1.94% of individuals 5 to 14 years of age and 0.67% of individuals 15 to 24 years of age as having communication disorders. The percentages for older students are still depressed significantly from those in the 6- to 11-year age range, perhaps due to intervention succeeding in ameliorating the language disorders of many young children, and perhaps due to the traditional focus on early child language as the time when services are most needed. Ironically, however, professionals have evidence that children who present with language disorders in early childhood often persist in having life-long disabilities (C.J. Johnson et al., 1999; Stothard, Snowling, Bishop, Chipchase, and Kaplan, 1998). This begs the question of why speech-language pathologists persist in terminating services at approximately age 11 (after fourth or fifth grade). In Chapter 7, we discuss the lifelong issues such students often face as a result of their communication disorder.

In addition to the sources already cited, federal data are available from which some trends and statistics can be deduced. For example, the Executive Summary of the Twenty-First Annual Report to Congress on the Implementation of the Individuals with Disabilities Education Act (IDEA; U.S. Department of Education, Office of Special Education, 1999) noted that students served under IDEA increased from 1988–89 to 1997–98 (see the sidebar that follows). Over the decade, the greatest increase was in the 12- to 17-year-olds.

According to a report by the American Speech-Language-Hearing Association (2001a), services provided for children with a speech or language impairment showed an overall increase of 10.5% between the 1988–89 and 1997–98 school years. In this same report, it was estimated that approximately 8 to 12% of preschool children had some form of language disorder. There were no statistics provided for older students with language disorders, but ASHA estimates are between 5 and 8%

Increase in the Number of Students Served under IDEA from 1988–89 to 1997–98

Age Range	Increase in Students Served
6–11 years	24.3%
12–17 years	37.58%
18–21 years	15.85%

Of these students, 90% were identified in 1 of 4 disability categories:

- Learning disabilities (51.1% or 2,676,299 students)
- Speech-language disability (20.1% or 1,050,975 students)
- Mental retardation (11.4 % or 594,025 students)
- Emotional disturbance (8.6% or 447,426 students)

Source: U.S. Department of Education, Office of Special Education (1999)

since the prevalence estimate for learning disabilities is around 5%. In this same report (ASHA, 2001a), it was noted that the average age for speech-language services was 8.6 years, whereas for learning disabilities, the average age for students receiving services was 12.5 years. Since many students with a learning disability also have a language disorder, it is apparent that speech-language pathologists should be involved with these older students. This assertion is made based on the legal definition of a specific learning disability under IDEA (1997; P.L. 105-17): "The term 'specific learning disability' means a disorder in one or more of the basic psychological processes involved in understanding or in using language, spoken or written, which disorder may manifest itself in imperfect ability to listen, think, speak, read, write, spell, or do mathematical calculations." (§ 602 (26) (A))

Unfortunately, wide discrepancies among school districts exist in the provision of services for preadolescents and adolescents with communication disorders. One program with which we have consulted has a full-time speech-language pathologist at a middle school with a school census of 1,200 students. Another school in the same geographical area has a school census of 1,800 students, but only 3 hours of services a week are provided for older students. The discrepancy is not due to vast prevalence swings, but rather is a reflection of the knowledge and commitment of the individual professionals within each of the buildings.

Unfortunately, wide discrepancies among school districts exist in the provision of services for preadolescents and adolescents with communication disorders.

Statistics for Adolescents in Juvenile Detention Centers

Each year, more than one million youth come into contact with some aspect of the juvenile justice system (Cocozza, 1997). In juvenile detention centers, a disproportionately large number of adolescents with communication disorders have been evident relative to those reported as served in public schools. Sanger, Moore-Brown, and Alt (2000) noted that in earlier studies (Cozad and Rousey, 1966; Falconer and Cochran, 1989; J. Taylor, 1969), the prevalence of communication disorders in juvenile delinquents ranged from 24 to 84%. Since prison populations are on the increase, current data are direly needed on the prevalence of communication disorders in incarcerated youth.

Sanger and her colleagues (Sanger, Hux, and Belau, 1997; Sanger, Creswell, Dworak,

and Schultz, 2000) studied female juvenile delinquents and found 14 to 22% were at risk and had not received language services. In a sequel study, Sanger, Moore-Brown, Magnuson, and Svoboda (2001) found that 19.4% of female juvenile delinquents (13 of 46) performed sufficiently low on two standardized tests to potentially qualify for services. Of these 13, IQ scores were available for 11. Using a discrepancy formula based on mental age, only 5 of the 11 would have met criteria for speech-language services; all 11 would have qualified based on a chronological age discrepancy formula. In reality, none of the adolescents had a history of speech-language assessment or intervention prior to incarceration, although 6 of the 13 had a history of special education (without speech-language services). Clearly, there is more that speech-language pathologists can offer to the educational teams who ultimately address the needs of incarcerated youth, and those at risk for such programs (Cimorelli, McCready, Brucke, and Bushur, 2000).

Characteristic Deficits in Older Students with Language Disorders

Using data reviewed for Part I of this text, extrapolating from curricular materials for youth, and drawing on our own clinical experiences with preadolescents and adolescents, we have constructed Table 6.1,

Characteristic Expectations and Problems of Older School-Age Students with Language Disorders

Table 6.1

	Expectations	Problems
Cognition	To be at the formal operational level	Often remain concrete operational thinkers
	To observe, organize, and categorize data from an experience	Make chaos out of order
	To identify problems, suggest possible causes and solutions, and predict consequences	May not recognize a problem when it exists; if so, do not view more than one solution
	To place concepts into hierarchical order	Often cannot place concepts in a hierarchy
	To find, select, and utilize data on a given topic	Have limited strategies for finding, selecting, and utilizing data
Metalinguistics	To demonstrate conscious awareness of linguistic knowledge	Have difficulty bringing awareness to categories and relations in all aspects of language
	To talk about and reflect on various linguistic forms	Do not know the labels for talking about language during formal education
	To assess communication breakdowns and revise them	Do not have an awareness of breakdowns; if so, lack repair strategies
Comprehension/Production of Linguistic Features	To comprehend all linguistic features and structures	Misunderstand advanced syntactical forms
	To follow oral directions of three steps or more after listening to them one time	May not realize that directions are being given and/or have difficulty following multistep (3+ step) directions
	To use grammatically intact utterances	Use sentences that are fragmented and that do not convey intended messages
	To have a vocabulary sufficient for expressing ideas and experiences	Have word-retrieval problems and often use low-information words
	To give directions with clarity and accuracy	Unclear and/or inaccurate directions leave listeners confused
	To get information or assistance by asking questions and to respond appropriately to questions	May know what questions or answers to give, but do not know how to do so tactfully
	To comprehend and produce the slang and jargon of the hour	Do not comprehend or produce slang/jargon, thus are ostracized from their most desired group

Continued on next page

133

Communication Solutions
for Older Students

Table 6.1–Continued

	Expectations	Problems
Discourse	To produce language that is organized, coherent, and intelligible	Use many false starts and verbal mazes
	To follow adult conversational rules for speakers (e.g., maintaining a topic, initiating a topic)	Consistently violate the rules of conversation
	To be effective listeners during conversation without displaying incorrect listening habits	Often have poor listening skills
	To make a report, tell or retell a story, and explain a process in detail	Fail to use organizational frameworks or narrative structure, thus leaving their listeners confused
	To listen to lectures and to select main ideas and supporting details	Often do not grasp the essential message of a lecture
	To analyze critically other speakers	Make arbitrary, illogical, and impulsive judgments
	To express attitudes, moods, and feelings and to disagree appropriately	Have abrasive conversational speech
Nonverbal Communication	To follow nonverbal rules for kinesics	Violate the rules for bodily movements and misinterpret gestures and facial expressions
	To follow nonverbal rules for proxemics	Violate the rules for social distance
Reading	To decode and comprehend from printed symbols in various academic, social, and vocational situations	Do not consistently and/or efficiently decode and comprehend words, sentences, and discourse in a meaningful way; may lack phonological awareness skills and alphabetic letter knowledge
	To read fluently across a variety of genres (e.g., narratives and expository text) and across a variety of disciplines	Do not alter reading strategies across genres and disciplines
	To read fluently for a variety of purposes (e.g., to be informed, to be persuaded, to be entertained)	Do not adjust reading strategies to accommodate the writer's purpose
Writing	To produce cohesive written language required in various academic, social, and vocational situations by organizing, planning, composing, and editing	Do not consistently and/or efficiently generate written language that conveys intended messages; tend not to plan or edit writing
	To spell fluently	Do not know and/or apply spelling rules or the exceptions to these rules

From *Language Disorders in Older Students: Preadolescents and Adolescents* (pp. 78–79), by V. Lord Larson and N.L. McKinley, 1995, Eau Claire, WI: Thinking Publications. © 1995 by Thinking Publications. Adapted with permission.

"Characteristic Expectations and Problems of Older School-Age Students with Language Disorders." We have listed language expectations within each of seven areas, followed by a summary of the data describing problems observed when these expectations are not met. The expectations are derived from the type of communication demands that educators, parents, and peers place on preadolescents and adolescents. The problems are derived from a review of the literature and from our clinical observations of older students with language disorders.

When reviewing Table 6.1, note that typically a single problem would not result in a student being placed on the caseload, although there may be exceptions (e.g., a severe word-retrieval problem). Usually, a number of concomitant problems must exist before a preadolescent or adolescent would become a candidate for speech-language services. Candidates for services must have communication deficits that interfere with achieving academic progress, developing personal-social skills, or reaching vocational potential (Larson and McKinley, 1987, 1995).

This book focuses on preadolescents and adolescents who display the problems listed in Table 6.1, regardless of etiology or setting. When professionals examine the multitude of problems that can interfere with the academic, social, and vocational well-being of a student, they cannot afford to ignore youth with communication disorders after the elementary years. Special

compensatory programs for elementary grades only make sense if sixth-grade level skills are the end goal of intervention. Some students, without continued intervention, will regress to previous levels of functioning by the time they enter middle school (M. Larson and Dittman, 1975). Other adolescents need continued assistance to learn the new and more complex language skills demanded for higher grade levels. Still other students surface for the first time during preadolescence, because they have not acquired the necessary communication skills to survive the verbal and social demands of higher grade levels. Early childhood and elementary speech-language programs are not ineffective, but by themselves, they perform only a portion of the task for some students.

Cognitive Deficits

Many researchers have found that preadolescents and adolescents with cognitive deficits often fail to attain high levels of abstract reasoning (Ellsworth and Sindt, 1991; Reuven Feuerstein, 1980; Hains and D. Miller, 1980; Havertape and Kass, 1978; Neimark, 1980; Seidenberg, 1988; Whitmire, 2000). In other words, these adolescents remain concrete thinkers and do not use organized, efficient strategies for solving problems.

Recall the range of cognitive levels found in each grade level discussed in Chapter 2 (see Table 2.2, on page 40). Secondary-level teachers are faced with providing instruction to many students who remain at the concrete level. Relatively few, however, are at the onset level (i.e., just transitioning into the concrete period) or below. These students would have particular difficulty with school curricula and would be at risk for concomitant language disorders and other related problems, discussed in Chapter 7.

Students with low cognitive levels struggle with conceptual development. Wiig and Secord (1992a) summarized two categories of concepts important for learning: spontaneous (intuitive [e.g., same, different]) and scientific (scholastic, disciplinary [e.g., molecule, isosceles triangle]). The latter category is especially at risk among students with language disabilities (Wiig and Secord). Scientific concepts are constantly being added throughout each grade level and often build on one another.

According to Stone and Forman (1988), preadolescents and adolescents with learning disabilities show patterns of general conceptual disorders, specific developmental delays, and poor awareness of the implicit demands of a research situation. Learning disabled adolescents tend to blame "inadequate ability" more for their failure than nondisabled students; they tend to believe that intelligence is fixed and static, thus promoting their negativeness when faced with obstacles to their achievement (Golumbia and Hillman, 1990).

While it might be tempting to blame hereditary or environmental factors, Reuven Feuerstein (1980) argues that errors in methods of teaching are frequently the cause of low levels of abstraction in adolescents. He cites a lack of mediated learning experiences

as the primary cause of cognitive deficiencies and sees all other potential causes (e.g., poverty of stimulation or low functioning level of parents) as secondary reasons for the deficit. His teaching methods designed to combat low levels of abstraction are summarized Chapter 12.

Metalinguistic Deficits

Three stages occur in metalinguistic development: intuitive use of linguistic knowledge, awareness and executive use of the knowledge in tasks that require such awareness, and automatic use of the knowledge (Menyuk, 1991). Youth with language disorders do progress in language development and, therefore, gradually and intuitively acquire knowledge of language, but they have great difficulty in achieving conscious awareness of that knowledge (Menyuk).

When the firm establishment of linguistic representations and automatic retrieval are delayed, language development is delayed (Menyuk, 1991). Children who have language disorders have difficulty bringing to awareness categories and relations in all aspects of language. Menyuk argued that a language delay might be "caused by metaprocessing difficulties since awareness of structures precedes and is necessary for comparison of what is known to what is still be learned and for automatic use of structures" (p. 395).

Kamhi (1987) summarized research that examined the meta-abilities in children with language disorders across six areas:

- Repairing communicative breakdowns
- Making listener judgments
- Making judgments of language content
- Analyzing language into linguistic units
- Understanding and producing rhymes, puns, and riddles
- Understanding and producing figurative language

A synthesis of the studies indicated that metalinguistic deficits exist in children with language disorders, but these deficits are not all-pervasive (Kamhi). For example, 9- to 14-year-old students with language disorders have been found to have more difficulty than language-age matched peers in identifying, revising, and justifying revisions of morphological errors, but they produce the same types of clarification requests.

In general, youth with language disorders have difficulty acquiring various linguistic forms and, once acquired, also have difficulty reflecting on these forms (i.e., they have difficulty with metalinguistic tasks). N. Nelson (1993) underscored the importance of older students' abilities to reflect consciously on language, to process it on more than one level simultaneously, and to know the labels and talk about language during formal education. Students with language disorders often have deficits that surface when engaging in such metalinguistic tasks.

In general, youth with language disorders have difficulty acquiring various linguistic forms and, once acquired, also have difficulty reflecting on these forms (i.e., they have difficulty with metalinguistic tasks).

Linguistic Feature Deficits

Comprehension

Comprehension deficits during adolescence are often marked by less understanding of the figurative uses of language when students are matched with same-age peers (Blackwell, Engen, Fischgrund, and Zarcadoolas, 1978; J. Jones and Stone, 1989; Nippold, 1991). For example, late adolescent males (16 to 18 years of age) with learning disabilities provide significantly fewer correct metaphor interpretations than do peers with typical achievement (Jones and Stone, 1989). Even after instruction has raised students' levels of literal language comprehension to within normal limits, individuals with histories of language disorders may demonstrate significant deficits in metaphor comprehension ability (Nippold and Fey, 1983).

Communication Solutions
for Older Students

Riedlinger-Ryan and Shewan (1984), using a series of standardized tests, investigated the auditory comprehension of linguistic features by learning disabled and academically achieving adolescents. This study supported the findings of previous studies that documented the persistence of auditory language comprehension deficits in adolescents with learning disabilities. While some deficits in auditory comprehension were clearly demonstrated, deficits in comprehension of supersegmental features remain controversial. For example, evidence conflicts regarding the ability of adolescents with learning disabilities to comprehend stress and intonation patterns (Vogel, 1974; Wiig, Kutner, Florence, Sherman, and Semel, 1977). Indeed, Cruttenden (1985) concluded that even typical 10-year-olds are very limited in interpreting utterances whose intonations are critical for comprehension to occur.

Little information exists on comprehension monitoring by youth with language disorders (Dollaghan, 1987). Some evidence suggests that they produce fewer spontaneous requests for clarification than do their peers with typical development (Donahue, 1984; Donahue, Pearl, and Bryan, 1980). Even when given instruction in making clarification requests, Donahue (1984) found that students with learning disabilities perform less well than their peers. This is in contrast to Kamhi's (1987) summation.

Interest in listening comprehension deficits has also been sparked by examining the differences between those who become poor readers and those who become skilled readers (B. Wong, 1991). A growing body of evidence indicates that poor readers do not comprehend sentences as well as good readers (Mann, Cowin, and Schoenheimer, 1989). They perform less well on spoken instructions, such as those in DiSimoni's (1978) Token Test for Children (e.g., touch the small red square and the large blue triangle; S. Smith, Mann, and Shankweiler, 1986). B. Wong stressed that poor readers do not have trouble with the grammatical structures involved in comprehension tasks so much as they have short-term memory problems: "It seems as if poor readers are just as sensitive to syntactic structure as good readers; they fail to understand sentences because they cannot hold an adequate representation of the sentence in short-term memory" (p. 146).

In summary, older students should not have any difficulty comprehending any type of syntax and yet students with language disorders do have problems with advanced language forms (Rhea Paul, 2001). In particular, older students with language disorders also have difficulty comprehending figurative language (Nippold, 1998).

Production

Production deficits during adolescence may be evident in agrammatical sentences (Wiig and Semel, 1975), sentences of shorter length (Donahue, Pearl, and Bryan, 1982; Wiig and Semel), sentences with insufficient cohesion (Lapadat, 1991), and sentences that are less syntactically complex than those of typically developing peers (Donahue, Pearl, and Bryan, 1982; Geers and Moog, 1978). Older students with language disorders often have longer response lags before producing sentences (Wiig and Semel, 1975). In addition, word-retrieval problems (difficulty calling up an intended word from memory) are common (Blalock, 1981; Wiig and Becker-Caplan, 1984; Wiig and Semel).

Lapadat (1991) analyzed the results of 33 studies that investigated the language of students with language disorders and learning disabilities. Some of these studies involved children between the ages of 3 and 8 years, while others involved students ranging in ages from 9 to 12 years. Lapadat's results indicated that students' difficulty with using sufficient cohesion to communicate intention led to problems that involved misunderstandings, confusion, and incomplete discourse.

Asking questions may be difficult (Bryan, Donahue, and Pearl, 1981) and may occur with low frequency in specific situations. Donahue (1984) found that teaching students to ask questions did not improve their use of questions when clarification was needed. Instead, students needed to be taught *how* and *when* to ask for appropriate clarification.

In addition, adolescents with language disorders often have problems expressing themselves concisely (Wiig and Semel, 1976), and they tend to overuse a limited and concrete vocabulary (Wiig and Semel,

1975, 1976). During referential communication tasks, oral descriptions of an item or activity by adolescents with learning disabilities tend to be less informative for listeners than those provided by normal adolescents (Knight-Arest, 1984; Noel, 1980; Spekman, 1981). Knight-Arest found that boys with learning disabilities talked more but conveyed less information than their peers with typical development. The boys with learning disabilities appeared more comfortable when doing a task than when describing a task to a listener. Furthermore, they were less effective at adapting messages to the needs of the listener than their peers with normal achievement (e.g., repeating rather than reformulating what they said). They often appeared to be oblivious to the listener's needs.

On the plus side, Bunce (1989) concluded that students with learning disabilities can benefit from training on referential communication tasks. Her trained subjects learned to provide specific information needed by the listener to complete a particular task, to generalize their newly learned skills to a different referential communication task, and to retain most of their skills when a follow-up check was completed seven months later.

In Loban's (1976) classic study, which investigated oral and written language development from grades K–12, differences between more effective and less effective oral language production were summarized (i.e., into a high-ability group vs. a low-ability group). The less effective subjects did not appear to have a plan for their talking that showed coherence and unity. Their vocabulary was meager, and they were not flexible in expressing their ideas. Speaking style was hesitant, faltering, and/or labored.

Rhea Paul (2001) noted that T-unit (i.e., a main clause with all the subordination clauses and nonclausal phrases attached to or embedded in it) length, use of subordination, and use of higher level structures (e.g., verb phrases, adverbial use, and complex sentence types) should be assessed in older students since it is not uncommon for these structures to present difficulty for older students with language disorders. Older students with language disorders tend to use simpler sentences and fewer structural complexities.

Older students with

language disorders tend to

use simpler sentences

and fewer structural

complexities.

Discourse Deficits
Conversation

Production deficits during conversational speech may include a lack of sustaining and monitoring conversations (Bryan, Donahue, and Pearl, 1981); a lack of

requesting clarification of inadequate or ambiguous messages (Donahue, Pearl, and Bryan, 1980); an inability to keep abreast of the verbal exchange (Donahue and Bryan, 1984); and a lack of arguing for or against a position (Bryan et al.). No significant differences have been found between adolescents with typical development and those with learning disabilities regarding the number of conversational turns (Bryan et al.), the number of times they engaged in conversations with peers (Schumaker, Sheldon-Wildgen, and Sherman, 1980), or the number of times they were targets of peer initiation (Schumaker et al.). Furthermore, some studies have found a lack of evidence that these adolescents, despite their social communication hindrances, are any more withdrawn, rejected, or isolated than adolescents with typical development (Bryan et al.; Deshler and Schumaker, 1983).

Donahue and Bryan (1984) suggested that there is a strong relationship between the knowledge and use of slang by adolescents with learning disabilities and their amount of interaction with and acceptance from their peer group with typical development. Thus, Donahue and Bryan believe that for students with learning disabilities, "failure to conform to peer group norms for appropriate language use may have increasingly negative consequences" (p. 18) and establishing and maintaining friendships and enhancing self-esteem may be difficult. Their misunderstanding of metaphors, jokes, puns, and sarcastic remarks, and their inadequate skills for rapid humorous verbal exchanges place older students with language disorders at a disadvantage when interacting with their peers.

Students with learning disabilities may lack basic social skills (e.g., they don't know how to use an appropriate tone of voice) or they may have knowledge of social skill strategies but fail to generalize them (Ellis and Friend, 1991). Other students are under inappropriate stimulus control (i.e., it is more reinforcing to act in a socially incompetent manner than to act competently; Kerr and C. Nelson, 1989). Some adolescents do not participate in class to avoid the risk of being humiliated for giving an inept answer (Ellis, 1989).

Blalock (1981) argued that the adolescent's oral language deficits and social imperceptions prevent quality interactions with others and impede close friendships. Nisbet, Zanella, and J. Miller (1984) found that adolescents with moderate disabilities are less talkative when conversing with peers who do not have disabilities. Their speech is typically "simple, direct, imperative, and informal, rather than subtle, complex, elaborate, or polite" (Bergman, 1987, p. 162).

According to Brinton and Fujiki (1999) and Fujiki, Brinton, Hart, and Fitzgerald (1999), both peer acceptance and friendship contribute to the school experience, but they do so in somewhat different ways. Peer

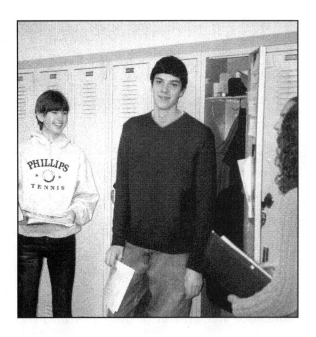

acceptance is the way others view the student with a language disorder and determines the general classroom social climate, in which the student works and plays. Friendship, however, requires mutuality. That is, to have a friend is to be a friend, and it is a way that students experience closeness, commitment, and support. These researchers go on to state that although both peer acceptance and friendship influence self-concept, school performance, and loneliness in school, friendship may have the stronger influence. It was found that students with language disorders between 6 and 12 years of age have problems in developing friendships since they do not have the social communication skills needed to develop and interact with peers. In turn, those who have fewer friends are less likely overall to be accepted by peers.

Communication Solutions
for Older Students

With our longitudinal study of typical development of conversational speech in students grades 7–12 (see Chapter 3 for a summary of these data), we attempted to document the development of conversational speech in adolescents identified as having language disorders from grades 7 through 12 (Larson and McKinley, 1998). We identified four boys and four girls in grade 7 and matched them with students of equivalent backgrounds but who had never been identified as having language disorders or special education needs. Part of our study involved having the students bring a peer of their choice, with whom they felt comfortable, to have a 10-minute conversation each year for the six-year duration of data collection. All eight students with language disorders succeeded in bringing a peer during 7th grade. By 8th grade, one of the boys failed to find a peer who would cooperate. By 9th grade, three of the students could find no peer who would agree to the conversational task, one student had now moved away from the community, and one student staunchly refused to participate any longer. When it was clear to us that we would have data for only 3 of the 8 subjects with language disorders in 9th grade, we abandoned our vision of a comparative longitudinal study of the two groups. The combination of no peers/friends for the study, family mobility, and uncooperativeness was too much to overcome.

One could speculate that some of the students with language disorders either had no close friends, or they had friends but none who would agree to participate in such a study, or they were inept in their social communication skills of asking for help and inviting a peer to participate. Whatever the underlying reason or reasons for not being able to find a cooperative peer, the experience of working with the group of adolescents with language disorders was very different from working with the group without disabilities. The latter group had no difficulties identifying a peer who would cooperate and who themselves chose to be cooperative even when they might have wanted to refuse. Several subjects in the study of the students without disabilities expressed displeasure midway through the study, but seemed to recognize the importance of participating all six years for the sake of research. (Or perhaps it was to continue to receive the McDonald's gift certificates we sent them each year as a thank-you gift!)

Schumaker and Hazel (1984) reported that students with learning disabilities who are in the speaker role are less likely to adapt their behaviors to meet the needs of their listeners and exhibit a lower occurrence of appropriate verbal and nonverbal skills than their peers without disabilities. Bergman (1987) was even more direct in her observations of adolescents with language-learning disabilities, noting that these individuals typically are not adaptive to their listeners and rarely express support, compliment them, or consider the feelings of others. For some adolescents, the skill of listening to conversational speech may also be impaired. In addition, Blalock (1981) observed that listening to fast-paced conversations is difficult for older students with learning disabilities and language disorders.

Adolescents with learning disabilities who have disturbed visual-spatial functioning also present conversational deficits (Bergman, 1987; Ratner and L. Harris, 1994). Unlike adolescents with language disorders, this group appears to have relatively intact language skills during early childhood and the elementary years. However, by adolescence, these individuals may exhibit speech and affect that are flat and stereotypical (Bergman). "Language emerges as grammatically precise, but also as loquacious, superficial, inappropriate, and tangential...nodes of relating are similarly automatized, perseverative, and meaningless" (Bergman, p. 164). This group of adolescents functions with extreme inconsistency during conversational exchanges in social situations.

Narration

Studies investigating story recall in children and adults with language disorders and learning disabilities have revealed that these individuals tend to preserve the order of events in a story and recall the patterns of story organization with the same degree of accuracy as their counterparts with normal achievement; however, they tend to recall significantly less information from stories

(P. Weaver and Dickinson, 1982; Worden, Malmgren, and Gabourie, 1982). Researchers found these same differences in quantity of information within spontaneous story production by learning disabled students (Roth and Spekman, 1986). Although some studies report no differences in storytelling or retelling between students with and without learning disabilities, these findings may be the result of applying story grammar analysis procedures that are insensitive to subtle developmental changes (Weaver and Dickinson).

Merritt and Liles (1987) investigated 9- to 11-year-olds and found differences between storytelling and retelling in children with and those without language disorders. The retelling task was less difficult for both groups than was the story generation task. In both groups of children, the retold stories were longer and contained more story grammar components and complete episodes. In the story-retelling task, the children with language disorders had shorter clause length and fewer complete episodes.

Differences have also been found when rating stories on the importance of their idea units (Worden and Nakamura, 1982). Older students with a learning disability had more difficulty rating stories on the importance of their idea units than did their counterparts with typical development. Worden and Nakamura suggested that the lower agreement on the ratings by students with learning disabilities may reflect a deficit in comprehension of the story or in remembering it.

Using another approach, MacLachlan and Chapman (1988) studied the communication breakdowns in children's conversations and narrations. They found that children with language-learning disabilities (LLD) between 9 years, 10 months and 11 years, 1 month incurred a significantly greater rate of communication breakdowns per communication unit in narrations than conversations compared to the control group of students without such disabilities. Also, they found that the mean length of the communication unit was significantly greater in narrations than conversations for the LLD group.

There is a growing body of research (C. Johnson, 1995; Scott, 1999; Westby, 1998a) demonstrating that older students with language disorders have difficulty using and understanding story-grammar elements relating to characters' internal responses, plans, and motivations; drawing inferences from narrative material; summarizing a story; and using cohesive markers within the text. Story elements such as internal responses to characters, including their intentions, goals, and plans for dealing with a problem central to the story's plot are particularly difficult for older students with language disorders (Westby, 1998a). Blalock (1982), summarizing persistent auditory language deficits, reported that young adults have difficulty with conveying extended narratives, with relating experiences, with retelling stories, and with organizing the narrative. And finally, according to Rhea Paul (2001), the use of advanced language structures (e.g., noun phrase elaboration and complex sentences) in stories is an area of difficulty for older students with language disorders.

Expository Text

As students reach fourth grade, many textbooks change from a narrative form to expository text. As students continue to advance through the grades, they encounter even more expository text (Rhea Paul, 2001). Paul found that students with language disorders have more difficulty with expository text than narrative forms because it:

- Falls at the most literate end of the language continuum

- Provides the least contextual support and relies most heavily on language processing

- Contains new information that explains and describes events, situations, etc.

- Requires the integration of new knowledge with what one already knows, thus taxing both short- and long-term memory

Much of the curriculum and the lecture style of teachers at the secondary level takes the form of expository text. Thus it is critical to know how the student with a language disorder processes this information. Adolescents with language disorders comprehend expository text, such as classroom lectures, less well than their peers with typical development (Blalock, 1981; Conte, Menyuk, and Bashir, 1992; N. Nelson, 1993).

Likewise, Scott (1999) noted that students with language disorders produce less mature expository structures in terms of both form and content.

Written expository text problems are likely to persist beyond the high school years. Gregg, Coleman, Stennett, and Davis (2002) examined the discourse complexity of college writers with and without disabilities. Three groups with disabilities were studied: those identified as having learning disabilities, those with Attention Deficit/Hyperactivity Disorder (ADHD), and those with a combination of the two. All the expository text samples were typed by the researchers—correcting spelling, handwriting, and punctuation errors, so these errors did not contribute to the evaluation of the students' writing. Even after eliminating these factors, the writing of all three groups with disabilities resulted in quality rating scores that were significantly below those of writers with no disabilities. Of particular interest is that the group with comorbidity (learning disabilities and ADHD) also rated significantly below the other two groups with disabilities with regard to quality of writing. Their dual disability places this population at greater risk for producing quality expository text. Some of the contributing factors to the quality ratings included significantly higher type-token ratios for the nondisabled writers and greater fluency in access to words and syntactical structures.

Persuasive and Argumentative Text

Nippold (1998) and Scott and Erwin (1992) identified persuasion and argumentation as a new discourse genre that confronts secondary students. They suggested that this genre may in fact develop later than expository text, and consequently may not become part of the student's repertoire until late in adolescence. It seems then that if students with language disorders are having problems with expository text, they would have even more serious problems with persuasion and argumentation, since these require a relatively high level of critical listening and thinking skills (Rhea Paul, 2001).

Nonverbal Communication Deficits

Although our clinical experiences indicate that many adolescents with language disorders have deficits in nonverbal behavior, little formal research confirms or refutes these observations. Wiig and S. Harris (1974) found that students with learning disabilities may have an inability to recognize nonverbal emotional expressions. Bryan (1977) found that students with learning disabilities were less skillful at understanding nonverbal behavior when compared with their peers with typical development. In addition, Blalock (1981) documented inappropriate use of proxemics (i.e., social distance) during conversational speech.

Adolescents (from ages 13 to 15 years) with emotional disturbances have been found to be significantly poorer at nonverbal encoding than adolescents developing typically (Feldman, White, and Lobato, 1982). Likewise, they are also less accurate in decoding nonverbal communication. Still, adolescents with emotional disturbances do have some nonverbal encoding and decoding skills in that they have been found to perform at levels greater than chance.

Our own observations of adolescents with language disorders have indicated these nonverbal communication problems:

- Frequent failure to interpret accurately the facial expression accompanying a spoken message

- Inconsistent understanding of gestures used by others

- Occasional failure to inhibit use of socially unacceptable gestures

- Significantly less eye contact (not related to cultural issues) than that of adolescent communicators with typical development

- Inappropriate maintenance of distance (not related to cultural issues) during conversational situations

Reading Deficits

Nationally, 30% of eighth graders and 25% of twelfth graders read below grade level (U.S. Department of Education, 1996, 1998). Approximately 74% of students identified as having a reading disability in the third grade remain disabled in the ninth grade (Lyon, 1996). Furthermore, fewer than

30% of middle-grade students comprehend their textbooks beyond a literal understanding (*Children's Literacy*, 1997). As McCray, Vaughn, and Neal (2001) observed, "(D)espite reading intervention programs during the primary grades, most students with reading disabilities continue to experience learning problems well into their adolescent years" (p. 17). At the same time, "What appears to be missing is sweeping agreement that high-quality and effective intervention programs in reading need to be in place for struggling middle school readers" (McCray, Vaughn, and Neal, p. 29).

Children with speech and language disorders encounter reading problems at least six times more often than controls do (Mason, 1976). Children with reading problems almost always have concomitant writing disorders. According to an American Speech-Language-Hearing Association report (2001b), it has been documented that a reciprocal relationship exists between students with language impairments and reading disabilities. In the report, it was noted that poor readers have problems with receptive and/or expressive vocabulary, semantic relations, comprehension and production of morphology and syntax, and text-level language.

Children with a reading disability show a significant lag in their development of grammatical sensitivity (i.e., the ability to correct grammatically incorrect sentences, the understanding of acceptable word order, control over regular and irregular morphological features of English, and the ability to remember sentences with varied grammatical structures; Siegel and Ryan, 1988). Additional research has documented that poor readers have deficits in phonological awareness, retrieval, memory, and production (American Speech-Language-Hearing Association, 2001b).

Catts and Kamhi (1999) noted that since spoken-language problems are both a cause and a consequence of reading disabilities, language problems will be a major component of the majority of cases of reading difficulties. Apel and Swank (1999) go on to state that the oral-written factors interact to such an extent that cause and consequence roles are obscured in older students who are poor readers. In summary, it is important to note that reading and writing problems may take various forms (Aaron, Joshi, and Williams, 1999) and that students with a history of reading problems may fail to develop higher level cognitive-linguistic skills (Cain and Oakhill, 1998; Stothard et al., 1998).

Writing Deficits

Students with oral language disorders almost always display written language deficits during preadolescent and adolescent years. Scott (1999) noted that students with language disorders produce written texts that are shorter, have more errors, are lower in overall quality, show less sensitivity to audience and genre, and contain less information. Computer-produced writing of students with language disorders contains more errors than handwritten products; while at the same time, it does not differ in length, structure, or amount of revision (Scott). A computer may make writing less laborious and messy; it does not, however, automatically improve the quality of the structure and content. Sturm and Koppenhaver (2000) differ with the view presented by Scott in that they have used selective software to help students plan a writing project using a mapping strategy (Inspiration, by Inspiration Software, 1997), and to help in editing or revising a project (IntelliTalk, by IntelliTools, 1996). They have noted that these software packages have been useful for improving the writing of students with developmental disabilities.

Hull (1987) summarized the error taxonomy for written language:

- **Production errors**—Errors that are traceable to the demands of writing a sentence, such as lost or abandoned patterns (e.g., "Tom's judgment, impaired by his lack of motivation, is fatigue, and his failure to remember directions")

- **Rhetorical errors**—Errors arising from the requirements of producing discourse rather than sentences, such as topic/comment structure mistakes (e.g., "His response to this story he felt he was talked into a different viewpoint")

- **Accidental errors**—Errors resulting from "slips of the pen" (or of the fingers on the keyboard; e.g., "Many people of out generation want to interact will older people")

- **Interference errors**—Errors caused by interference from a second register, dialect, or language (e.g., "I and him are going fishing")

- **Systematic errors**—Errors signifying an idiosyncratic or unstable rule system (e.g., "They had to designed everything they made")

Those students considered inexperienced writers share many of the same characteristics as students with writing deficits. Inexperienced writers do not integrate their writing plans like competent writers do (Hayes and Flower, 1987). They write significantly shorter essays with fewer words per sentence part (7.3 words per part vs. 11.2 words per part; Hayes and Flower). Also, novices see revision largely as a sentence-level task in which the goal is to improve individual words and phrases without modification of the text structure (Hayes and Flower). Experts detect about 1.6 times as many problems in a faulty text than do novices (Hayes, Flower, Schriver, Stratman, and Carey, 1985). Abundant evidence exists that those identified as having a learning disability have difficulty with editing (Gregg, 1983). Scott and Erwin (1992) reported that students with language disorders spend less time in the planning and revising process than their peers without disabilities.

When Gillam and Johnston (1992) compared the written and spoken narratives of 9- to 12-year-old children who were language and learning impaired with three groups matched for age, or spoken language, or reading, they found that spoken narratives were superior to written narratives in the organization of textual form for all groups. Conversely, written narratives were superior to spoken narratives in the organization of textual content. Sentences were longer in spoken narratives than in written narratives, but not necessarily more complex. The group with language and learning impairments performed appreciably worse on a measure of complex sentence usage. They also produced a large percentage of grammatically unacceptable sentences, especially in their written narratives, making errors in both simple and complex sentences.

Spelling Deficits

Spelling will predictably be affected when students have difficulties in segmenting words into phonemes (Nation and Hulme, 1997). Typically, individuals with poor word segmentation skills will delete letters and/or syllables when they spell words (e.g., *cos* for *cost*, or *penlize* for *penalize*).

Spelling error patterns can be determined by looking at which rules are and are not being followed across the following language knowledge domains critical for spelling (Masterson, Apel, and Wasowicz, 2002):

- Phonological awareness
- Orthographic knowledge
- Semantic knowledge
- Morphological knowledge
- Mental orthographic memory

Initially, phonological awareness skill deficits play a large role in spelling errors, but the other domains also become critical as the student gains additional language experience.

Berninger et al. (2000) noted that some students have no difficulty learning to read, but they have poor spelling skills that are masked or ignored until written assignment requirements increase, usually in the upper-elementary grades and beyond. Other students overcome their reading disability only to struggle with persistent spelling problems (Berninger et al.). As Sipe, Walsh, Reed-Nordwall, Putnam, and Rosewarne (2002) observed, "For students who struggle with spelling, poor spelling too often translates to a sense of hopelessness about their writing" (p. 23). They identified four categories of challenged spellers, which are described in the sidebar.

Explicit training in the alphabetic principle has been effective in preventing reading disability (Foorman, Francis, Fletcher, Schatschneider, and Mehta, 1998), and it may be effective in preventing spelling disabilities as well, because written English is an alphabetic system (Berninger et al., 2000). Unfortunately, virtually no research has been completed on how to best prevent spelling deficits. As Apel and Masterson (2000) so aptly pointed out, "Spelling has not received the degree of respect it warrants; many professionals do not understand the factors involved in spelling. It is (our) contention that spelling instruction must be provided by professionals with knowledge of the phonological, semantic, syntactic, morphological, and pragmatic aspects of language" (p. 83). The professional they described fits the description of a speech-language pathologist.

Challenged Spellers: Descriptive Categories

Category One: Full Literacy Lives

- Exhibits strong reader behaviors; enjoys specific types of books
- Exhibits strong writer behaviors; writes for a variety of purposes; writes outside of school
- Exhibits a strong sense of personal control over reading and writing; knows own strengths/ weaknesses
- Uses multiple self-correction strategies, both internally and externally based
- Sees spelling as secondary to meaning and as an editing issue
- Impact of visual memory unclear
- Enjoys language
- Actively uses and advocates multiple drafts in writing

Continued on next page

Communication Solutions
for Older Students

Continued

Category Two: Literacy at Arm's Length

- Exhibits average reader behaviors; can read but often chooses not to
- Exhibits average writer behaviors; does school assignments but little personal writing outside of school
- Demonstrates little sense of personal control over language
- Uses few strategies for spelling; relies mostly on external resources like spell checkers, peers, or mom
- Tends to spell known words correctly; has few strategies for spelling unknown words
- Exhibits many gaps in learning about spelling rules, patterns, and generalizations
- Exhibits weak visual memory recall and very weak delayed visual memory recall
- Seeks assistance with editing

Category Three: Literacy Resistance

- Exhibits reluctant reader behaviors; reads when told to
- Exhibits weak writer behaviors; does not write outside of school
- Demonstrates minimal sense of control over language or learning
- Uses external spelling strategies like spell checkers, peers, or adult editors
- Seeks editing help from external sources
- Exhibits little personal ownership for own writing/spelling
- Demonstrates minimal motivation to achieve in spelling
- Exhibits weak visual memory
- Demonstrates over-reliance on phonics

Category Four: Literacy Avoidance

- Exhibits weak reader behaviors; actively doesn't like reading
- Exhibits weak writer behaviors; does no writing out of school; may not complete school writing
- Demonstrates no sense of personal control over language or learning
- Uses few spelling strategies; spelling happens or it doesn't
- Identifies self as "bad" at spelling; does not appear to have any ideas on how to improve spelling
- Views spelling as important only for grades
- Demonstrates over-reliance on phonics
- Equates poor spelling with being poor at writing and at English

From "Supporting Challenged Spellers," by R. Sipe, J. Walsh, K. Reed-Nordwall, D. Putnam, and T. Rosewarne, 2002, *Voices from the Middle*, 9(3), p. 27. © 2002 by the National Council of Teachers of English. Reprinted with permission.

Points of Discussion

1. Study the list of expectations and problems in Table 6.1 (on pages 133–134). Which have you observed? Should any be added? If so, which ones?

2. Why do you think the prevalence of communication disorders in incarcerated youth is so elevated compared to their nonincarcerated peer group? What preventative measures might be implemented?

Suggested Readings

McCray, A.D., Vaughn, S., and Neal, L.I. (2001). Not all students learn to read by third grade: Middle school students speak out about their reading disabilities. *The Journal of Special Education, 35*(1), 17–30.

Sanger, D., Moore-Brown, B., and Alt, E. (2000). Advancing the discussion on communication and violence. *Communication Disorders Quarterly, 22*(1) 43–48.

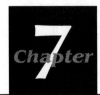

7

Frequent Concomitant Problems with Language Disorders

Goals

- Present information on TBI, ADD, FAS, ASD, and learning disabilities as they relate to language disorders

- Describe problems facing youth at risk

- Discuss language disorders as a lifelong disability

Problems confronting youth are increasing in the number of students diagnosed with a traumatic brain injury (TBI) resulting from automobile crashes and other accidents, attention deficit disorder (ADD), and fetal alcohol syndrome (FAS). Likewise there is an increased number of students diagnosed as having autism spectrum disorders (ASD). We mention these problems here because ADD may not be diagnosed until preadolescence or adolescence and a TBI may not occur until adolescence. FAS and ASD are present from birth, but the symptoms persist into preadolescence and adolescence. Learning disabilities remain a critical problem as they relate to adolescents with language disorders.

Before describing each of these concomitant problems facing students with language disorders, it is important to discuss two of them in light of executive function disorders.

According to Ylvisaker and DeBonis (2000), "For some disability categories, including traumatic brain injury (TBI) and attention deficit/hyperactivity disorder (ADHD), impaired executive functions may be at the core of the disability" (p. 29). They go on to state that executive functions have been noted to include the following:

- Self-awareness of strengths and limitations (in any domain of functioning), and associated understanding of the difficulty level of specific tasks

- Ability to set reasonable goals

- Ability to plan and organize behavior designed to achieve the goals

- Ability to initiate behavior toward achieving goals and inhibit behavior incompatible with achieving those goals

- Ability to monitor and evaluate performance in relation to the goals

- Ability to flexibly revise plans and strategically solve problems in the event of difficulty or failure (that is, efficiently profit from feedback) (p. 31)

Furthermore, they go on to state that the communication ramifications of someone with an executive function problem are:

- Reduced social-interactive competence (pragmatic language disorders)

- Difficulty with the demands of discourse in terms of organizational aspects

- Inefficient strategic word memory and retrieval

- Overall impaired strategic thinking

- Reduced ability to take the perspective of the listener

- Difficulty with abstract thinking and indirect language

- Difficulty transferring newly acquired language skills from the context of acquisition to application

- Difficulty learning from context

Executive functions are metacognitive processes that cross all content and context domains. Executive functions allow for self-regulation, interpretation of ongoing behavior, and controlling of psychological, physiological, and physical interference (Farmer, 2000).

Traumatic Brain Injury (TBI)

Normal development of executive functions begins in infancy, continues throughout childhood, and reaches its peak during adolescence and young-adult years. Table 2.1 (see page 36) outlines three generally distinct phases of adolescent development, corresponding to early, middle, and late stages of adolescence. In Table 7.1, Ylvisaker and

Immediate and Delayed
Consequences* of TBI in Adolescence

Table 7.1

Stage of Adolescence	Key Development Issues	Common Concerns with TBI at This Stage	Common Delayed Symptoms Related to Earlier Injury
Early	**Social-emotional-behavioral issues** Emerging personality identity associated with short-term future goals, often involving physical accomplishments Emphasis on following a rigid code of behavior and on punishment in moral thinking Development of a cognitive map of social networks with primary emphasis on same-sex peers Emergence of fixed friendships, along with crowds and cliques External locus of control, with deference to the approval or disapproval of peers	**Social-emotional-behavioral issues** Social vulnerability, related to separation from clique; socially awkward behavior (associated with frontal lobe injury) Physical changes caused by the injury may precipitate role confusion and psychogenic problems ("I am not who I was") Likelihood of behavior problems associated with vulnerability to environmental stressors (especially with frontal lobe injury)	**Social-emotional-behavioral issues** Behavior problems associated with decreasing external control and an inability to meet the expectation for increasing behavioral self-regulation Inability to meet increasing social demands associated with puberty
	Cognitive-academic issues Increase in abstract thinking and hypothetico-deductive reasoning Increase in ability to use organizing schemes deliberately to process large amounts of information (e.g., for reading texts and writing essays)	**Cognitive-academic issues** Increasing concerns with the academic curriculum associated with cumulative effects of new learning problems; difficulty organizing large amounts of information; difficulty with increasingly abstract information	**Cognitive-academic issues** Increasing academic problems, associated with cumulative effects of new learning problems; difficulty organizing large amounts of information; difficulty with increasingly abstract information

Continued on next page

155

Communication Solutions
for Older Students

Table 7.1—Continued

Stage of Adolescence	Key Development Issues	Common Concerns with TBI at This Stage	Common Delayed Symptoms Related to Earlier Injury
Middle	**Social-emotional-behavioral issues** Increasing awareness of changes associated with puberty; increasingly heterosexual social networks Increasing need to experiment and take risks Increasing ability to manage environmental stressors, profit from feedback, and make flexible and autonomous decisions Increasing ability to read social cues	**Social-emotional-behavioral issues** Discontinuity of personal identification as a result of physical and cognitive changes; breakdown in social grouping associated with communication and other changes Difficulty managing increasing environmental stressors; ongoing rigidity in responding; inability to profit from feedback Experimentation and risk taking at dangerous levels Possible "hyper-egocentrism," with focus on the injury Difficulty reading social cues	**Social-emotional-behavioral issues** Continued rigidity and dependence on external control while peers become increasingly flexible and autonomous Hypersexuality Social withdrawal
	Cognitive-academic vocational issues Decreasing egocentrism, resulting in increasing ability to communicate varied thoughts and feelings competently in varied social settings Emerging vocational goals and long-range goal planning	**Cognitive-academic vocational issues** Difficulty with increasingly demanding curriculum Possibly increasing incongruity between vocational goals and vocational potential after the injury	**Cognitive-academic vocational issues** Increasing academic failure because of cumulative effect of new learning problems Difficulty achieving communicative effectiveness in varied social settings requiring varied social registers General difficulty with divergent thinking and flexible problem solving

Table 7.1—Continued

Stage of Adolescence	Key Development Issues	Common Concerns with TBI at This Stage	Common Delayed Symptoms Related to Earlier Injury
Late	**Social-emotional-behavioral issues** Social networks loosen and shift, based on vocational and social needs Reduction in risk taking Increasing ability to identify source of stress and adjust behavior accordingly (self-management) Continued reduction in egocentrism and growth in attention to the needs of others (a life-long process) Sexual relations move toward an increasing interest in companionship and love Solidification of communication styles **Cognitive-academic-vocational issues** Solidification of vocational and academic goals; organization of behavior in pursuit of these goals Increasingly mature understanding of academic and vocational potential	**Social-emotional-behavioral issues** Regression to rigid behavior, egocentric perspective, and dependence on external control; difficulty considering alternative perspectives Inability to anticipate and recognize stressors and alter behavior accordingly Loss of social networks; possible dependence on old social networks Sexual relations continue to focus on physical aspects **Cognitive-academic-vocational issues** Regression to rigid and concrete communication; loss of subtlety, abstractness, and flexibility in communication Incongruity of previous academic vocational goals and current abilities	**Social-emotional-behavioral issues** Retention of concrete thinking and rigid responding Immature social skills; continued dependence on cliques while peers move on Continued dependence on same sex peers for support; relations with opposite sex may be characterized by hypersexuality Possible perception of differences between self and others as representing a psychiatric problem **Cognitive-academic-vocational issues** Possible failure in college or on the job due to the elimination of the supports provided in high school

From "Traumatic Brain Injury in Adolescence: Assessment and Reintegration," by M. Ylvisaker and T. Feeney, 1995, *Seminars in Speech and Language, 16*, pp. 36–37. © 1995 by Thieme Medical. Reprinted with permission.

*"Delayed consequences" refer to symptoms associated with an earlier injury, usually incurred at a previous developmental stage, that are observed in individuals whose recovery had appeared to be generally good.

Freeney (1995) note key developmental issues in each of these stages as well as common concerns with TBI at each of these stages as they relate to social-emotional-behavioral issues and cognitive-academic-vocational issues.

TBI occurs with an increased incidence in preadolescents and adolescents, particularly

Communication Solutions
for Older Students

in the latter group as a result of automobile accidents resulting in closed head injury (CHI). According to Blosser and DePompei (1989), the student with CHI is not a "peer" of other students with disabilities. Characteristics of students with CHI that make them different from other students with language disorders are listed in the sidebar.

> *(T)he student with CHI is not a "peer" of other students with disabilities.*

When working with students who have CHI, it is important to keep in mind how they

---

Characteristics of Students with Closed Head Injury

• A sense of being normal that persists from the premorbid period

• Discrepancies in ability levels

• A previous history of successful experiences in academic and social settings

• Inconsistent patterns of performance

• Variability and fluctuation in the recovery process, resulting in unpredictable and unexpected spurts of recovery

• More extreme problems with generalizing, integrating, or structuring information

• Poor judgment and loss of emotional control, which cause the student to appear to be emotionally disturbed at times

• Cognitive deficits that, although present in other handicaps, are more uneven in extent of damage and rate of recovery

• Combinations of handicapping conditions that do not fall into usual categories of disabilities

• Inappropriate behaviors that may be more exaggerated than the behaviors of students with other handicaps (e.g., greater impulsivity or distractibility)

• A learning style that requires the use of a variety of compensatory and adaptive strategies

• Some intact high-level skills (making it difficult to understand why the student will have problems in performing lower-level tasks)

From "The Head-Injured Student Returns to School: Recognizing and Treating Deficits," by J. Blosser and R. DePompei, 1989, *Topics in Language Disorders*, 9(2), p. 69. © 1989 by Lippencott. Reprinted with permission.

are similar to and different from other older students with language disorders. According to Gruen and Gruen (1994), numerous cognitive-linguistic disorders are common in these individuals: "These impairments include deficits in concentration, sustained attention, memory, nonverbal problem solving, part/whole analysis and synthesis, conceptual organization and abstraction" (p. 3).

The student with CHI may suffer from psychological difficulties as well as physical impairment and cognitive-communication problems. Psychological difficulties may include depression, anger, and behavior inappropriate to the situation. The National Institutes of Health (1984) cited three types of personality change in individuals with CHI. One common personality change is apathy—a reduced interest in life's activities and challenges. This can be devastating for a student, since such apathy may lead to teachers and family members ignoring these individuals because they are not behavior problems in the classroom or home. This lack of attention only reinforces the adolescent's or young adult's apathy. Another personality change common among individuals with CHI is to become overly optimistic (i.e., believing that things are better than they are or underestimating their disabilities). A third common personality change is loss of social restraint and judgment. Some clients with CHI become tactless, talkative, and hurtful, and they may have outbursts of rage in response to trivial frustrations.

Attention Deficit Disorder (ADD)

ADD is a cluster of syndromes that includes a short attention span, difficulty concentrating, poor impulse control, distractibility, sudden mood changes, and sometimes a learning disability and hyperactivity (resulting in the label of ADHD). Frequently, students with ADD have oral and written language disorders; are poorly organized; and scramble information, which leads to reaching wrong conclusions. Many of these students have executive function disorders and exhibit the types of behaviors and communication skills listed at the outset of this chapter (Ylvisaker and DeBonis, 2000; Ylvisaker and Feeney, 1995).

The American Psychiatric Association's *Diagnostic and Statistical Manual-IV (DSM-IV;* 2000) defines characteristics of ADD under two relatively separate behavior dimensions: inattention and hyperactivity-impulsivity (see the sidebar on page 160).

According to Westby and Cutler (1994), "many of the behaviors described in the *DSM-IV* list can easily be analyzed as pragmatic deficits (difficulty in using communication patterns appropriate to persons and situations) and metacognitive deficits (difficulty in organizing, planning, monitoring, and evaluating behavior)" (p. 60). Since pragmatic and metacognitive behaviors are language-based, rule-governed behaviors, it is critical that the student with ADD be

DSM-IV Diagnostic Criteria for Attention-Deficit/Hyperactivity Disorder

A. Either (1) or (2):

(1) Six (or more) of the following symptoms of **inattention** have persisted for at least 6 months to a degree that is maladaptive and inconsistent with developmental level:

Inattention
   (a) often fails to give close attention to details or makes careless mistakes in schoolwork, work, or other activities
   (b) often has difficulty sustaining attention in tasks or play activities
   (c) often does not seem to listen when spoken to directly
   (d) often does not follow through on instructions and fails to finish schoolwork, chores, or duties in the workplace (not due to oppositional behavior or failure to understand instructions)
   (e) often has difficulty organizing tasks and activities
   (f) often avoids, dislikes, or is reluctant to engage in tasks that require sustained mental effort (such as schoolwork or homework)
   (g) often loses things necessary for tasks or activities (e.g., toys, school assignments, pencils, books, or tools)
   (h) is often easily distracted by extraneous stimuli
   (i) is often forgetful in daily activities

(2) Six (or more) of the following symptoms of **hyperactivity-impulsivity** have persisted for at least 6 months to a degree that is maladaptive and inconsistent with developmental level:

Hyperactivity
   (a) often fidgets with hands or feet or squirms in seat
   (b) often leaves seat in classroom or in other situations in which remaining seated is expected
   (c) often runs about or climbs excessively in situations in which it is inappropriate (in adolescents or adults, may be limited to subjective feelings of restlessness)
   (d) often has difficulty playing or engaging in leisure activities quietly
   (e) is often "on the go" or often acts as if "driven by a motor"
   (f) often talks excessively

Impulsivity
   (g) often blurts out answers before questions have been completed
   (h) often has difficulty awaiting turn
   (i) often interrupts or intrudes on others (e.g., butts into conversations or games)...

314.01 Attention-Deficit/Hyperactivity Disorder, Combined Type: if both Criteria A1 and A2 are met for the past 6 months

314.00 Attention-Deficit/Hyperactivity Disorder, Predominantly Inattentive Type: if criterion A1 is met but Criterion A2 is not met for the past 6 months

314.01 Attention-Deficit/Hyperactivity Disorder, Predominantly Hyperactive-Impulsive Type: if Criterion A2 is met but Criterion A1 is not met for the past 6 months

From *Diagnostic and Statistical Manual of Mental Disorders* (4th ed., text revision; pp. 92–93), by the American Psychiatric Association, 2000, Washington, DC: Author. © 2000 by the American Psychiatric Association. Reprinted with permission.

assessed for language, cognitive, and communication problems as they relate to academic, personal-social, and vocational needs.

The prevalence of ADD in children with learning disabilities ranges from 9% to 92% (Shaywitz, Fletcher, and Shaywitz, 1994). While not all students with ADD have language disorders, the research indicates that they engage in excessive talking, and they may be more dysfluent in situations when they must organize and generate language (known as executive function problems; Shelton and Barkley, 1994).

Fetal Alcohol Syndrome (FAS)

Abel (1990) noted that confirmed heavy and frequent drinking of alcoholic beverages by a mother during pregnancy can be responsible for the pattern of abnormalities known as FAS. FAS includes such features as unusual facial formation; prematurity; low birth weight; postnatal growth retardation; malformation, especially of the heart, limbs, and palate; delayed intellectual development; and delayed language development (Ratner and L. Harris, 1994). Infants who are exposed to alcohol in utero may exhibit some but not all the characteristics associated with FAS. They are known as children with fetal alcohol effects (FAE). Sparks (1993) estimated that FAE occurs at two or three times the frequency of FAS. Ratner and Harris

(1994) described characteristic behaviors of children with FAS and FAE as follows:

- Lack of social skills
- Hyperactive, distractible, inattentive, and impulsive
- Delayed motor development
- Uninhibited behavior
- Lack of attachment or indiscriminate attachment
- Difficulty making transitions to new activities
- Poor judgment and poor recognition of cause-effect relationships
- Inappropriate language use in context
- Conceptual confusion
- Temper tantrums and defiance of authority

Ratner and Harris (1994) also present characteristics of FAS and FAE in adolescents. These include sexual difficulties, depression (due to social isolation), restlessness, and the tendency to be truant or drop out of school.

In discussing academic behaviors of FAS and FAE students, Ratner and Harris (1994) state that academic difficulties occur in such areas as listening and reading comprehension; abstract thinking; memory (visual and spatial); basic problem solving; and time, space, and causal concepts. The types of communication difficulties noted are poor pragmatic language skills; difficulty comprehending social language rules and expectations; and ineffective communication because it lacks substance, cohesion, meaning, and relevance. FAS and FAE affects adolescents in that they seem to plateau in daily and academic functions. Later, their behaviors (such as attention deficits, poor judgment, and impulsiveness) make successful employment difficult (Ratner and Harris, 1994). It is not uncommon for children with FAS and FAE to become alcoholic themselves, and the cycle repeats itself.

Autism Spectrum Disorders (ASD)

One of the most demanding areas of school-based speech-language services is in meeting the needs of students with autism spectrum disorders (ASD), formerly known as autism (Moore-Brown and Montgomery, 2001). What the term *ASD* suggests is a range of related qualities or activities that overlap but are clinically distinct and separately diagnosed. A similar term, *pervasive developmental disorders (PDD)*, has also been used to describe this broad classification of disorders. PDD is a general classification for a group of severe and pervasive impairments affecting social interaction and communication, often accompanied by stereotyped behaviors, interests, and activities (American Psychiatric Association, 2000; Fahey and Reid, 2000; Rhea Paul, 2001). There are five disorders within the PDD category. They are listed and explained in the sidebar that follows. It should be noted that the most common types are

autism and PDD-NOS (pervasive developmental disorder not otherwise specified), with Asperger's syndrome becoming more and more prevalent.

The IDEA 1992 definition of autism (as cited by the Council for Exceptional Children (CEC), 2003) states the following:

(i) Autism means a developmental disability significantly affecting verbal and nonverbal communication and social interaction, generally evident before age 3, that adversely affects a child's educational performance. Other characteristics often associated with autism are engagement in repetitive activities and stereotyped movements, resistance to environmental change or change in daily routines, and unusual responses to sensory experiences. The term does not apply if a child's educational performance is adversely affected primarily because the child has an emotional disturbance, as defined in paragraph (b)(4) of this section.

(ii) A child who manifests the characteristics of "autism" after age 3 could be diagnosed as having "autism" if the criteria in paragraph (c)(1)(i) of this section are satisfied. (§ 300.7 (c) (1))

Although autism is commonly thought of as occurring in infants, it is a lifelong disability in more than 95% of the people diagnosed (Rhea Paul, 2001). Lord and Rhea Paul (1997) reported that 80% of children-

The Pervasive Developmental Disorders

Autistic Disorder

A. A total of six (or more) items from (1), (2), and (3), with at least two from (1), and one each from (2) and (3):

   (1) qualitative impairment in social interaction, as manifested by at least two of the following:

      (a) marked impairment in the use of multiple nonverbal behaviors such as eye-to-eye gaze, facial expression, body postures, and gestures to regulate social interaction

      (b) failure to develop peer relationships appropriate to developmental level

      (c) a lack of spontaneous seeking to share enjoyment, interests, or achievements with other people...

      (d) lack of social or emotional reciprocity

   (2) qualitative impairments in communication as manifested by at least one of the following:

      (a) delay in, or total lack of, the development of spoken language (not accompanied by an attempt to compensate through alternative modes of communication such as gesture or mime)

      (b) in individuals with adequate speech, marked impairment in the ability to initiate or sustain a conversation with others

      (c) stereotyped and repetitive use of language or idiosyncratic language

      (d) lack of varied, spontaneous make-believe play or social imitative play appropriate to developmental level

   (3) restricted repetitive and stereotyped patterns of behavior, interests, and activities, as manifested by at least one of the following:

      (a) encompassing preoccupation with one or more stereotyped and restricted patterns of interest that is abnormal either in intensity or focus

      (b) apparently inflexible adherence to specific, nonfunctional routines or rituals

      (c) stereotyped and repetitive motor mannerisms (e.g., hand or finger flapping or twisting, or complex whole-body movements)

      (d) persistent preoccupation with parts of objects

Delays or abnormal functioning in at least one of the following areas, with onset prior to age 3 years: (1) social interaction, (2) language as used in social communication, or (3) symbolic or imaginative play...

Rett's Disorder

A. All of the following:

   (1) apparently normal prenatal and perinatal development

   (2) apparently normal psychomotor development through the first 5 months after birth

   (3) normal head circumference at birth

B. Onset of all of the following after the period of normal development:

   (1) deceleration of head growth between ages 5 and 48 months

   (2) loss of previously acquired purposeful hand skills between ages 5 and 30 months with the subsequent development of stereotyped hand movements...

   (3) loss of social engagement early in the course (although often social interaction develops later)

   (4) appearance of poorly coordinated gait or trunk movements

   (5) severely impaired expressive and receptive language development...

Continued on next page

Communication Solutions
for Older Students

Continued

Childhood Disintegrative Disorder

A. Apparently normal development for at least the first 2 years after birth...

B. Clinically significant loss of previously acquired skills (before age 10 years) in at least two of the following areas:

(1) expressive or receptive language

(2) social skills or adaptive behavior

(3) bowel or bladder control

(4) play

(5) motor skills

C. Abnormalities of functioning in at least two of the following areas:

(1) qualitative impairment in social interaction...

(2) qualitative impairments in communication...

(3) restricted, repetitive, and stereotyped patterns of behavior, interests, and activities, including motor stereotypes and mannerisms...

Asperger's Disorder

A. Qualitative impairment in social interaction, as manifested by at least two of the following:

(1) marked impairment in the use of multiple nonverbal behaviors...

(2) failure to develop peer relationships appropriate to developmental level

(3) a lack of spontaneous seeking to share enjoyment, interests, or achievements...

(4) a lack of social or emotional reciprocity

B. Restricted repetitive and stereotyped patterns of behavior, interests, and activities as manifested by at least one of the following:

(1) encompassing preoccupation with one or more stereotyped and restricted patterns of interest that is abnormal either in intensity or focus

(2) apparently inflexible adherence to specific, nonfunctional routines or rituals

(3) stereotyped and repetitive motor mannerisms...

(4) persistent preoccupation with parts of objects

C. The disturbance causes clinically significant impairment in social, occupational, or other important areas of functioning.

D. There is no clinically significant general delay in language (e.g., single words used by age 2 years, communicative phrases used by age 3 years).

E. There is no clinically significant delay in cognitive development...

Pervasive Developmental Disorder Not Otherwise Specified (Including Atypical Autism)

This category should be used when there is a severe and pervasive impairment in the development of reciprocal social interaction associated with impairment in either verbal or nonverbal communication skills or with the presence of stereotyped behavior, interests, and activities, but the criteria are not met for a specific Pervasive Developmental Disorder, Schizophrenia, Schizotypal Personality Disorder, or Avoidant Personality Disorder.

From *Diagnostic and Statistical Manual of Mental Disorders* (4th ed., text revision; pp. 75, 77, 79, 84), by the American Psychiatric Association, 2000, Washington, DC: Author. © 2000 by the American Psychiatric Association. Reprinted with permission.

with autism function in a range considered as mental retardation on intelligence and adaptive behavior measures. Some individuals with autism have what is called *splinter skills* (i.e., unusually high levels of ability in one or two areas, such as math or music, but low levels of abilities in other areas).

Autism, as with the other PDD classifications, is primarily a disorder in communication and social functioning, rather than specific language behaviors. Individuals with autism have sparse verbal expressions; lack spontaneity; and display problems in adapting what they say to the needs of the listener, distinguishing existing information from new information, following rules of politeness, making relevant comments, maintaining topics outside of their own obsessive interests, and giving listeners their fair share of conversational turns (Lord and Rhea Paul, 1997).

The other PDD classification receiving increased attention in recent years is that of Asperger's syndrome, which is determined on the basis of autisticlike deficits in social and pragmatic skills in the presence of a history of more or less typical cognitive development and language form (see the previous sidebar). According to personal communication with the Heath Director (Barr, November 15, 2000), there is an increase in the number of college-age students who have been diagnosed with Asperger's syndrome and who want to attend postsecondary education institutions. They often do not know how to accommodate these students who are usually very intelligent but do not have strategies to navigate the social world of postsecondary educational institutions.

Gallagher (1999) noted some of the frequently cited pragmatic language problems among those identified as having behavioral/emotional problems to be:

"• Language output not adapted to listener needs

• Difficulty introducing, maintaining, and changing topics

• Fewer socially positive utterances produced within interactions

• Insufficient verbalization during tasks requiring planning and organization" (p. 2).

She goes on to state that these students have difficulty using language to explain emotions and using language for social interactions. These language problems can result in the preadolescent or adolescent becoming more aggressive in his or her day-to-day activities.

Learning Disabilities

According to Hammill (1990), there have been 11 definitions of *learning disabilities* since 1962. He maintains that one of the most influential definitions is that put forth by the National Joint Committee on Learning Disabilities in 1991, which reads as follows:

> Learning disabilities is a general term that refers to a heterogeneous group of disorders manifested by significant

difficulties in the acquisition and use of listening, speaking, reading, writing, reasoning, or mathematical abilities. These disorders are intrinsic to the individual, presumed to be due to central nervous system dysfunction, and may occur across the life span. Problems in self-regulatory behaviors, social perception, and social interaction may exist with learning disabilities but do not by themselves constitute a learning disability. (p. 19)

However, the definition of *specific learning disability* used by federal law P.L. 105-17, the 1997 Individuals with Disabilities Education Act (IDEA) Amendments, is as follows:

The term "specific learning disability" means a disorder in one or more of the basic psychological processes involved in understanding or in using language, spoken or written, which disorder may manifest itself in imperfect ability to listen, think, speak, read, write, spell, or do mathematical calculations. (§ 602 (26) (A))

The definition goes on to state that the "term does not include a learning problem that is primarily the result of visual, hearing, or motor disabilities, of mental retardation, of emotional disturbance, or of environmental, cultural, or economic disadvantage" (§ 602 (26) (C). Definitions of learning disabilities differ from state to state. Confusion still abounds about the causes and the various types of learning disabilities.

The prevalence (i.e., the proportion of cases in a population at any moment in time) of learning disabilities ranges from 4% to as high as 20% of the U.S. population. In the school-age population, it appears to be closer to 5 to 10% (Rhea Paul, 2001).

It is critical that speech-language pathologists understand the types of language disabilities frequently encountered by students with learning disabilities (Fahey and Reid, 2000; Ratner and Harris, 1994). They are summarized in the sidebar that follows.

The classroom and the pragmatic issues are of particular concern to older students with language disorders. Through appropriate assessment and intervention protocols these problems can be discerned and delivery models chosen that will be most effective for each student.

Problems Facing Youth at Risk

A myriad of problems face youth at risk (see the sidebar on page 168). One of the major problems is juvenile delinquency. "Eighty-five percent of teenagers appearing in juvenile court are functionally illiterate, as are 79 percent of welfare dependents, 85 percent of dropouts, 72 percent of the unemployed" (Schubert and Gates, 1990, p. 9).

Language, Social-Emotional, and Classroom Problems in Students with Learning Disabilities

Language, Syntax, Semantics, and Pragmatics

- Problems with speech sounds, intelligibility, morphological endings of words
- Limited syntax with use of simple sentences and few complex sentences
- Difficulty with directions and questions
- Paucity of vocabulary
- Difficulty with figurative language, humor, slang, and double meanings of words
- Literal interpretation of words and concepts
- Confusion with concepts and ideas
- Difficulty initiating, maintaining, and terminating conversational exchanges
- Immature turn-taking strategies
- Inadequate code-switching
- Pauses, word fillers, word repetitions, and circumlocutions
- Difficulty taking the listener's perspective
- Difficulty using language to revise language
- Inappropriate comments and responses to questions and ideas
- Provision of insufficient information for the listener

Social-Emotional Problems

- Poor eye contact
- Poor sense of fair play (e.g., sharing, win/lose rules)
- Difficulty with new situations
- Difficulty expressing wants, needs, and ideas
- Inappropriate clowning
- Poor self-concept
- Limited repertoire of emotions
- Impulsive
- Need for immediate gratification
- Inability to accept responsibility
- Gullible; easily led
- Sensitive to criticism
- Poor coping strategies
- Unpredictable

Classroom Issues

- Poor retention of material; need for constant repetition
- Problems in organization and planning
- Difficulty problem solving
- Left/Right confusion
- Reversal of symbols, letters, numbers
- Short- and long-term memory problems
- Poor integration of information
- Poor generalization of information to novel situations
- Inability to verbalize about academic tasks
- Distraction by visual and auditory stimuli
- Attentional deficits
- Auditory and visual perceptual difficulty

Sources: Fahey and Reid (2000); Ratner and Harris (1994)

Problems Facing Youth at Risk

- Delinquency and violence

- Adolescent injury (from motor vehicle accidents, drowning, sport and recreational activities)

- Substance abuse (experimentation with drugs, tobacco, and alcohol)

- Sexual activity, pregnancy, and disease (frequent sexual activity resulting in pregnancy and sexually transmitted diseases)

- Nutrition, activity, and fitness (too much junk food, too little activity, and too much obesity)

- Depression and suicide (many suffer depression and are driven to suicide by some combination of substance abuse, trouble with the law, intense anxiety in the face of social or academic challenges, feelings of personal worthlessness, impulsivity, guilt, and shame)

Source: Hamburg (1992)

One report summarized the issue this way:

While illiteracy and poor academic performance are not direct causes of delinquency, empirical studies consistently demonstrate a strong link between marginal literacy skills and the likelihood of involvement in the juvenile justice system. Most incarcerated youth lag two or more years behind their age peers in basic academic skills, and have higher rates of grade retention, absenteeism, and suspension or expulsion.... In other words, the prevalence of youth with disabilities is three to five times greater in juvenile corrections than in public school populations. (National Center on Education, Disability, and Juvenile Justice, 2002, ¶ 3,7)

While illiteracy and poor academic performance are not direct causes of delinquency, empirical studies consistently demonstrate a strong link between marginal literacy skills and the likelihood of involvement in the juvenile justice system.

A glimmer of "good news" is that crime and violence by all youths, and especially Black youths, are declining. The number of juveniles arrested for violent crime declined 23% between 1996 and 2000. This decline is largely due to the nearly 43% decline in violent-crime arrests of Black youths, which was the largest decline among those racial groups represented (Children's Defense Fund Action Council (CDFAC), 2002). In 1993, the number of juveniles murdered peaked at approximately 2,900 young lives. By 2000, the murder figure had dropped by more than half to 1,300 juveniles, but a disturbing 45% were Black youths (CDFAC, 2002).

Many incarcerated youth are in prison systems from drug-related charges. In 1986, nearly at the height of the drug war, 31 out of every 100,000 youth were admitted to state prisons for drug offenses. By 1996, 122 youth per 100,000 were entering prison on drug convictions. This represents an astounding 291% increase in the rate at which young people of all races were incarcerated because of drug involvement (Beatty, Holman, and Schiraldi, 2000). In 1996, the young White rate of incarceration had doubled from 15 per 100,000 White youth in 1986 to 30 per 100,000 White youth, and the young Black rate had grown nearly six and one-half times, to 511 per 100,000 Black youth (Beatty et al.). Is this because drug use is greater for the latter group? Or is it because of inequitable treatment of the two races with regard to drug

enforcement? Perhaps it is a combination of both.

Hechinger (1992), noting the crisis proportions that adolescent health in America has reached, claimed:

> Large numbers of ten- to fifteen-year-olds suffer from depression that may lead to suicide; they jeopardize their future by abusing illegal drugs and alcohol, and by smoking; they engage in premature, unprotected sexual activity; they are victims or perpetrators of violence; they lack proper nutrition and exercise. (p. 21)

Hechinger viewed these needs for health services as largely ignored. The leading cause of death among White youth in the 1980s was automobile accidents that were frequently related to drug or alcohol abuse (Schubert and Gates, 1990). Still in 2001, the leading cause of death among all youth was motor vehicle crashes (i.e., 31% of all deaths in 2001; National Center for Chronic Disease Prevention and Health Promotion (NCCDPHP), 2002). Homicide is the second leading cause of death for adolescents aged 15–19 years and the third leading cause of death for adolescents aged 10–14 years (National Women's Health Information Center (NWHIC), 2000). However, among Black males aged 15 to 24 years, homicide is the leading cause of death, and the firearm death rate for Black males aged 15–19 years is four times that of White males of the same age (CDFAC, 2002).

Communication Solutions
for Older Students

In an article written by U.S. Senator Dan Coats (1991), he stated that "suicide is now the second leading cause of death among adolescents, increasing 300 percent since 1950" (p. 1). In the early 2000s, it was the third ranking killer of adolescents aged 15–19 years and the fourth leading killer of younger adolescents (NWHIC, 2000). This younger group is particularly troubling to caring professionals: The Los Angeles Suicide Prevention Center found that 50% of young victims (10 to 14 years of age) were diagnosed as learning disabled—specifically as hyperactive, perceptually impaired, and dyslexic. Some researchers suggest that being learning disabled is accompanied by feelings of low self-esteem—another reason for placing this population in a high-risk category (Peck, 1982).

Furthermore, the majority of case studies have shown that suicide victims feel they have no one with whom they can talk. This lack of a friend, or someone who will listen, can be a major concern for adolescents with learning or language disorders. Their communication problems often interfere with making and keeping friends (Donahue and Bryan, 1984) and with expressing their feelings; both are potential contributing factors in the total despair preceding suicide (Peck, 1982). Major attempts at preventing suicide rely on talking and listening as evidenced by the number of hot lines available across the country. When oral language skills are impaired, and the adolescent is suicide-prone, there is cause for concern.

One more health issue that remains at the forefront for adolescents is AIDS (acquired immune deficiency syndrome). AIDS has presented a new and increasingly serious risk to adolescents since it was publicly diagnosed in 1981. Because of no curative therapy, AIDS ranked as the most serious epidemic of the past 50 years (Gray and House, 1989). It was projected that the number one killer of youth during the 1990s (exceeding the number of deaths resulting from automobile accidents in White adolescents and homicides in Black adolescents) might be AIDS unless preventive measures were taken. Fortunately this prediction did not come true: Just 1% of youth from ages 10 to 24 years died of HIV infection in 2001

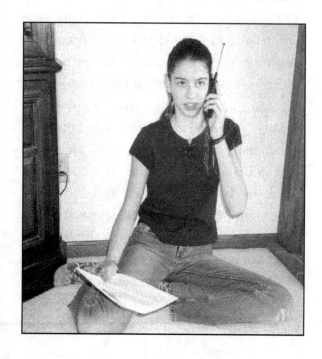

(NCCDPHP, 2002). Nonetheless, the issue cannot be dismissed as irrelevant since 46% of youth surveyed in 2001 reported they had sexual activity (NCCDPHP) and about 3 million adolescents contract a sexually transmitted disease annually (NWHIC, 2000).

Finally, professionals need to consider why some youth have such violent and risk-filled adolescent years. One consideration is child neglect and abuse.

In 1999, nearly 2.9 million children were reported as suspected child abuse or neglect cases, and an estimated 826,000 of them were confirmed victims of maltreatment. Approximately 25 per 1,000 Black children were confirmed victims of maltreatment, more than double the national average, and the highest victimization rate among racial groups represented (CDFAC, 2002, ¶ 4).

Healthy youth are more likely to come from healthy families. Perhaps professionals should marvel that so many youths survive the ages of 9 to 19, are not incarcerated, and want to transition into the world of work or postsecondary education. And those youth who do not survive, or remain in our prison systems, should teach professionals valuable lessons about how they need to adjust their interventions to help more children safely through adolescence and into adulthood.

Language Disorders Viewed as a Lifelong Disability

Children who were language impaired during their early years experience a "continuum of failure" as they mature into adolescents (Aram, Ekelman, and Nation, 1984; Aram and Hall, 1989; De Ajuriaguerra et al., 1976; Garvey and Gordon, 1973; Griffiths, 1969; C.J. Johnson et al., 1999; King, C. Jones, and Lasky, 1982; Stothard, Snowling, Bishop, Chipchase, and Kaplan, 1998; Strominger and Bashir, 1977; Weiss, Hansen, and Heubelein, 1979). Some considerations of this "continuum of failure" are noted in the sidebar on page 172.

A 15-year follow-up study of 50 speech-language students ranging in age from 13 years, 10 months to 20 years, 5 months was conducted by King et al. (1982). At the time of the investigation, 42% of the students still had some form of a communication problem. These students' spoken language disabilities frequently underlie and interact with reading failures that persist into adolescence and adulthood (Allington and Fleming, 1978; Johnston, 1985; Lewis and Freebairn, 1992; Rees, 1974; Snyder and Downey, 1991; Velluntino, 1978). Lewis and Freebairn, using a cross-sectional study, suggested that remnants of preschool phonology disorders are detectable past grade school and into adulthood; and that subjects with a history of language problems in addition to the

The "Continuum of Failure"—Some Considerations

Byers Brown and Edwards (1989) reinforced the notion of a "continuum of failure." They responded to questions first posed by Byers Brown and Beveridge (1979).

Q. **"Is there a continuum of language disturbances seen initially in the acquisition of the spoken word and later revealed as deficits in the secondary systems of reading and writing?" (p. 19)**

A. Authorities are inclined to answer yes.

Q. **"Can we assume that all children with initial disorders of language must be at risk educationally?" (p. 19)**

A. The answer to this second question is yes if the initial disorder was correctly diagnosed as affecting language.

Q. **"Is there an underlying factor which is causal and thereby links all language manifestations? Or, are the skills all related by factors in the child's disposition, neurological, emotional, or environmental but not causally linked?" (p. 19)**

A. The answers to these questions are not readily available. Nonetheless, the questions are important to consider.

Q. **"Are different language and learning problems occurring independently in vulnerable children rather than being bound together by one definable disability?" (p. 19)**

A. Likewise, the answer to this question is not yet available. The complexity and diversity of conditions cast under the broad heading of "language disorders" suggest a homogeneity that does not exist. The same can be said of "learning disability."

Sources: B. Byers Brown and Beveridge (1979); Byers Brown and Edwards (1989)

phonology disorders performed more poorly on reading and spelling measures than subjects with a history of preschool phonology disorders alone.

Lahey (1990) spoke to the diversity of procedures for identifying children with language disorders and the resultant confusion about the meaning of the term *language disorder*. The clinical forum on specific language impairment as a clinical category (Kamhi, 1991; Leonard, 1991) also stressed that language disorder is not a homogenous category and debated the nature of specific language impairment. Leonard (1991) argued that "children with language limitations are not simply late in reaching early language milestones, but have limitations that are long standing, at least in the absence of intervention" (p. 67), and he proposed the concept of a continuum of language ability.

In her extensive review of the literature, N. Nelson (1998) noted that prognostic data from longitudinal studies for children with language disorders indicate that the disorders persist but change in their characteristics. As children grow older, they may have more problems with written communication, such as reading, and the complexity of oral communication. Statistics on the persistence of language or speech disorders as the student gets older range from 40 to 80%. In spite of these statistics, Nelson cautions us to use them carefully since none of us knows exactly what will be the prognostic outcome for a particular individual with a language disorder.

Stothard et al. (1998) concluded that if a child's language problems persist to age 5 or 6, language, literacy, and educational difficulties are likely to be evident throughout childhood into adolescence. Even children who had early language problems that were resolved by age 5 to 6 appeared to be weaker than peers with typical development in literacy skills and phonological processing.

C.J. Johnson et al. (1999) studied 5-year-old children with speech and/or language impairments over 14 years, specifically at ages 12 and 19 years. At each of these three age levels, the students' cognitive, academic, behavioral, and psychiatric areas were assessed. The results indicated that (1) high rates of communication problems persisted into adulthood; (2) language performance was stable over time; (3) long-term outcomes for those with speech impairments were better than those with language impairments; and (4) progress was more favorable for those with specific language impairments than for those with impairments secondary to sensory, structural, neurological, or cognitive deficits. Overall, these findings are consistent with earlier follow-up studies noting that language impairments persist over time.

Points of Discussion

1. Compare and contrast the various types of frequent concomitant problems that exist for older students with language disorders.

2. Discuss how "the continuum of failure" concept might influence your analysis of the students' abilities and prognosis for success.

Suggested Readings

Fahey, K., and Reid, K. (2000). *Language development, differences, and disorders: A perspective for general and special education teachers and classroom-based speech-language pathologists.* Austin, TX: Pro-Ed.

Johnson, C.J., Beitchman, J.H., Young, A., Escobar, M., Atkinson, L., Wilson, B., et al. (1999). Fourteen-year follow-up of children with and without speech/language impairments: Speech/language stability and outcomes. *Journal of Speech, Language, and Hearing Research, 42*(3), 744–760.

Ylvisaker, M., and DeBonis, D. (2000). Executive function impairment in adolescence: TBI and ADHD. *Topics in Language Disorders, 20*(2), 29–57.

Part

Language Assessment of Adolescents

8 *Chapter*

Assessment— A Comprehensive Process

Goals

- Provide an overview of the assessment process
- Describe the five characteristics that make assessment comprehensive
- Explain factors to consider in the assessment of educational and environmental systems
- Present assessment issues as they relate to a pluralistic society

Assessment is an ongoing process in which the examiner selects and administers appropriate measurement instruments (formal tests and informal procedures) and observes and records the student's communication behaviors—as well as the behaviors of the members in the student's environment—to determine the existence, type, nature, and severity of a communication disorder. Before beginning the assessment process, the exact purpose should be determined. Is the purpose to:

- Determine the existence of a problem?
- Establish appropriate intervention goals?
- Decide if dismissal is warranted?

This purpose must be established first to select appropriate procedures and subsequently to obtain the information needed to accomplish the desired task.

In this chapter, we provide an overview of assessment for an initial speech-language evaluation or for periodic retesting.

The assessment process begins with a referral for a suspected problem. Note that prior to a referral, IDEA 1997 requires a student study team or similar decision-making group to converse periodically to determine classroom modifications for individual students. It is critical that the speech-language pathologist be part of this team (Moore-Brown and Montgomery, 2001). Some of the observational and interview tools for assessing the educational and environmental systems, which are discussed later in this chapter, might prove to be helpful during this student study team process as well. For example, see the questionnaire regarding classroom routines on page 190. Someone on the student study team might ask these questions of a student even before a referral for assessment is made. Answers to these questions will provide insight regarding a student's understanding of classroom rules and routines while simultaneously providing information on the teacher's behaviors and expectations. Should a referral for assessment come from the student study team, the pertinent data from observations and interviews can and should be used in determining whether a language disorder or a language difference exists.

Identification of Students Needing Assessment

The first area to address is how the student came to be identified. In earlier times (i.e.,

before the mid-1970s), routine school-based mass screening programs were conducted periodically (e.g., in kindergarten, first, third, sixth, and ninth grades) to identify students with language disorders. This approach was not very efficient or cost-effective. A more efficient and effective process is to inform potential referral sources (such as teachers, parents, and students themselves) about the signs of both oral and written language disorders (Larson and McKinley, 1987). This is more effective because these referral sources have spent the greatest amount of time with the student, resulting in more in-depth knowledge across a variety of communication situations. This is a more efficient process because new observational situations do not need to be created since information can be gleaned from existing situations. Also, mass screening takes a great amount of time that does not need to be spent when using a referral system. A sample secondary-level referral form is presented in Appendix A and can be used for determining which students might need to be referred for assessment. To obtain the most appropriate referrals, speech-language pathologists should share this form with colleagues who interact frequently with students with suspected langauge disorders.

It is possible that a referral system may not work for all adolescents. A selective screening process may be needed for high-risk groups such as:

- Adolescents in special programs (e.g., a classroom for students with autism)

- All middle school or junior high students receiving or in need of reading services

- Individuals about to drop out of school

- Students who have failed minimal competency testing for graduation one or more times

- Adolescents with academic difficulties not related to attitude or motivation

Likewise, selective screening as routine intake activities should be undertaken in juvenile detention centers, adolescent psychiatric institutions, and alternative high schools (Larson and McKinley, 1987). Once determined that a problem exists, it should be established if it is a language difference or a suspected language disorder. Recall from Chapter 5 that a language difference exists when a student does not have a problem within his or her primary language system, but rather within a secondary language system.

Assessment as a Comprehensive Process

A number of paradigm shifts (see the sidebar) have changed behaviors that speech-language pathologists assess and how those behaviors are assessed (Westby and Erickson, 1992). The assessment process recommended for older students is one that is descriptive/explanatory, authentic, dynamic, student centered, and multidimensional (J. Damico, 1993; Larson and McKinley, 1988). This

Shifts in Assessment Paradigms

FROM	TO
• Discrete point, decontextualized, standardized tests	• Authentic, functional, descriptive, naturalistic assessment
• A totally client-centered approach	• A more multidimensional approach that takes into account the student's social systems
• Exclusively assessing spoken communication	• Including written communication and problem-solving skills; the interaction between spoken and written language in older students is acknowledged
• Focus on student similarities	• An awareness of cultural and linguistic diversity among students
• Exclusively using quantitative data and procedures	• Including qualitative data and procedures

Source: Westby and Erickson (1992)

comprehensive approach will result in collecting the most cogent data about the student so that dismissal or programming can be focused on assisting the student in achieving the highest academic progress, enhancing personal-social needs, and reaching vocational/post-secondary potential. The five facets of a comprehensive assessment model are not mutually exclusive, but rather interact and help determine if the student is an effective communicator within and across various situations. Each of the five dimensions are discussed briefly in the sections that follow.

Descriptive/Explanatory Assessment

In descriptive/explanatory assessment, the clinician's evaluation documents and describes the student's communication problem and its underlying causes, if possible. A bilevel analysis paradigm is required, including a descriptive analysis of the communicative performance and a detailed explanatory analysis of language proficiency (J. Damico, 1993).

A *descriptive analysis* focuses on directly observing and recording behaviors that (1) have been found to be necessary for successful communication in selected contexts in which the student is likely to communicate and in selected modalities that the student is likely to use, and (2) are believed to be valid indices of communicative difficulty.

An *explanatory analysis* determines the causal factors for the communication disorder

that was observed during the descriptive analysis. The explanatory phase does not involve more data collection (J. Damico, 1993), but is a deeper interpretation of the data collected in the descriptive analysis. The examiner needs to sort out the communication behaviors that were successful and those that were not under the descriptive analysis.

For those communication behaviors that were not successful, it is important to ask, "Why not?" Was it because of the student's social/cultural experiences, cognitive abilities, emotional abilities, physical abilities (e.g., hearing or fine motor abilities), or a combination of the above?

For those communication behaviors that were not successful, it is important to ask, "Why not?"

J. Damico (1993) generated a set of questions that could be used in analyzing those variables that might have contributed to the communicative difficulties. These two general sets of questions (i.e., extrinsic explanatory factors and intrinsic explanatory factors) are listed in Table 8.1.

Questions to Ask to Determine Explanatory Factors Contributing to Communication Disorders

Table 8.1

Factor Type	Questions
Extrinsic	1. Are there any overt variables that immediately explain the observed communicative difficulties? Among the potential considerations: • Are the documented problematic behaviors occurring at a frequency that would be considered within normal limits or in random variation? • Were there any procedural mistakes in the descriptive analysis phase that account for the problematic behaviors? • Is there an indication of extreme test anxiety during the observational assessment in one context but not in the subsequent ones? • Is there significant performance inconsistency between different contexts within the targeted manifestations? 2. Is there evidence that the problematic behaviors noted in the descriptive analysis phase can be explained according to normal second language acquisition or dialectal phenomena? 3. Is there any evidence that the problematic behaviors noted in the descriptive analysis phase can be explained according to cross-cultural interference or related cultural phenomena? 4. Is there any evidence that the problematic behaviors noted in the descriptive analysis phase can be explained according to differences in the student's past history or experience? 5. Is there any evidence that the problematic behaviors noted in the descriptive analysis phase can be explained according to any bias effect that was in operation before, during, or after assessment? • Is the student in a subtractive language learning environment? • Is the student a member of a disempowered community? • Are negative or lowered expectations for this student held by the student, the student's family, or the educational staff? • Were specific indications of bias evident in the referral, administrative, scoring, or interpretative phases of the evaluation? NOTE: If the communicative difficulty cannot be accounted for by asking the first five questions, then the final question aimed at intrinsic explanatory factors should be conducted.
Intrinsic	6. Is there any underlying linguistic systematicity to the problematic behaviors noted during the descriptive analysis phase? This can be determined by completion of the following steps: • Ensure that no overt factors account for the problematic behaviors (first five questions); • Isolate the turns or utterances that contain the problematic behaviors; and • Perform a systematic linguistic analysis on these data points, looking for consistency in the appearance of problematic behaviors.

From "Language Assessment in Adolescents: Addressing Critical Issues," by J. Damico, 1993, *Language, Speech, and Hearing Services in Schools, 24*(1), p. 33. © 1993 by the American Speech-Language-Hearing Association. Adapted with permission.

Authentic Assessment

Authentic assessment has been of major interest to classroom teachers and administrators who are concerned about standardized measures and feel there is a need to develop new kinds of testing measures based on performances. Authentic assessment evaluates the actual behaviors professionals want students to be able to do. If clinicians judge "students to be deficient in writing, speaking, listening, artistic creation, research, thoughtful analysis, problem posing, and problem solving" (Wiggins, 1989, pp. 41–42), then the tests should measure how students "write, speak, listen, create, do original research, analyze, pose, and solve problems" (Wiggins, pp. 41–42). Authentic tests have four basic characteristics (Wiggins):

1. They are designed to be representative of performance in the field; problems of scoring reliability and logistics of testing are considered after that.

2. Attention is paid to the teaching and learning of the criteria to be used in the assessment.

3. Self-assessment plays a much greater role than in conventional testing.

4. Students frequently are "expected to present their work and defend themselves publicly and orally to ensure that their apparent mastery is genuine" (p. 45).

Table 8.2 presents a more thorough list of characteristics of authentic tests.

The data collected for assessment should be actual utterances that serve to transmit ideas or intentions as a speaker/writer to a listener/reader in real communication situations (J. Damico, 1993). Authentic assessment possesses both linguistic realism and ecological validity. *Linguistic realism* means that assessment must be meaning based and integrative as opposed to fragmenting language into discrete components. *Ecological validity* means that assessment must be accomplished in naturalistic/realistic settings (J. Damico).

According to Silliman, Wilkinson, and Hoffman (1993), "authentic assessment should be approached as a dynamic, evolving, social process jointly constructed over time through the multiple perspectives of students, their families, educational staff, administrators, and researchers" (p. 71). Contrived language data (e.g., in a testing situation with discrete point testing) will be of little value in determining what type of communicator the student is in actual communication situations. The examiner should evaluate the preadolescent or adolescent across and within a variety of natural communication situations (e.g., in the classroom, at home, and during sports activities) and with both familiar and unfamiliar listeners. Communication styles change as a function of the situation and the listener. These changes must be taken into account during an authentic assessment process.

Table 8.2

Characteristics of Authentic Tests

Authentic Test	Characteristics
Structures and Logistics	Are more appropriately public; involve an audience, a panel, and so on. Do not rely on unrealistic and arbitrary time constraints. Offer known, not secret, questions or tasks. Are more like portfolios or a season of games (not one-shot). Require some collaboration with others. Recur—and are worth practicing for, rehearsing, and retaking. Make assessment and feedback to students so central that school schedules, structures, and policies are modified to support them.
Grading and Scoring Standards	Involve criteria that assess essentials, not easily counted (but relatively unimportant) errors. Are not graded on a "curve" but in reference to performance standards (criterion-referenced, not norm-referenced). Involve demystified criteria of success that appear to students as inherent in successful activity. Make self-assessment a part of the assessment. Use a multifaceted scoring system instead of one aggregate grade. Exhibit harmony with shared schoolwide aims—a standard.
Intellectual Design Features	Are "essential"—not needlessly intrusive, arbitrary, or contrived to "shake out" a grade. Are "enabling"—constructed to point the student toward more sophisticated use of the skills or knowledge. Are contextualized, complex intellectual challenges, not "atomized" tasks, corresponding to isolated "outcomes." Involve the student's own research or use of knowledge, for which "content" is a means. Assess student habits and repertoires, not mere recall or plug-in skills. Are representative challenges—designed to emphasize depth more than breadth. Are engaging and educational. Involve somewhat ambiguous ("ill-structured") tasks or problems.
Fairness and Equity	Ferret out and identify (perhaps hidden) strengths. Strike a constantly examined balance between honoring achievement and native skill or fortunate prior training. Minimize needless, unfair, and demoralizing comparisons. Allow for appropriate room for student learning styles, aptitudes, and interests. Can be—should be—attempted by all students, with the test "scaffolded up," not "dumbed down," as necessary. Reverse typical test-design procedures: they make "accountability" serve student learning (Attention is primarily paid to "face" and "ecological" validity of tests.)

From "Teaching to the (Authentic) Test," by G. Wiggins, 1989, *Educational Leadership, 46*(7), p. 45. © 1989 by the Association for Supervision and Curriculum Development (ASCD), Alexandria, VA. Reprinted with permission. All rights reserved.

Dynamic Assessment

Dynamic assessment, sometimes referred to as *learning potential assessment*, focuses on learning processes rather than products, which are the focus of traditional assessment procedures (Lidz, 1991). When the focus of assessment is on the product, no information is gathered regarding the reason(s) for failure or success on a given test item.

According to Lidz (1991), there are variations in the interpretation of the dynamic assessment model. However, there are defining characteristics on which all proponents appear to agree. Dynamic assessment:

- Follows a test-intervene-retest format

- Focuses on learner modifiability (i.e., assessing the amount of learner change as a response to the intervention and the learner's increased implementation of relevant metacognitive processes in problem solving)

- Provides useful information for developing intervention

- Documents the intensity of intervention needed to produce change

Examiners using dynamic assessment procedures are interested in the metacognitive processes of problem solving, and in the extent to which the learner's metacognitive abilities can be enhanced. However, dynamic assessment is more than a model with procedures; it also represents an attitude. According to Lidz (1991), dynamic assessors are:

convinced that children can learn if sufficient time and effort is expended to discover the means by which they can profit from intervention. Dynamic assessors are also more interested in spending this time to derive ideas for intervention rather than for placement or classification decisions.... The focus of dynamic assessment is on the assessor's ability to discover the means of facilitating the learning of the child, not on the child's demonstration of ability to the assessor. (p. 9)

The theoretical underpinnings for dynamic assessment go back to Vygotsky's (1962) concept of the zone of proximal development (ZPD). "The ZPD is the difference between the child's level of performance when functioning independently and the child's level of performance when functioning in collaboration with a more knowledgeable partner. This can also be viewed as a definition of potential" (Lidz, 1991, p. 7).

We have elected to apply Reuven Feuerstein's (1979) learning potential philosophical approach when assessing older students because it emphasizes process over product. This dynamic assessment approach, based on a theory of structural cognitive modifiability, involves three core concepts, highlighted in the sidebar that follows.

Core Concepts of Dynamic Assessment

1. The learner's behavior may be characterized by a series of cognitive functions and deficiencies that are organized according to an input-elaboration-output model of the mental act.

2. The assessor's behavior is characterized in terms of the components of the mediated learning experience (e.g., the assessor might bridge a current experience to a previous experience or might attribute value and highlight the importance of the content through voice modulation and affect).

3. The task is conceptualized in terms of a cognitive map that reveals the features that distinguish one task from another. The cognitive map comprises seven dimensions on which the mental act can be described. These dimensions are content, modality, phase of the mental act, cognitive operations, level of complexity, level of abstraction, and level of efficiency; all dimensions are part of the Language Potential Assessment Device (LPAD).

Source: Reuven Feuerstein (1979)

Student-Centered Assessment

In student-centered assessment, the student directs and assesses the language/communication process along with the diagnostician (Boyce and Larson, 1983; Larson and McKinley, 1987, 1995; Tattershall, 2002). Oftentimes, adolescents provide unique insights into their problems. Many students engage in meta-awareness tasks such as thinking about their thinking (metacognition), using language to analyze their language (metalinguistics), and revising communication breakdowns (metacommunication), which provides important information about how students perceive their own performance. Other preadolescents and adolescents may be oblivious to their own communication disorders.

By asking for an explanation of the problem, the examiner can determine whether there are discrepancies among examination results, the adolescent's perspective, and the perspectives of persons within the educational and environmental systems. If a discrepancy exists among any of these dimensions, it may suggest the need for further evaluation, educational inservice, or family counseling.

In the student-centered assessment process, the examiner should explain to the adolescent—before the evaluation procedure—what behaviors are to be assessed, how they are to be assessed, and the reason for the various procedures. This is in contrast to what is typically done—simply administering tests without explanation. By explaining the testing process, the examiner will usually find the adolescent is a more cooperative and active participant. The adolescent should be encouraged to challenge and to question what is being done. After all, who should be more interested in what is happening than the person to whom it is happening?

Likewise, in a student-centered assessment process, we strongly recommend that adolescents, in conjunction with the professionals and parents present, participate in the evaluation results and recommendations. If that is too threatening or otherwise undesirable, separate meetings could be held with adolescents to discuss evaluation performance and its implications for their academic, social, and vocational goals.

Adolescents should be told about their strengths as well as their weaknesses. Whenever possible, examiners should illustrate how students may use strengths to overcome or to compensate for weaknesses. If intervention is not indicated, this interaction will provide insight into the inconsistencies in performance that the older student may have been experiencing. If the student is scheduled for intervention, these comments can prepare him or her for that.

Whenever possible, examiners should illustrate how students may use strengths to overcome or to compensate for weaknesses.

Multidimensional Assessment

In multidimensional assessment, all aspects of the preadolescent's or adolescent's environment are assessed. That is, the student is evaluated, but so are the school, home, and work settings. An analysis of the student's educational and environmental systems may reveal that:

- One or both systems may be contributing to the student's suspected language disorder

- One or both systems may be supportive of the student with a suspected language disorder

- One or both systems, not the student, may be the primary "problem" (i.e., the student does not have a language disorder)

To determine precisely the relationship among students and their educational and environmental systems, careful assessment procedures are needed. The next two sections highlight critical factors to consider during multidimensional assessment. Although multidimensional assessment may be time consuming, it will give a more comprehensive perspective of students' capabilities as they interact with their school, family, and community.

Educational System Considerations

The educational system consists of a variety of professionals, but for the purpose of this chapter, the assumption is made that teachers are involved in the majority of professional interactions with older students. Major areas of assessment needing to be considered include the structure of the educational system, teacher language and classsroom routines, curriculum variables, and post-secondary education options.

Structure of the Educational System

The structure of the educational system is important to assess because it indicates how flexible administrators and teachers might be when modifications to the system are proposed. The checklist of questions in the sidebar can be used to quickly assess the structure of the educational system. This checklist will also allow for better insight into the history of speech-language programs within the educational system in question. Those speech-language pathologists who have initiated programs in the past, and who are now in the maintenance phase, may use the checklist as a summary of the current status of the educational system.

Responses to the questions should be analyzed to determine what variables within the educational system might be changed (e.g., modification of criteria for entrance and exit; an increase in the number of inter-disciplinary teams to which speech-language pathologists are assigned). When armed with this information, speech-language patholo-gists are better able to engage in program

Questions to Ask to Assess the Structure of the Educational System

- Is there a willingness to implement new programs or alternative programs for older students with communication disorders?

- Are there concerted efforts to find ways to reduce the dropout rate?

- Are minimum competency tests required of all adolescents to graduate?

- Is the organizational framework the same as it has been for decades (i.e., teachers teach as they were taught (lecturing, monitoring, and quizzing); high schools continue to be horizontally struc-tured by age group (freshmen, sophomores, juniors, seniors) and vertically organized by program track (e.g., college-bound, vocational education, special education))?

- Is the educational system aware of the speech-language pathologist and the role this professional plays in the interdisciplinary evaluation team?

- What are the state's and region's entrance and exit criteria for speech-language programs? Do these criteria need to be revised and, if so, is there a willingness on the part of administrators to do so?

From *Language Disorders in Older Students: Preadolescents and Adolescents* (p. 90), by V. Lord Larson and N.L. McKinley, 1995, Eau Claire, WI: Thinking Publications. © 1995 by Thinking Publications. Adapted with permission.

planning and to initiate modifications in the educational system that are beneficial to older students.

Teacher Language and Classroom Routines

Assessment of teacher language and routines in the classroom is essential to determine if modifications are necessary to meet the needs of students. The language of the classroom teacher directly and indirectly influences students' responses (Gruenewald and Pollak, 1984). Teacher language is comprised of an instructional mode (explanations/directions and questions), a syntactical mode (word order and sentence complexity), and a speaking mode (length, rate, and intonation; Gruenewald and Pollak, 1984).

Assessment of teacher language and routines in the classroom is essential to determine if modifications are necessary to meet the needs of students.

Some adolescents may find rapid speech, lengthy directions, or complex questions too difficult to process. Therefore, failure in that teacher's classroom continues until modifications are made. Assessment of the teacher's rate of speech, tone of voice, length of directions, complexity of directions, level of vocabulary, and organization of ideas, as well as the ease of listening by others, should be documented to determine where communication breakdowns occur. Is the breakdown in the teacher's messages or in the student's comprehension of those messages?

One method for evaluating the teacher's language is to use a self-evaluation technique. While teacher language might be analyzed best by speech-language pathologists, teachers who welcome such professionals into their classrooms for the purpose of evaluating their language during instruction are rare. More common reactions include feelings of anxiety, fear, and invasion of privacy or academic freedom. Yet most teachers are interested in improving their classroom instruction, and many are receptive to self-evaluating their language, if data remain confidential.

Appendix B contains a self-evaluation form for classroom teachers. Speech-language pathologists should train teachers in this technique of self-evaluation. Alternatively, a student evaluation of teacher language designed for use in the classroom is provided in Appendix C. Each student is given a form by the teacher immediately following a 10- to 15-minute lecture or some detailed instructional situation. Students should be assured that there are no "wrong" answers and that their answers will not influence their grades for the course.

The request for the student's name on the form is to encourage taking the evaluation seriously and to discourage "silly" responses. The requirement of names, is, however, at the discretion of the teacher. If there are a number of poor readers in the classroom, the teacher should read the form aloud for all students before, or during, their completion of the form. Explanations of the characteristics of the teacher's language to be rated should be provided, whether or not students ask for them. Honesty of answers should be stressed.

Teachers should collect the forms, study responses to each item on the form, and compute the mean for the class. Forms containing responses that are on the extreme low end of the rating scale—for example, only one student evaluating the level of vocabulary as very hard—should be analyzed carefully. If, however, several students react negatively to the difficulty level of vocabulary being used, there may be cause to further analyze this issue. Teachers who notice a significant number of students (e.g., 20%) negatively assessing various aspects of their language of instruction might wish to consider modifications in their language.

It is particularly helpful for a teacher to use the evaluation technique when a student in his or her classroom has been referred for testing for a suspected communication disorder. The evaluation form will allow a comparison of that student's perception of the teacher's language with the perceptions of peers in the classroom. If the referred student was unique in his or her responses or was more negative than the other students were, the teacher's language within that course may be problematic for that student.

In addition to evaluating teacher language, Creaghead and Tattershall (1991) developed a questionnaire to be used with students to assess teachers' classroom routines and rules. These questions can be found in the sidebar on page 190. When asking students to answer the questions, watch for two main types of responses: (1) answers that seem to indicate the student does not know the routines and rules, and (2) answers that seem to indicate the teacher has unpredictable routines and rules. A combination of response types may also exist.

Ideally, the speech-language pathologist can directly observe teacher language and classroom routines in relationship to the students' completed questionnaires. However, classroom observations at the secondary level are more challenging than in the younger grades, because adolescents have multiple teachers and classrooms each day. Also, adolescents are easily embarrassed by the presence of an outsider in the classroom observing their and their teacher's behaviors. Therefore, having a set of questions like those in the sidebar on page 191 can help guide an interview with a teacher when observation is not advisable.

Whether interviewing the secondary teacher or observing in the classroom, it is critical that the student be assessed in relationship to these important educational

Questionnaire to Use with Students
Regarding Classroom Routines and Rules

- What does your teacher do or say when he or she is angry with the class?

- What really makes your teacher mad or angry?

- What is the most important thing that you should always do in class?

- What is the most important thing that you should never do in class?

- How do you know when it is time to go... [to your next class]?

- What is the first thing that you should do when class begins?

- What does your teacher do or say when she is going to say something really important?

- What is the last thing you should do before you go home at the end of the day?

- When is it OK to talk out without raising your hand at school?

- How do you know when your teacher is joking or teasing?

- What does your teacher do when it is time for a lesson to begin?

- When is it all right to ask a question in class?

From "Observation and Assessment of Classroom Pragmatic Skills," by N.A. Creaghead and S.A. Tattershall in *Communication Skills and Classroom Success: Assessment and Therapy Methodologies for Language and Learning Disabled Students* (p. 110), edited by C.S. Simon, 1991, Eau Claire, WI: Thinking Publications. © 1991 by Thinking Publications. Reprinted with permission.

components. Likewise, classroom assessment should be authentic in that it should be "an integrated continuous and natural part of the everyday activities of the classroom, because any teaching-learning interaction contains potential assessment information" (Silliman, Wilkinson, and Hoffman, 1993, p. 71)

Curriculum Variables

The types of curriculum variables that might be interfering with a student's academic success constitute another area to be assessed within the educational system. Several of the curriculum variables to be considered are shown in the sidebar on page 192.

Examiners should keep in mind that it is plausible that several problems will be identified. The student might be having difficulty in a course because of an underlying language disorder, but at the same time there may be problems in the curriculum (e.g., the readability of the text is not at grade level or the course has spiral organization and the student has been "lost" for months). Also consider whether negative attitude and poor

Interview Questions to Ask Teachers of
Secondary Students with Suspected Language Disorders

- How is the student doing academically in your class?

- What are the student's strengths in your class?

- How well organized is the student?

- How does the student do with these school routines?

    - Following directions
    - Answering questions
    - Completing assignments
    - Understanding written material
    - Getting along with peers
    - Listening to lectures and classroom conversations

- How would you rate the student's vocabulary?

- What problems is the student having in your class?

- Are there classroom routines that the student has difficulty with?

- Describe a classroom activity that the student has recently had problems with.

- What aspects of the curriculum present the greatest problems for the student?

- What changes would you like to see in the student's classroom performance?

- What is the student's realistic potential in this class?

- What expectations do you have for this student succeeding?

Sources: N. Nelson (1998); Rhea Paul (2001); Work, Cline, Ehren, Keiser, and Wujek (1993)

motivation are contributing factors to the student's failure in the course.

Appendix D is an example of a curriculum analysis form that could help examine curriculum variables. The intent of this analysis is that it be completed whenever one or two content areas are particularly troublesome to the student undergoing an initial assessment (rather than for every student in every content area). Completion of the curriculum analysis form may help identify the problem (i.e., may determine if it is within the adolescent and/or within the educational system). Such identification is necessary for appropriate program planning.

Curriculum analysis may also be helpful once older students with language disorders begin intervention. The form then serves as an organized, coherent approach to studying their abilities within existing curricula and as a reference point for needed modifications in the classroom, if a consultation model is used.

Curriculum Variables That Could Interfere with Academic Success

Comprehension of Spoken Information: Is the older student having difficulty understanding what is said in many different situations or primarily in one course? What is the nature of the comprehension problem?

Organization of the Course: Is the course organized sequentially, as though there is little interaction among units (e.g., one topic is "geology" and the next is "electricity") or in a spiral fashion, as though there is major interaction among units (e.g., parts of speech are taught to provide the background for sentence diagramming)? If the course is organized sequentially, have all units been problematic for the student, or only some?

Requirements in the Course: Does the course demand significantly different requirements than other courses in which the student is not struggling (e.g., excessive reading, lengthy term papers, or public speaking)?

Textbooks and Tests in the Course: Is the readability of the textbook appropriate for the preadolescent or adolescent? Is it organized like other texts that the student is using? Are the course tests significantly different from those in other courses (e.g., essay questions or objective questions that demand synthesis of information)?

From *Language Disorders in Older Students: Preadolescents and Adolescents* (pp. 92–93), by V. Lord Larson and N.L. McKinley, 1995, Eau Claire, WI: Thinking Publications. © 1995 by Thinking Publications. Adapted with permission.

An alternative procedure for curriculum assessment includes curriculum-based language assessment and intervention (N. Nelson, 1989, 1992, 1998). Nelson's (1998) curriculum-based language assessment focuses on whether the student is using language knowledge, skills, and strategies effectively to learn the course content. Nelson describes six curricular types (see the sidebar that follows). Analysis of the student's reading, writing, speaking, and listening skills should be qualitatively and quantitatively undertaken. According to Nelson (1998):

> Curriculum-based language assessment involves several kinds of data collection. The primary tools and strategies, in addition to ethnographic interviews, are artifact analysis (e.g.,)...classroom lecture notes and written assignments; onlooker observation (e.g.,)...sitting in the classroom at a distance and observing signs of participation including evidence of attention, listening, and communicative expressions; and participant observation...the specialist sits beside the student while the student attempts a targeted curricular task...and provides scaffolding (for the student). (p. 402)

Curricular Types

The speech-language pathologist needs to be aware of all of these curricular types to adequately assess the student's ability to interact with the curriculum.

1. **Official:** What is produced by curriculum committees

2. **Cultural:** The unspoken expectations of the mainstream culture that serves as a backdrop to the official curriculum

3. **Defacto:** The use of textbook selections that determines the curriculum

4. **School Culture:** The set of rules, both spoken and unspoken, about the classroom interactions, such as when to talk and when not to talk, and how to request a turn

5. **Hidden:** The teacher's subtle expectations for determining who are the good students

6. **Underground:** The rules for social interaction among peers that determine who is accepted and who is not

---

Source: N. Nelson (1998)

Postsecondary Education Options

Too often we assume that if adolescents have a language or learning disability, they are not capable of university-level work. Aune and Friehe (1996) are adamant about the need for educators to encourage the adolescent with a language and/or learning disability to take college preparatory courses during the high school years and to pursue a college education. In addition, they advocate that the transition from high school to college be carefully prepared for, starting at age 16, and understood by the student:

> In high school, which operates under IDEA, school personnel are responsible for identifying students with disabilities, determining their needs and providing services to meet those needs. Students are passive recipients of these services. In college, which operates under Section 504, students are expected to identify themselves, determine their own needs and request accommodations. Students here are active participants in obtaining the accommodations they need. Secondary education is oriented to providing services to ensure success. Postsecondary education is oriented to providing accommodations to ensure equal access. (p. 7)

Communication Solutions
for Older Students

Given these differences, it is critical that students be assessed to determine their understanding of their rights under the law and if they are capable of being a self-advocate. If not, this concept must be taught if they are to succeed at the postsecondary level. At a minimum, adolescents who are college-bound must deal with issues of "self-development, knowledge of their disability, self-advocacy, networking, disclosure, and accommodations" (Aune and Friehe, 1996, p. 11). During the assessment phase, students should gain knowledge of their disability and take responsibility for compiling a transition portfolio (see the sidebar). Such a portfolio would inform school personnel about the type and extent of the disability and the accommodations needed.

J. Simon (2001) noted that there are numerous legal issues surrounding postsecondary students' services, such as definition and documentation of the disability and access to standardized testing. The most pervasive arguments are the definition of a disability and what is considered to be a "reasonable accommodation." The various issues of whether a reasonable accommodation has been provided are still being tested in the courts. From a "best practices" point of view, all stakeholders should be involved and they should leave their preconceived notions at the door (J. Simon). All stakeholders should understand the continuum of accommodations and who is primarily responsible for what when. An excellent diagram (by Aune and Friehe, 1996) of what the continuum of accommodations might look like is presented in Figure 8.1.

Measuring the academic performance of the postsecondary student with a language disorder is an essential component of the educational process in universities and colleges, including vocational technical colleges. It is true that taking a test under typical standard conditions (usually written, timed tests) requires certain skills apart from those areas

Contents of a Transition Portfolio

- Description of recent assessment documents

- Test-taking strategies

- Vocational rehabilitation resources, if appropriate

- Sample scripts for how to disclose and request information

- Writing samples of assignments

- Effective accommodations

- Academic transcripts

- Entrance examination data

- Speaking skills

- Listening strategies used

Sources: Aune and Friehe (1996); Rhea Paul (2001)

Continuum of Accommodations
and Responsibilities

Figure 8.1

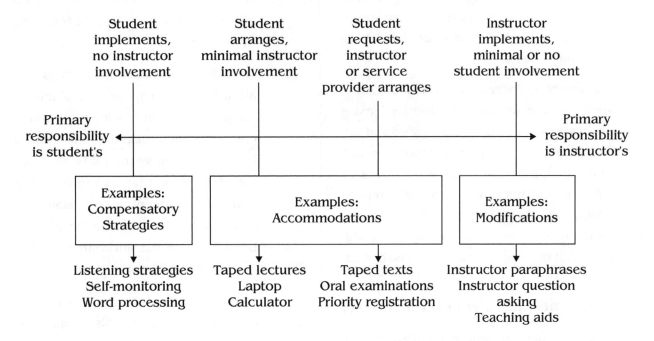

From "Transition to Postsecondary Education: Institutional and Individual Issues," by B. Aune and M. Friehe, 1996, *Topics in Language Disorders, 16*(3), p. 16. © 1996 by Lippencott. Reprinted with permission.

being assessed on the test (Heath Resource Center, 1985). The speech-language pathologist should simulate the assessment situations in which the student is likely to be placed within the postsecondary environment. Students need to be assessed under "typical" conditions likely to be found in postsecondary settings; then an analysis should be conducted and interpretation presented so that students understand what their strengths and weaknesses are within a standard test-taking format.

Students whose situations fall under Section 504 of the Rehabilitation Act of 1973 have the right to request adaptations to the testing situation. For example, if the student has a severe speech disorder, written examinations might be substituted for oral recitation exams. The student may write responses for oral recitation and have that presentation read by an interpreter. If the student has a language disorder and is easily distracted, the student may request that the test be given individually in a quiet room. If writing is difficult, the student may arrange for alternative methods of recording answers, such as taping the responses or word-processing them.

Thus, the student may need a different test environment, an exam proctor, and/or additional test time. Whatever the adaptation needed, based on analysis of the situation, it is critical that the student and teachers know that adaptation does not mean changing or lowering standards for the course or admission requirements.

Ganschow, Philips, and Schneider (2001) pointed out that as part of the decision-making process to pursue postsecondary education, the student should carefully select the university that can best accommodate his or her needs. There are large differences among universities as to their ability and desire to accommodate the needs of students with language and learning disabilities.

Environmental System Considerations

Evaluating the environmental system consists of assessing the family situation, the peer group to which the older student belongs, and the employment setting (if appropriate). Examination of these areas is critical to determine if the preadolescent or adolescent has a language disorder.

Family

Examiners assessing the environmental system should realize that the American "family" has changed dramatically over the past decade. The American family of father and mother and 2.5 children does not exist. It is important for the examiner to know about the preadolescent's or adolescent's family situation because it provides the foundation for language and communication. Major purposes for assessing the family unit are these:

- To understand the family members' perceptions of the older student's communication disorder, or suspected disorder, including past history and future goals

- To gather information on feelings and attitudes of family members toward the preadolescent or adolescent with a communication disorder and toward the educational system; this may indicate how supportive and tolerant the home environment is of disabilities and how amiable the relationship has been between the environmental and educational systems

- To obtain information about the family's communication style; this permits the speech-language pathologist to determine if a language difference exists

Data obtained from the family regarding previous speech-language services and the importance of improving speaking, listening, and thinking should be compared with the preadolescent's or adolescent's responses for agreement. Data should also be gathered from families to address the issues suggested in the sidebar that follows. This information is also captured in the case history interview form in Appendix E.

In addition, the examiner should investigate the family's attitudes toward educational services and toward professionals providing services. Family members of adolescents being assessed may have experienced many years of professionals trying to help, and still

Family Members' Perceptions of the Student's Communication Problem

• Do the family members feel that a problem exists, or do they feel that the school or someone else is fabricating the problem?

• If the family members feel a communication disorder exists, is it a primary or secondary concern?

• If the family feels that a problem exists, do they feel frustrated, embarrassed, guilty, and ashamed, or are they accepting of the adolescent's communication?

• How does or doesn't the family attempt to cope with the child with a communication disorder (e.g., by talking for the adolescent, by excluding the preadolescent from the mainstream of family life and decision making, by ignoring the disorder)?

• What are the goals and expectations of the family for the preadolescent or adolescent with a communication disorder or a suspected disorder? Are they realistic?

From *Language Disorders in Older Students: Preadolescents and Adolescents* (p. 95), by V. Lord Larson and N.L. McKinley, 1995, Eau Claire, WI: Thinking Publications. © 1995 by Thinking Publications. Adapted with permission.

the youth may have problems. As adolescents grow older, parental involvement often lessens, but not parental concern.

Determining the family's communication style/behaviors is important in evaluating whether the older student has a communication disorder or difference. If the older student's communication style is similar to that of other family members, probably a communication difference, and not a disorder, is present. This decision is complicated when English is not the primary language spoken in the preadolescent's or adolescent's home. Communication style must be assessed from the perspective of the first language in the family, even if that language is not English. Through the use of an interpreter, the examiner should determine whether the older student understands and produces the primary language similarly to other family members who are approximately the same age or older. Langdon and Cheng (2002) offer excellent guidelines for use of interpreters during assessment.

Peer Group

It is important to obtain the peer group members' perceptions of the preadolescent's or adolescent's communication behavior and to determine whether they have difficulty understanding the individual. Peers' feelings and attitudes toward the preadolescent's or adolescent's communication should also be evaluated. If they feel a problem exists, do they reject or accept the person as a friend or a member of the group? Do they avoid talking or listening to the individual? What is most disturbing to them about their peer's communication? Answers to these questions will help to document the amount of social isolation that the student being assessed may or may not be experiencing.

In addition, the peers' communication styles should be assessed to determine the typical communication behaviors for this age group. By analyzing the peers' communication styles, the examiner can determine how the peers may be requiring the youth being assessed to comprehend or produce social-interactive language (e.g., idiomatic expressions or slang).

The procedures used to assess family and peer members' perceptions of the preadolescent or adolescent, their feelings and attitudes, and their communication styles involve a combination of interviewing,

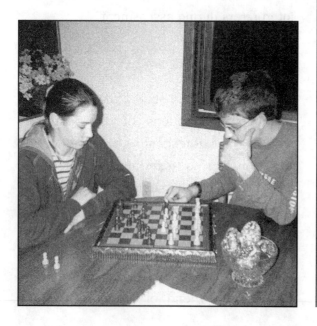

observing, and recording behaviors (Larson and McKinley, 1987). Interviewing is a directed conversation in which the examiner seeks to get information and to give information that will be helpful to the student and others in the student's environment in either solving or preventing problems. The observing and recording of behaviors should document communication styles of family members and peers. As discussed previously, if family members or peers and the youth being assessed speak similarly, the problem may not be a communication disorder but a communication difference, and should be evaluated accordingly.

Employment Setting

As older students with language disorders graduate from school and plan to enter the workforce, the transition may be easier on everyone if students are assessed to determine whether they have adequate skills to enter the workplace.

Table 8.3 summarizes a series of employability skills that were found by Stemmer, B. Brown, and C. Smith (1992) to be needed for an individual to be successful within the workplace. Stemmer et al. suggest the implementation of a portfolio assessment model that uses the skills listed in Table 8.3 as indicators to recognize successes, to seek opportunities to fill gaps in skill areas needed for employment, and to assist the student in gaining confidence in preparing for work.

Table 8.3
Employment Skills Profile

Skills	Profile
Academic Skills	Read and understand written materials Understand charts and graphs Understand basic math Use mathematics to solve problems Use research and library skills Use specialized knowledge and skills to get a job done Use tools and equipment Speak in the language in which business is conducted Write in the language in which business is conducted Use scientific method to solve problems
Personal Management Skills	Attend school/work daily and on time Meet school/work deadlines Develop career plans Know personal strengths and weaknesses Demonstrate self-control Pay attention to details Follow written and oral instructions Follow written and oral directions Work without supervision Learn new skills Identify and suggest new ways to get the job done
Teamwork Skills	Actively participate in a group Know the group's rules and values Listen to other group members Express ideas to other group members Be sensitive to the group members' ideas and views Be willing to compromise if necessary to best accomplish the goal Be a leader or a follower to best accomplish the goal Work in changing settings and with people of differing backgrounds

Of the employability skills listed in Table 8.3, the speech-language pathologist should carefully assess the student's ability to speak and write in the language needed for the business setting in which the student desires employment. Can the student engage in basic problem-solving skills? Can the student follow written and oral instructions? Can the student listen to other employees and attempt to accommodate their suggestions? This means that the speech-language pathologist will need to talk with the company's human resource person or personnel director to determine the communication and problem-solving skills required to do the job. At the same time, accommodations under the 1990 Americans with Disabilities Act (P.L. 101–336) that might be made for the youth can be discussed.

The Individuals with Disabilities Education Act (IDEA; 1997; P.L. 105–17) requires that students with language/learning disabilities between the ages of 16 and 21 years have developed an Individualized Transition Plan (ITP), similar to an Individualized Education Program (IEP). For some students, initial planning for the ITP is begun at age 14. The ITP may include such issues as the student's progress toward high school graduation and an outline of post-secondary options (e.g., college or employment or community-living arrangements).

It is important that the students' communication abilities are assessed to determine their communication needs for vocational success. Lunday (1996) noted that half of America's high school students do not have the basic communication skills for employment. Before entering an on-the-job employment setting, the student should be assessed for listening, speaking, and interaction skills; vocational vocabulary; and writing skills needed

for employability. A checklist (see Figure 8.2) to ascertain communication skills essential to occupational success can be used by teachers and speech-language pathologists as a guide for observation and as a way to determine needs for transition planning.

Assessment Issues in a Pluralistic Society

Changing demographics must be taken into account when establishing assessment procedures. Cultural and linguistic factors require that a wide array of assessment procedures be used when assessing students from culturally and linguistically diverse populations.

The speech-language pathologist must be aware of the legal mandates for service to linguistically and culturally different students. The historical bases for assessment of linguistically and culturally different clients "reside in Section 504 of the Rehabilitation Act of 1973 (29 USC 794 et seq.), in Title VI of the Civil Rights Act of 1964 (20 USC 200d et seq.), and in PL 94-142 (20 USC 1401 et seq.)" (Carpenter, 1990, p. 72). Collectively, these legal mandates require nondiscriminatory practices. The examiner cannot discriminate on the basis of race, national origin, or handicap if receiving federal funds. Furthermore, assessment materials and procedures must not be racially and culturally discriminatory and must be administered in the language or mode of communication in which the client is most proficient.

Figure 8.2

Checklist of Communication Skills Considered Essential to Classroom and Occupational Success

I. Vocabulary:

Does the student need to:

	Teacher's Expectations yes no n/a	Student's Success pos +/- neg
understand technical terms/jargon?	☐ ☐ ☐	☐ ☐ ☐
use technical terms/jargon?	☐ ☐ ☐	☐ ☐ ☐
use terms in question form?	☐ ☐ ☐	☐ ☐ ☐
comprehend abstract or figurative expressions?	☐ ☐ ☐	☐ ☐ ☐
read terms in manuals or textbooks?	☐ ☐ ☐	☐ ☐ ☐
read terms on diagrams, charts, and graphs?	☐ ☐ ☐	☐ ☐ ☐
write terms in notes, reports, or tests?	☐ ☐ ☐	☐ ☐ ☐
spell terms accurately?	☐ ☐ ☐	☐ ☐ ☐
summarize project in written report?	☐ ☐ ☐	☐ ☐ ☐
identify abbreviations/symbols?	☐ ☐ ☐	☐ ☐ ☐

II. Use:

Is the student required to:

	Teacher's Expectations yes no n/a	Student's Success pos +/- neg
converse with others in group settings?	☐ ☐ ☐	☐ ☐ ☐
request tools, supplies, or parts from a stock depot?	☐ ☐ ☐	☐ ☐ ☐
follow a step-by step procedure?	☐ ☐ ☐	☐ ☐ ☐
plan or design a schedule/procedure?	☐ ☐ ☐	☐ ☐ ☐
explain a procedure to instructor/other student?	☐ ☐ ☐	☐ ☐ ☐
ask for specific help?	☐ ☐ ☐	☐ ☐ ☐
verbally detail equipment malfunction?	☐ ☐ ☐	☐ ☐ ☐
identify and report safety hazards?	☐ ☐ ☐	☐ ☐ ☐
orally report assignment/ project completion?	☐ ☐ ☐	☐ ☐ ☐
attend lecture presentations?	☐ ☐ ☐	☐ ☐ ☐
maintain a topic focus?	☐ ☐ ☐	☐ ☐ ☐

III. Function:

Is the student required to verbally:

	Teacher's Expectations yes no n/a	Student's Success pos +/- neg
participate in classroom discussions?	☐ ☐ ☐	☐ ☐ ☐
define technical terms?	☐ ☐ ☐	☐ ☐ ☐
sequence step-by-step procedures?	☐ ☐ ☐	☐ ☐ ☐
report progress?	☐ ☐ ☐	☐ ☐ ☐
paraphrase information?	☐ ☐ ☐	☐ ☐ ☐
formulate specific questions?	☐ ☐ ☐	☐ ☐ ☐
respond to procedural questions?	☐ ☐ ☐	☐ ☐ ☐
express/support ideas?	☐ ☐ ☐	☐ ☐ ☐
provide suggestions?	☐ ☐ ☐	☐ ☐ ☐
give detailed advice?	☐ ☐ ☐	☐ ☐ ☐
acknowledge others?	☐ ☐ ☐	☐ ☐ ☐
describe equipment breakdown?	☐ ☐ ☐	☐ ☐ ☐
explain errors?	☐ ☐ ☐	☐ ☐ ☐
retrieve previously learned information?	☐ ☐ ☐	☐ ☐ ☐

IV. Organization:

Does the student need to:

	Teacher's Expectations yes no n/a	Student's Success pos +/- neg
keep an organized note book?	☐ ☐ ☐	☐ ☐ ☐
follow (a) prescribed schedule or routine?	☐ ☐ ☐	☐ ☐ ☐
anticipate direction from the classroom routine?	☐ ☐ ☐	☐ ☐ ☐
manage time based on a syllabus?	☐ ☐ ☐	☐ ☐ ☐
use classroom materials independently?	☐ ☐ ☐	☐ ☐ ☐

V. Form:

Does the student need to:

	Teacher's Expectations yes no n/a	Student's Success pos +/- neg
comprehend multilevel directions in complex syntax?	☐ ☐ ☐	☐ ☐ ☐
listen for organizational cues or signal words?	☐ ☐ ☐	☐ ☐ ☐
decipher complex information?	☐ ☐ ☐	☐ ☐ ☐
understand test directions independently?	☐ ☐ ☐	☐ ☐ ☐
use writing mechanics correctly?	☐ ☐ ☐	☐ ☐ ☐
relate worksheet information to test format?	☐ ☐ ☐	☐ ☐ ☐

VI. Pragmatics:

Is the student expected to:

	Teacher's Expectations yes no n/a	Student's Success pos +/- neg
differentiate speech/register when interacting (e.g., peers, teachers, authority figures, general public)?	☐ ☐ ☐	☐ ☐ ☐
use language appropriate to various settings (e.g., classroom, private conversations, group project activities)?	☐ ☐ ☐	☐ ☐ ☐
give and react to nonverbal cues?	☐ ☐ ☐	☐ ☐ ☐
listen for content importance transmitted by prosody?	☐ ☐ ☐	☐ ☐ ☐
modify communication based on feedback?	☐ ☐ ☐	☐ ☐ ☐
initiate, take turns, and terminate interactions?	☐ ☐ ☐	☐ ☐ ☐
display responsive and appropriate language behavior?	☐ ☐ ☐	☐ ☐ ☐
handle concerns and complaints appropriately?	☐ ☐ ☐	☐ ☐ ☐
provide and support an opinion?	☐ ☐ ☐	☐ ☐ ☐

Other comments:

From "A Collaborative Communication Skills Program for Job Corps Centers," by A.M. Lunday, 1996, *Topics in Language Disorders, 16*(3), p. 29. © 1996 by Lippencott. Adapted with permission.

Communication Solutions
for Older Students

The Committee on the Status of Racial Minorities (1983) stated, "no dialectal variety of English is a disorder or a pathological form of speech or language" (p. 23). Thus, some students will have language differences and not disorders. Language differences are defined as communication behaviors that meet the norms of the primary linguistic community but that do not meet the norms of standard English.

It is possible, though, for dialectal speakers to have speech and language disorders within the native language. To determine if the adolescent has a dialectal difference or a communication disorder, speech-language pathologists must have the following competencies (L. Cole, 1983):

1. knowledge of the particular dialect as a rule-governed linguistic system;

2. knowledge of nondiscriminatory testing procedures;

3. knowledge of the phonological and grammatical features of the dialect;

4. knowledge of contrastive analysis procedures;

5. knowledge of the effects and attitudes toward dialects; and

6. thorough understanding and appreciation for the community and culture of the nonstandard speaker. (p. 25)

Recall that considerable information on dialectal differences can be found in Chapter 5 of this text. The purposes of assessment with culturally and linguistically diverse children are (1) to determine if academic difficulties, inappropriate personal-social interactions, or limited vocational potential are due to a language disorder or a language difference, and (2) to determine if instructional programming is needed and, if so, what programming is the most appropriate. To accomplish these two purposes, examiners must engage in bias-free assessment (Chamberlain and Medinos-Landurand, 1991) by:

- Increasing their knowledge and awareness about students with different cultural and linguistic backgrounds

- Determining the student's level of acculturation

- Determining how to control for cultural variables that interfere with testing outcomes

- Determining the language to be used in testing

- Knowing when an interpreter is needed and whom to use as an interpreter

- Being aware of problems resulting from the examiner's cultural insensitivity, such as miscommunication attempts; cross-cultural stereotyping; misperceptions; and not understanding that some cultures are based on cooperation and collaboration, not competition

According to Snow, Burns, and Griffin (1998), "the literacy risk is considerably higher for children with cultural and linguistic differences.... Fourth graders with such differences (are) almost twice as likely as their peers to lack 'basic' reading skills" (as cited in ASHA, 2001b, p. 39).

Assessing students from culturally different populations may include some of the same methods as used for White students, such as standardized tests, developmental scales, criterion-referenced procedures, dynamic assessment, and behavioral observations (Rhea Paul, 2001). In recent years, a variety of standardized tests have been developed in non-English languages, primarily Spanish. Table 8.4 lists a sample of these standardized tests.

Criterion-referenced tests are usually administered with the aid of an interpreter, if necessary, to establish baseline function, identify goals for intervention, and document progress in programming (Rhea Paul, 2001). When gathering a language sample, it has been found helpful to use ethnographic methods like those presented in Table 8.5.

Obtaining a language sample from the student has long been felt to be one of the most viable assessment procedures for culturally/linguistically diverse students. Stockman (1996) discussed the advantages and disadvantages of using such a procedure to assess language differences. They are summarized in the sidebar on page 206. Overall, collecting a sample is advantageous, especially to increase the possibility of being culturally sensitive and unbiased.

According to Bernstein (1989), appropriate identification and assessment of bilingual/bicultural children require: "(1) the use of appropriate assessment instruments and techniques, and (2) the use of appropriate personnel in the assessment process" (p. 16). When using standardized tests with these students, the tests need to have certain characteristics (i.e., they should have a solid theoretical underpinning, be valid and reliable, and be standardized on the population for which the test will be used). These are also appropriate criteria for monolingual students. Whenever possible, the examiner should use a naturalistic assessment approach (i.e., informal procedures that allow the speech-language pathologist to describe specifically the communication behaviors of the student across and within a wide array of communication situations).

Bernstein (1989) also confronted the need to use appropriate personnel in the assessment process. Federal law mandates that the abilities of limited English proficient (LEP) children be assessed in their native language. Since few speech-language pathologists are bilingual, and even those who are may not be proficient in the language of a particular student, it is necessary to implement this federal mandate by applying several alternative approaches to using linguistically qualified personnel. Bernstein recommended using a trained interpreter/native speaker during the assessment process so that the assessment materials and procedures are as culturally and linguistically relevant as possible.

Communication Solutions
for Older Students

Table 8.4

A Sample of Standardized Multicultural Tests

Test	Age Range	Primary Areas Assessed	Measurement Interpretations
Ber-Sil Spanish Test, Secondary Level (Revised) Beringer, M., 1984, Rancho Palos Verdes, CA: The Ber-Sil Company	5–17 years	• Listening	Norm-referenced
Clinical Evaluation of Language Functions (CELF)–3 (Spanish) Semel, E., Wiig, E., and Secord, W., 1997, San Antonio, TX: The Psychological Corporation	6–21 years	• Listening • Speaking	Norm-referenced
Expressive One-Word Picture Vocabulary Test (Spanish) Brownell, R., 2000, Oceanside, CA: Academic Communication Associates	2 to 18;11 years	• Speaking	Norm-referenced
Receptive One-Word Picture Vocabulary Test (Spanish) Brownell, R., 2000, Oceanside, CA: Academic Communication Associates	2 to 18;11 years	• Listening	Norm-referenced
Test of Auditory Reasoning and Processing Skills (TARPS) Gardner, M., 1993, Oceanside, CA: Academic Communication Associates	5 to 13;11 years	• Listening • Thinking	Norm-referenced
Test of Auditory Perceptual Skills–Upper Level (TAPS: UL) Gardner, M., 1994, Oceanside, CA: Academic Communication Associates	12–18 years	• Listening	Norm-referenced

Another approach recommended by Bernstein (1989) is to use bilingual teacher aides. The advantage to this approach is, again, that the aide is familiar with the student's cultural/linguistic background. The disadvantage is that it takes the aide away from instructional tasks that he or she has been hired to do, and thus some educators

Communication Dimensions to Assess
Using Ethnographic Methods

Table 8.5

Dimension	Considerations
Conversational Partners	• How often does the student interact with other peers, adults? • How many are involved in a conversation?
Mode	• How much of an interaction is verbal vs. nonverbal? • How is silence used? How is eye contact used?
Duration	• How long do conversations last?
Structure	• Who starts, continues, ends conversations? • How does the student request a turn?
Topics	• What topics are acceptable? Rude?
Speech Acts	• Are certain types of acts (e.g., questions, stories) used by certain speakers? • Who can give orders or make requests to whom?
Social Beliefs	• How does the culture view disabilities?

Sources: Crago and E. Cole (1991); Rhea Paul (2001)

may resist the aide being used in this way. Likewise, some aides may find it difficult to shift roles between being part of the assessment process and assisting with intervention procedures.

Langdon and Cheng (2002) designed several excellent checklists that speech-language pathologists and interpreters should use before, during, and after assessment. They emphasized the importance of the speech-language pathologist and the interpreter briefing before the testing time and debriefing afterward to maximize the information obtained on the student and to ensure the collection of valid data. Langdon (2002) also created a 5-session educational program for interpreters and translators so that they become adequately trained to assist speech-language pathologists during the assessment and intervention processes. Together, the Langdon and Cheng and the Langdon resources provide a wealth of ideas for the best use of interpreters.

Advantages and Disadvantages for Using Language Samples for Culturally/Linguistically Diverse Students

Advantages

- Cultural sensitivity is enhanced

- Validity is increased because all aspects of language (phonology, morphology, syntax, and semantics) are observed within a communication context

- Accessibility to a language sample is readily available because it occurs during natural events

- Flexibility is ensured because regardless of the student's linguistic or cultural system, a language sample is not tied to a rigid set of response conditions like in standardized testing

Disadvantages

- Managing context variation is difficult, since language samples can vary depending on the person and on the situational context the student is in and can vary from one time period to another, so one cannot conclude with great validity that a particular language feature is absent

- Observing and transcribing the flow of speech can be very challenging given the rapidity of speech, and it can have natural false starts and verbal mazes, making it difficult to observe and transcribe

- Evaluating the language sample can be challenging since little data may be available on a student from a particular culture and in a given age group, like early, middle, or late adolescence

- Finding the time to do language sample analysis can be difficult because it is extremely time consuming, and to increase validity and reliability, a number of utterances need to be analyzed

Source: Stockman (1996)

Points of Discussion

1. What issues arise when assessing the communication behaviors of bilingual students vs. students with dialectal differences?

2. Explain the comprehensive, five-faceted model of assessment. Why is it important to take such a comprehensive, multifaceted approach to assessment?

Suggested Readings

Damico, J. (1993). Language assessment in adolescents: Addressing critical issues. *Language, Speech, and Hearing Services in Schools, 24*(1), pp. 29–35.

Langdon, H.W., and Cheng, L.-R.L. (2002). *Collaborating with interpreters and translators: A guide for communication disorders professionals.* Eau Claire, WI: Thinking Publications.

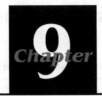

Chapter

Procedures for Direct Assessment

Goals

- Describe the 10 aspects to assess in older students (ages 9–19)

- Discuss how to assess cognitive and communication behaviors using informal procedures

- Summarize formal assessment instruments that might be used with older students

Who to Assess

This chapter focuses on assessing 10 aspects within the preadolescent or adolescent whether in an early, middle, or late stage of development. Figure 9.1 provides an overview of the who, the what, and the how involved in the process of direct assessment. This process assumes that the initial screening of the student has occurred (or a child study team has attempted interventions), that a language difference has been ruled out, and that further investigation is warranted to determine the existence and degree of a communication disorder. Assessment of the 10 aspects can be accomplished through use of informal and formal testing procedures.

What to Assess

History

Relevant data on the older student's history, current status, and future goals should be obtained during the initial part of the

Figure 9.1 **Direct Assessment of Older Students**

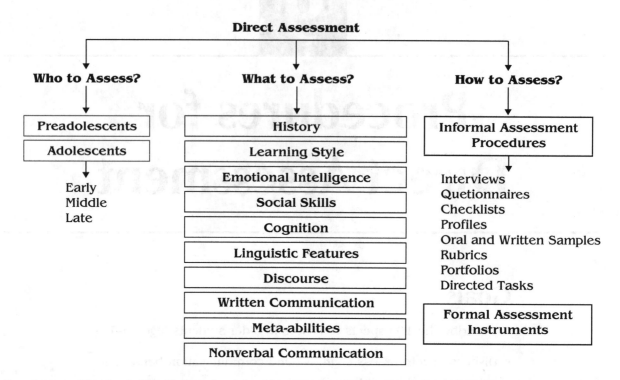

From *Language Disorders in Older Students: Preadolescents and Adolescents* (p. 104), by V. Lord Larson and N.L. McKinley, 1995, Eau Claire, WI: Thinking Publications. © 1995 by Thinking Publications. Adapted with permission.

evaluation process. Only in this way can an accurate assessment battery be planned.

As discussed in Chapter 8, the examiner should obtain information about the student's environmental, educational, and vocational systems. This information gathering should begin with the student's initial evaluation and be updated during any re-evaluations. The history of the individual's environmental system should be accumulated based on family members and peers. Educational and vocational histories should be gathered to document specific strengths and weaknesses in academic subject areas and current and future vocational goals. In addition, health

data that might affect performance should be collected (e.g., past and present medications, allergies, and seizures). Irrelevant data collection should be avoided (e.g., the age at which the student first walked or the age at which the student was toilet trained). However, any records of past speech, hearing, and language services should be reviewed, regardless of the age of the student when services were received.

Another critical area to investigate is the student's feelings and attitudes toward current thinking, listening, speaking, reading, and writing abilities, and the willingness to modify these skills. This investigation will reveal the student's perspective of the suspected communication problem. It will also assist in documenting metacognition, metalinguistics, and metacommunication.

Feelings and Attitudes toward Thinking

Reuven Feuerstein (1980) emphasized that adverse affective-motivational factors can result in deficient cognitive functioning or thinking. Furthermore, a negative attitude may affect general involvement with cognitive tasks that are demanded in academic and real-life situations.

Learned helplessness describes the phenomenon of individuals who, when faced with a problem, act helplessly. Youth with learned helplessness view outcomes as uncontrollable. Other effects of learned helplessness are passivity, negative beliefs about oneself, severe reduction in persistence, and depression (Greer and Wethered, 1984). Older students with learned helplessness have no strategies, or ineffective ones, for solving problems, and they perceive few alternatives. By high school, they have made so many mistakes and have failed so often that they mistrust their own thinking. Thus, students who could have intact cognitive functions believe they cannot think and, therefore, they do not.

Feelings and Attitudes toward Listening

Feelings and attitudes toward listening may be influenced by the following barriers: calling the subject dull; criticizing the speaker's looks, actions, or speaking style; getting overstimulated and emotionally involved; listening for isolated facts; outlining everything; wasting the extra time available between normal speaking speed (175 words per minute (wmp) and thinking speed 450 wpm); listening only to what is easy to understand; allowing personal prejudices and biases to impair understanding; letting emotionally laden words get in the way; and allowing distractions to interfere (Nichols and Stevens, 1957).

In addition to asking older students about their listening, the examiner should investigate whether they have any misconceptions about listening that may interfere with their learning to be a better listener. Ten major misconceptions about listening are listed in the sidebar on page 212. They were adapted by Schreiber and McKinley (1995) into student-oriented statements in the listening questionnaire provided in Appendix F. If desired, the questionnaire can be administered orally, requiring the student to listen rather than read.

Professionals can use this questionnaire to examine the student's listening habits and determine whether the adolescent holds any misconceptions about listening. By realizing that these beliefs are erroneous, more efficient and effective listening abilities can be developed.

Feelings and Attitudes toward Speaking

The feelings and attitudes of older students toward their oral language production can

211

Misconceptions about Listening

1. **Listening is a matter of intelligence.** Intelligence is not a criterion for listening, and there appears to be no strong relationship between intelligence and efficient listening. Efficient listening is more a result of training.

2. **Good hearing and good listening are closely related.** Although there is a relationship between hearing and listening, good hearing does not guarantee good listening. Hearing is a physical activity, whereas listening is a mental activity.

3. **Listening is an automatic reflex.** Listening is not an innate skill, but one that is learned.

4. **Daily practice eliminates the need for training in listening.** Practice does not necessarily mean a skill becomes better, especially if it is not practiced correctly. Therefore, to be a better listener, one must be trained to practice the skill correctly.

5. **Learning to read will automatically improve listening.** This is a false assumption, since the two activities place different demands on the individual. Listening may actually be a more difficult activity because a listener cannot reread a passage and thus cannot control the rate of the message as one can in reading.

6. **Learning to read is more important than learning to listen.** This is not true, since most people listen three times more than they read.

7. **The speaker is totally responsible for success in oral communication.** Successful communication is a 50/50 proposition. Equal importance must be given to the role of listening, and listeners should not assume that the speaker is 100 percent responsible for successful oral communication.

8. **Listening is essentially a passive activity.** This is an erroneous assumption, since the only way successful communication can occur is if the listener is actively engaged in the process.

9. **Listening means agreement.** Good listeners do not necessarily agree with the speaker, but they listen first and then agree or disagree as a result of listening to what the speaker has to say.

10. **Consequences of careless listening are minimal.** This is a misconception, since careless listening can be time consuming, costly, and socially destructive.

Sources: Wolff, Marsnik, Tacey, and Nichols (1983); Wolff and Marsnik (1992)

reveal their awareness of communication, their ability to take another's perspective, and their motivation to change behaviors. Preadolescents and adolescents may be marginal communicators who have a "defective" attitude toward communication, but who may not qualify for speech-language services (Blue, 1975). Marginal communicators do not initiate conversations; they respond with minimal, faint but intelligible utterances in a one-to-one situation. For these students, the assessment procedure will need to determine if it is their attitude toward communication that is defective, or their communication system, or both.

Attitudes and feelings about speaking may differ, contingent upon the listener (e.g., a friend, a group of peers, or a teacher) and the setting (e.g., school or home). Therefore, the professional should explore both the student's general feelings and attitudes toward his or her own communication, as well as variations that occur during specific communicative contexts.

Feelings and Attitudes toward Reading

Paratore (1995) recommended that the student engage in self-evaluation to assess literacy. Students should ask themselves questions such as these:

- What types of books do I like to read best? Why?

- Which type of book is easiest for me to read? Why?

- Which type of book is hardest for me to read? Why?

- What would I like to do better in reading? What do I find my greatest reading challenge to be?

Students must answer these questions to determine their feelings and attitudes toward reading. Students' expressed feelings and attitudes help determine what motivates them to engage (or not engage) in the reading process.

Feelings and Attitudes toward Writing

Roth (2000) noted that students must spend substantial time writing to derive appreciable gains and develop a positive attitude toward the writing process. She recommended engaging in writing at least 4 days a week. Paratore (1995) recommended that students evaluate their writing abilities by reviewing the pieces of writing they did, selecting their best piece, and asking:

- Why is this my best piece?

- When is writing difficult for me? Why?

- What topic do I like to write about most?

- How do I plan my writing, by outlining?

- How do I revise and edit my writing before considering it finished?

- What would I like to do better in my writing?

It is important that adolescents ask themselves these questions to become aware of their feelings and attitudes toward writing. Again, by analyzing students' responses to these questions, professionals can determine what motivates them to participate (or not participate) in writing activities.

Learning Style

It is important to obtain data on how pread-olescents and adolescents best learn certain tasks. These data can help them use their strengths to overcome their weaknesses and thus be more successful in school or on a job. Some factors to investigate that might affect how the student learns a new or difficult subject are captured in the sidebar.

In addition to the factors in the sidebar, the professional should investigate the student's strategy for learning materials presented via lectures or textbooks, inside and outside the classroom. Collectively, this information can be analyzed to determine how the individual learns best in school and at home, and it should be shared with teachers and parents. Obtaining this information may also provide older students with some insight into their own behaviors, and thus increase their awareness levels and their willingness to change their attitude toward learning new tasks.

Emotional Intelligence

Drawing from the work of Goleman (1995, 1998), we believe the concept of human intelligence shared by speech-language pathologists and their colleagues has been far too narrow. For years intelligence quotients (IQs), as measured by standardized tests, have been used to project how well someone will do in life. Goleman has argued that this restricted definition of intelligence ignores a crucial range of abilities known as *emotional intelligence.*

Goleman (1995) noted that "At best, IQ contributes about 20 percent to the factors that determine life success, which leaves 80 percent to other forces" (p. 34). The greatest

Factors Involved in Learning Style

- The best time of day to learn a task (e.g., morning, afternoon, evening)
- The level of noise in the room (e.g., quiet, music, TV, conversation)
- The level of light in the room (e.g., dim, moderate, or bright)
- The temperature in the room (e.g., cold, warm, or very warm)
- The presence or absence of food or drink
- The best place to learn (e.g., home, school, library)
- The best location to learn (e.g., desk, floor, sitting, reclining)
- The reasons that motivate the adolescent to complete a task (e.g., I want to; My parents expect/want me to; I get money)
- The desire to work alone or with other people

Sources: Dunn, Dunn, and Price (1989); Larson and McKinley (1995)

percentage of those other forces is emotional intelligence, which can be taught. Emotional intelligence includes five domains: self-awareness, self-regulation, motivation, empathy, and social skills (Goleman).

Goleman (1998) defined *emotional competence* as "a learned capability based on emotional intelligence that results in outstanding performance at work" (p. 24). Emotional intelligence determines one's potential for learning the emotional competencies necessary for being successful in the workplace. Just because a person has high emotional intelligence does not guarantee

that he or she will use the emotional competencies; he or she simply has the potential to do so. Emotional intelligence capacities build on one another (i.e., they are hierarchical). "Self-awareness is crucial for self-regulation and empathy; self-regulation and self-awareness contribute to motivation; all the first four are at work in social skills" (Goleman, pp. 27–28).

Presented in Table 9.1 are the 5 dimensions and 25 emotional competencies. The 25 emotional competencies and their definitions are presented in Appendix G.

Emotional Intelligence Dimensions and Competencies

Table 9.1

Dimension	Competencies	
Self-Awareness	Emotional awareness	Accurate self-assessment
	Self-confidence	
Self-Regulation	Self-control	Trustworthiness
	Conscientiousness	Adaptability
	Innovation	
Motivation	Achievement	Commitment
	Initiative	Optimism
Empathy	Understanding others	Developing others' abilities
	Advancing a service	Leveraging diversity
	Being politically aware	
Social Skills	Influence	Communication
	Conflict management	Leadership
	Change catalyst	Building bonds
	Team capabilities	Collaboration & cooperation

Source: Goleman (1995)

Social Skills

As noted in the section above on emotional intelligence, social skills are one of the dimensions of emotional intelligence. Social skills are so critical to the success of adolescents with language disorders that we have created a separate section here to emphasize this point.

According to Walker, Schwarz, Nippold, Irvin, and Noell (1994), competent social skills allow students to develop positive relationships with others; cope successfully with the demands and expectations of various settings; communicate one's desires, needs, and preferences effectively; and perform in a range of academic, personal, vocational, and community contexts. Gajewski, Hirn, and Mayo (1998a, 1998b) noted a number of important social skills that students with language disorders need to be taught, which students with typical development learn incidentally, such as using manners, making a positive first impression, offering help, asking for help, developing friendships, maintaining friendships, asking permission, controlling anger, accepting no, and making an apology, to name only a few of the more than 50 skills they have isolated.

Cognition

As with any assessment, examiners can look for functions that are present and intact, or they can look for functions that are weak, deficient, or absent. Ideally, both methods are used, and a pattern of strengths and weaknesses surfaces. The cognitive functions in the input, elaboration, and output phases (see Table 9.2) have proven to be an effective guide for what to assess during preadolescence and adolescence (Reuven Feuerstein, 1979). The input phase involves gathering needed information; the elaboration phase involves using the information that was gathered; and the output phase involves expressing the solution to a problem.

A cognitive function that is consistently applied across a variety of contexts is a strength for that adolescent. Cognitive functions may be deficient if they do not appear spontaneously, regularly, and predictably in an individual's behavior. Deficient cognitive functions can provide a method for profiling weaknesses within adolescents.

Cognitive functions that should be assessed are taken from Reuven Feuerstein (1979) and are listed in Table 9.2 in question form. The interaction of language and cognition becomes obvious when the list of cognitive functions is examined. Many language disorders present during adolescence have underlying cognitive deficits. Professionals should be concerned not only with which cognitive functions are intact or deficient during assessment, but also with the student's awareness of these functions (i.e., metacognition). A greater awareness of cognitive functions produces more control over applying those functions when appropriate situations present themselves (Reuven Feuerstein, 1980).

Table 9.2

Assessment of Cognitive Functions

Phase	Questions to Help Assess Cognitive Functions
Input	• Is the student using senses (e.g., hearing, seeing) to gather clear and complete information? • Is a plan being used so that important information is not being skipped or missed? • Is the student consistently naming objects and events so that they can be remembered and talked about clearly? • Are events and objects being described in terms of where and when they occur? • Are characteristics of objects and events recognized as the same even when changes take place? (E.g., Is a square tilted onto its corner still recognized as a square?) • Can the student organize information by several characteristics simultaneously (e.g., by date and time of day; by size and by shape)? • Does the student know when and how to be precise and accurate (e.g., when reporting data about an emergency to the appropriate authorities)?
Elaboration	• Can the student define problems and determine what needs to be done? • Is the student using only the information that is relevant to the problem and ignoring the rest? • Does the student form "good pictures in the mind" about what must be done to solve the problem? • Is the student making a plan that includes steps needed to reach a goal? • Are the various pieces of information needed to solve the problem being remembered? • Is the student looking for relationships by which separate objects, events, and experiences can be tied together? (E.g., A flat tire, a sick child, and an overdrawn checkbook have made my mother very upset today; therefore, this is not the time to ask for a new jacket.) • Are objects and experiences being compared to others to determine what is similar and what is different? • Is the student finding the class or set to which new objects or experiences belong? • Is the student thinking about different alternatives and what would happen if one or another were chosen? • Is logic being used to prove answers and to defend opinions?
Output	• Is the student being clear and precise in language so that the listener understands the message? • Is the student thinking through the response instead of immediately trying to answer and making a mistake? • Is restraint being used before saying or doing something that will be regretted later? • Is a strategy being used to help find answers rather than panicking when stuck on a problem?

Source: Reuven Feuerstein (1979)

Linguistic Features

A select number of linguistic features should be assessed in the older student with a suspected language disorder. Nippold (1998), N. Nelson (1998), and Rhea Paul (2001) all conveyed the need to look at linguistic features (e.g., word relations, word definitions, comprehension and production of linguistically complex sentences, and figurative language) in real-life situations and especially within linguistic contexts in which students are likely to engage (e.g., textbooks used in a class, classroom lectures, and activities that are more toward the literate end of the continuum, such as narrations and expository text, as opposed to conversations).

Both oral and written samples should be taken. Scott and Stokes (1995) recommended analyzing:

- T-units

- The use of the subordination index (i.e, clause density)

- The presence of high-level, low-frequency structural markers, such as noun phrases, verb phrases, adverbials, and complex sentences with multiple clauses

- Morphological features, such as prefixes and suffixes, nominalization, and later developing conjunctions (e.g., *instead, nevertheless, furthermore*)

In addition, the examiner should assess the student's ability to engage in a variety of informational listening tasks (Boyce and Larson, 1983; Larson and McKinley, 1987, 1995). Informational listening requires the ability to listen for main ideas and significant details and to listen for oral directions or a sequence of events. This type of listening also assumes the ability to identify and recall main ideas and to take notes on orally presented information. Table 9.3 presents questions to be answered during assessment concerning linguistic features.

Arwood (1983) argued against looking at the comprehension of linguistic features in isolation from the speech act, because professionals may end up assessing products rather than processes. To determine, for example, that a student does not understand comparative adjectives tells the examiner nothing about why comprehension is absent or what impact this has on the speech act. While it is important to assess the student's ability to comprehend language features, examiners cannot lose sight of the reason for doing so (i.e., to determine the impact on communication).

Production of linguistic features must also be considered during assessment. Unlike younger children, who may have extremely limited output, older students generally have a production repertoire, albeit inefficient and often redundant. For example, they may start the majority of their question forms with *what*, using a variety of forms (e.g., "What time..." rather than "When..." and "What

Table 9.3

Assessment of Linguistic Features

Area	Questions to Help Assess Linguistic Features
Comprehension	Does the student: • Identify morphological structures, such as compound words, prefixes, and suffixes? • Differentiate grammatical phrases, clauses, and sentences as incorrect or incomplete? • Comprehend various sentence transformations? • Comprehend sentences of various lengths and complexity? • Comprehend various semantic features (e.g., multiple-meaning words, verbal analogies, inclusion-exclusion, idioms)?
Informational Listening	Does the student: • Comprehend factual information (e.g., directions and dates)? • Concentrate attention on the speaker? • Use advantageously the time differential between thinking and speaking speed (i.e., people think two times faster than they listen)? • Understand and differentiate between main ideas and supportive details? • Formulate questions of clarification?
Production	Does the student: • Use simple and complex sentences? • Use appropriate sentence fragments (e.g., a response of "eleven o'clock" to the question, "What time will you be home tonight?")? • Avoid an excessive number of run-on sentences that are strung together with *and* or *and then*? • Use a variety of question forms, such as *wh-* questions, tag questions, interrogative reversals, and questions marked by rising intonation? • Use figurative language such as slang, jargon, idioms, metaphors, similes, and language for the purpose of entertainment or humor? • Avoid overuse of nonspecific language such as low-information words (e.g., *things, stuff, everybody)*? When requested to do so, can the student rephrase, using more specific language? • Display few, if any, word-retrieval problems?

From *Language Disorders in Older Students: Preadolescents and Adolescents* (p. 109), by V. Lord Larson and N.L. McKinley, 1995, Eau Claire, WI: Thinking Publications. © 1995 by Thinking Publications. Adapted with permission.

place..." rather than "Where...."). Thus, when assessing production features, focus is on the flexibility of the language system. To document flexibility, questions such as those posed in the sidebar should be kept in mind.

Unlike younger children,

who may have extremely

limited output, older

students generally have

a production repertoire,

albeit inefficient and

often redundant.

Discourse

During assessment of discourse, specific aspects of conversations, narrations, and expository text need to be analyzed: cohesion devices, critical listening, and verbal mazes. Table 9.4 summarizes the discourse parameters that should be assessed in the older student across any discourse type. Subsequent sidebars in this section will summarize additional aspects to assess within conversations (see page 222), narrations (see page 225), and expository text (see page 227), respectively.

Cohesion devices should be analyzed to determine whether they contribute to or disrupt the continuity of meaning. Cohesive devices that contribute to continuity are the *referent* (i.e., a word whose meaning is apparent from the context), the *conjunction* (i.e., a linking word whose meaning is appropriate to

Determining Flexibility of the Adolescent's Language System

- How much variation is used?

- Are complex sentences used, or just simple sentences?

- Is figurative language used?

- Does the student clarify the meaning of nonspecific words?

- Does the student use a variety of clauses and later developing conjunctions, thus increasing the complexity of the language used?

- Does the student use similar or different linguistic features when writing as when speaking?

- Does the student use different linguistic features during conversations vs. narration or expository text?

Table 9.4

Assessment of Discourse

Parameter	Questions to Help Assess Discourse Features
Cohesion Devices	Does the student: • Use cohesion devices that contribute to the continuity of meaning in the conversation, narration, or expository text? • Use cohesion devices in a way that avoids the disruption of continuity?
Critical Listening	Does the student: • Identify and recognize the credibility of the source or speaker? • Recognize and use inductive and deductive reasoning? • Detect false reasoning (e.g., does he or she discriminate between fact and opinion)? • Recognize propaganda devices (e.g., loaded words)? • Draw inferences and judge statements heard?
Verbal Mazes	Does the student: • Avoid an excessive amount of verbal mazes that interfere with communication? • Avoid an excessive amount of false starts that interfere with communication?

From *Language Disorders in Older Students: Preadolescents and Adolescents* (p. 111), by V. Lord Larson and N.L. McKinley, 1995, Eau Claire, WI: Thinking Publications. © 1995 by Thinking Publications. Adapted with permission.

the words being linked), and the *ellipsis* (i.e., a redundant word or words that are eliminated from the context but can be determined). Disruptive cohesion devices are *referent errors* (i.e., using a word to refer to elements that are absent from the context), *conjunction errors* (i.e., using linking words that are inappropriate to the context), and *ellipsis errors* (i.e., eliminating elements whose referents cannot be determined from the context).

Critical listening is essential to the older student's comprehension during discourse. A critical listener must be a critical thinker (i.e., capable of engaging in higher level thought when required by the situation).

Verbal mazes (i.e., words or unattached fragments not necessary to the message) can impair communicative intent. While all speakers engage in some verbal mazes, the expectation is not to exceed significantly what is normal for a given grade level (Loban, 1976). Some students use verbal mazes with such high frequency that it is impossible to comprehend their spoken message. Along with verbal mazes, the speech-language pathologist should assess the presence of an excessive number of false starts at the beginnings of utterances (e.g., "You know what?," "Guess what?"). Both verbal mazes and false starts can be distracting to listeners and can interfere with the clarity of the speaker's message.

Conversations

Numerous rules govern conversational exchanges. In conversation, one person selects a topic that is maintained until a topic shift is initiated. When assessing students' use of conversational rules, speech-language pathologists should observe the student conversing, while asking the questions listed in the sidebar.

Switching topics can be accomplished abruptly with no warning provided for the listener, or it can be cued directly (e.g., "Can I talk with you about something else for a

Assessment of Conversations

Does the student:

- Know the rules of conversation?
- Initiate conversations in a variety of situations?
- Select appropriate topics?
- Maintain a topic over a number of speaker-listener exchanges?
- Switch topics in an appropriate and orderly manner?
- Terminate conversations in a timely manner?

To what extent does the student use the communication function of:

- Giving information?
- Getting information (i.e., asking questions)?
- Describing an ongoing event?
- Getting the listener to do, believe, or feel something (i.e., persuading)?
- Expressing his or her own intentions, beliefs, and feelings (i.e., practicing self-disclosure)?
- Indicating a readiness for further communication?
- Using language to solve problems?
- Using language to entertain?

Source: Larson and McKinley (1995)

minute?") or indirectly (e.g., "That reminds me of..."). During conversation, the speaker and listener take turns. Turn-taking should occur with a minimum of interruptions; repairs and revisions should be made when necessary (Rees and Wollner, 1982).

As stated in Chapter 3, Grice (1975) proposed four fundamental rules of conversation that summarize expectations held by speakers and listeners. We hypothesize that these rules are intact by late adolescence, but they may emerge even earlier and therefore should be evaluated to determine the student's knowledge and application of the rules.

Wiig (1982, 1983) and Fahey and Reid (2000) have stressed the importance of the adolescent's ability to switch registers, or codes, during conversational speech. While talking with peers, an informal register is acceptable. However, when talking with adults, a more formal register is used. A formal register contains more noun phrase elaborations and verb phrase complexity, and it assumes that the speaker and listener do not share mutual information; thus, it necessitates more precise descriptions and explanations. A formal register also uses more polite forms than an informal register. Failure to discriminate which register to use for each communicative situation is a significant problem for some adolescents.

Failure to discriminate which register to use for each communicative situation is a significant problem for some adolescents.

Communication functions have been described by a variety of taxonomies (Austin, 1962; Chapman, 1972, 1981; Dore, 1974, 1975; Greenfield and J. Smith, 1976; Halliday, 1975; Hymes, 1972; Searle, 1965). The taxonomies developed by Austin and Searle were primarily designed to analyze adult speech acts, whereas the taxonomies developed by Dore and Halliday were created to analyze child-based speech acts. The system for the older student population to which we adhere was extrapolated from the work of Austin.

Our extrapolated taxonomy includes eight communication functions (Boyce and Larson, 1983; Larson and McKinley, 1987, 1995, 1998). The eight functions are listed in the bottom half of the sidebar on page 222. All eight communication functions should be present within the language of the preadolescent and adolescent. Missing functions limit the communicative intents that can be expressed by older students.

Communication Solutions
for Older Students

Narrations

The student's ability to comprehend and to produce narratives should be investigated, because this task demonstrates whether information can be integrated. Also, "narratives are structurally midway between the language of the oral tradition and the language of the essayist literary tradition" (Westby, 1984, p. 124). Thus, knowing the student's ability to generate narratives should allow the examiner to determine readiness to develop a more literary language structure and to learn the written form of language. The generation may be either a storytelling or retelling task (Hughes, McGillivray, and Schmidek, 1997).

When analyzing story grammar units, the speech-language pathologist can use either a developmental approach (Applebee, 1978) or a story grammar taxonomy (Roth and Spekman, 1986). When using a developmental approach during assessment, the professional should keep in mind the developmental hierarchy leading up to the true narrative (Applebee), as explained in detail in Chapter 3 (see page 74). The sidebar that follows lists the questions that should be answered and, therefore, the narrative behaviors to be assessed in the preadolescent and adolescent.

The other type of story grammar analysis is that of using a taxonomy that identifies the elements common to stories and specifies a formal set of rules underlying the construction of any story (Mandler and N. Johnson, 1977; Rumelhart, 1975; Stein and Glenn, 1979; Thorndyke, 1977). All story grammars have a setting in which the main character is introduced, and a description of the social, physical, or temporal context of the story is presented. All story grammars have a goal that is met in an episode system. Episodes have a beginning, which is an initiating event; an action, or attempt by the characters to deal with the initiating event; an outcome, or consequence of the attempt; and an ending. All the elements of a story grammar taxonomy should be present in the older student's narration.

Expository Text

ASHA's position paper on reading and writing (2001b) noted that "at least from the third grade on, the expository text genre becomes an important element of the general education curriculum and a major medium for acquiring content knowledge about academic subjects" (p. 36). This is supported by Fahey and Reid (2000), who stated that expository text is the most dominant form of discourse used in the classroom after the fourth grade. Whereas elementary programs involve students in expressive and narrative activities, secondary programs require more formal and expository forms of writing—reports, explanations, arguments, essays, research writing, and term papers.

Furthermore, N. Nelson (1998) stated that expository discourse is critical to academic success since most textbooks and teachers' lectures are based on expository text. She

Assessment of Narrations

Developmental Assessment

- At what stage of narration is the student functioning:

  - Heap stories?
  - Sequence stories/Macrostructure?
  - Primitive narratives?

  - Unfocused chains?
  - Focused chains?
  - True narratives? (5–7 years of age)

- Does the student summarize stories? (7–11 years of age)

- Does the student categorize stories both subjectively and objectively? (7–11 years of age)

- Does the student understand and produce complex stories with multiple embedded narratives? (11–12 years of age)

- Does the student analyze stories? (13–15 years of age)

- Does the student generalize from the meaning of the story, formulating abstract statements about the theme or message, and focus on reactions to the story? (16 years–adulthood)

Story Grammar Taxonomy Assessment

- Is a setting provided?

- Are the characters identified and described?

- Are the events of the story presented sequentially?

- Is a goal present?

- Is there an initiating event?

- Is there a causal relationship between events?

- Is an internal response present?

- Is there an attempt to attain the goal?

- Is there a consequence?

- Are multiple plans used to meet the goal?

- Is a partial or complete episode embedded in another episode?

- Are there two characters with separate goals and actions that influence each other's actions?

Sources: Applebee (1978); Larson and McKinley (1995); Roth and Spekman (1986)

goes on to state that expository text consists of (1) oral classroom discourse, such as following directions, taking notes, and making transitions between activities; and (2) textbooks, worksheets, and handouts that present information about theories, persons, facts, dates, generalizations, limitations, and conclusions.

Westby (1994) summarized the seven most commonly used forms of text in Standard American English (SAE) as follows:

- **Description**—telling what something is

- **Enumeration**—providing a list that is related to a topic

- **Sequential/Procedural**—telling what occurred or how to do something

- **Comparisons and contrasts**—noting similarities and differences

- **Problem solving**—stating a problem and solutions

- **Persuasion**—taking and trying to justify a position

- **Cause-effect explanation**—giving reasons why something happened

These seven forms of expository text structures are important to the older student's academic and possibly employment success. The types of questions that the assessment process should answer when determining the student's ability to engage in activities that require a knowledge of expository text are listed in the sidebar that follows.

Written Communication

As the student becomes older, there is an interaction between oral and written communication. It appears that oral communication can enhance written communication skills and vice versa. Both reading and writing skills need to be assessed in the older student with a language disorder.

Reading

During the high school years, students are expected to read using several activities,

> including (a) text scanning exercises, (b) implicit self-questioning, (c) examination of text structures, (d) elaboration of texts, (e) drawing inferences, (f) finding the main ideas and supporting points (and also outlining), (g) summarizing text in their own words, (h) using several sources to research topics, and (i) relating information verbally or in written reports. (Fahey and Reid, 2000, pp. 154–155)

According to Greene (1996), assessing reading should entail five interdependent areas:

- Single-word identification (check at least 20 basic sight words per grade level)

- Contextual word identification (in sentences, paragraphs, passages)

Assessment of Expository Text

Does the student:

- Shift focus of attention from one question to another?

- Shift from one perspective to another?

- Integrate verbal and visual information?

- Integrate old and new information?

- Reason logically?

- Predict outcomes?

- Construct and explain inferences?

- Use abstract vocabulary?

- Use grammatical complexity to reflect conceptual complexity?

- Justify a decision or position?

- Determine and explain causes and consequences?

- Describe what something is?

- List items relevant to a topic?

- Compare and contrast topics?

- State a problem and solutions?

- Tell what occurred and how to do something?

Sources: Gillam, Pena, and L. Miller (1999); Westby and Clauser (1999)

- Cuing systems that use graphophonemic, semantic, syntactic, and schematic cues

- Miscue analysis at the phonological, morphological, syntactic, semantic, and pragmatic levels

- Comprehension of oral and silent reading of sentences, paragraphs, and longer passages

Table 9.5 lists the types of questions that need to be asked when assessing reading skills.

Writing

According to Greene (1996), it is important to assess the following components in a student's writing:

- Phonological and linguistic awareness and awareness of word juncture

- Vocabulary usage

- Generation and organization of ideas in a precise, sequential, and systematic way

- Morphological usage (inflectional and derivational endings, compounding, affixes)

Table 9.5

Assessment of Reading

Level	Questions to Help Assess Reading Skills
Early Elementary (K–3)	Does the student have: • Phonological awareness skills using such tasks as rhyming, syllable and phoneme segmentation, and syllable and phoneme blending? • Rapid automatic naming of visually presented symbols, such as letters, digits, and common objects? • Phonological memory skills to repeat strings of digits, words, or letters presented auditorily? • Letter identification skills, such as naming the alphabet? • Speech to print letter skills in terms of spelling? • Single-word decoding skills? • Oral reading fluency? • Reading comprehension as measured through questions, paraphrasing, and story retelling tasks?
Later Elementary (4th grade and above)	Does the student have: • Knowledge of derivational morphology and orthographic patterns of irregularly spelled words? • Knowledge of different text structures and genres, such as narratives and expository passages? • Knowledge of the different purposes of text, such as to persuade, negotiate, inform, and entertain? • Strategies for different styles of reading, such as skimming, overview, analytic, and critical? • Strategies for facilitating comprehension, storage, and retrieval of information, such as using headings and subheadings, table of contents, summaries, and end-of-chapter questions?

Source: ASHA (2001b)

• Variation of syntactic usage

• Variation of semantic usage

In advanced levels, it is important to evaluate the student's ability to engage in narrative writing, such as developing characters, plot, and setting, as well as evaluating their implementation of such literary devices as theme, voice, and mood. "In expository writing, components such as organization, development, transition, and clarity and non-literal, pragmatic, and figurative language usage are broad areas for concern" (Greene, p. 55). Also, notetaking is a critical writing skill for academic success, as is the ability to summarize written material. N. Nelson (1998) noted five summarization rules that develop from fifth grade to college level: (1) deleting unimportant information, (2) deleting redundant information, (3) substituting category names for lists, (4) selecting a topic sentence, and (5) inventing a topic sentence.

Recall that Hayes and Flowers (1987) view the complex task of writing as three major stages: planning, sentence generation, and revising. We have simplified these terms for students as prewriting, composing, and editing.

Table 9.6 lists the questions that need to be answered about each stage. Stewart (1991) noted that those who are poor writers tend not to plan (i.e., not to gather and organize data before writing), but just begin writing; dwell on mechanical concerns, such as spelling and punctuation, which stifles their writing process; and frequently do not see their own errors and revise passages appropriately.

N. Nelson (1998) recommended that written language samples be analyzed for six knowledge modules. They are listed in the sidebar on page 230.

Table 9.6

Assessment of Writing

Stage	Questions to Help Assess Writing Skills
Prewriting	Does the student: • Develop ideas in written form? • Gather information about a topic? • Organize content? • Take the reader (audience) into consideration? • Consider the purpose for writing (e.g., to tell a story, to explain a process, to give directions)?
Composing	Does the student: • Use planning information to write the draft? • Use appropriate syntax and semantics to write a passage? • Spell and punctuate appropriately?
Editing	Does the student: • Edit the written product? • Find errors and make revisions?

From *Language Disorders in Older Students: Preadolescents and Adolescents* (p. 114), by V. Lord Larson and N.L. McKinley, 1995, Eau Claire, WI: Thinking Publications. © 1995 by Thinking Publications. Adapted with permission.

Knowledge Modules to Analyze in Written Language Samples

- Graphophonemic knowledge (e.g., spelling accuracy)

- Semantic knowledge (e.g., appropriate words, cohesive and transition devices)

- Syntactic knowledge (e.g., subject-verb agreement, parallel sentence structures)

- Discourse knowledge (e.g., organization, formatting, and cohesion)

- Pragmatic knowledge (e.g., considering the audience's informational needs, topic clarity, and ability to use different writing strategies)

- World and prior knowledge (e.g., accurate and appropriately organized and elaborated information about the world)

Source: N. Nelson (1998)

Written language samples should also be assessed for evidence of patterns in spelling errors. Masterson and Apel (2000) noted three basic methods that can be used by examiners to identify a student's spelling abilities/disabilities:

- **Dictation**—The examiner reads aloud a list of words and the student writes each

- **Connected writing**—The student writes a response to a picture or story retelling task

- **Recognition**—The student is given a group of words that have correct and misspelled words and the student identifies the correctly spelled words

They recommend that a student spell 50 to 100 words using these three methods to capture patterns of spelling errors. To determine the nature of the student's spelling errors, the speech-language pathologist will need to analyze the student's phonological and morphological awareness skills, as well as the student's orthographic knowledge and visual storage.

Meta-abilities

Van Kleeck (1987) defined students' various *meta-abilities*, or their abilities to "know that they know" as "awareness of strategies and mental activities while carrying out various cognitive processes such as memory, comprehension, learning, and attention" (p. vi). She further defines *metalinguistic ability* as "being able to consciously reflect on the nature of language—that it is meaningful, arbitrary, conventional, and made up of elements (words, sounds, and bound morphemes) that are combined by rules (grammar)" (p. vi). Furthermore, *metapragmatic skill*, according to van Kleeck (1987), "consists of the child's conscious awareness of the cultural rules for using language effectively in various social contexts" (p. vi).

Developing meta-abilities is critical to students being able to reflect on the effectiveness of their current communication behaviors (i.e., to determine current communication breakdowns and correct them by adapting to the needs of the listener) and to consciously incorporate new communication behaviors. Therefore, as part of the assessment process, determination of the adolescent's or young adult's ability to engage in metalinguistic, metacognitive, metapragmatic,

metanarrative, and metacommunication behaviors is important (N. Nelson, 1998; Rhea Paul, 2001; Schuele and van Kleeck, 1987). Table 9.7 lists the types of questions to ask when assessing the student's meta-abilities.

Developing meta-abilities is critical to students being able to reflect on the effectiveness of their current communication behaviors.

Table 9.7

Assessment of Meta-abilities

Area	Questions to Help Assess Meta-abilities
Metalinguistic	• Does the student show evidence of metalinguistic skills (e.g., the ability to talk about grammatical rules and to use language terms such as *paragraph* and *sentence)?*
Metacognitive	• Does the student show metacognitive skills (i.e., the ability to assess thinking or to think about thinking)?
Metapragmatic	• Does the student show metapragmatic skills (i.e., the ability to be aware of cultural rules for using language appropriately across and within various social contexts)?
Metanarrative	• Does the student show metanarrative skills (i.e., the awareness of story elements and structure so as to manipulate intentionally the various story elements)?

From *Language Disorders in Older Students: Preadolescents and Adolescents* (p. 115), by V. Lord Larson and N.L. McKinley, 1995, Eau Claire, WI: Thinking Publications. © 1995 by Thinking Publications. Adapted with permission.

Nonverbal Communication

Research indicates that people will believe nonverbal messages over verbal messages; when the two may contradict each other, it is frequently the nonverbal communication behavior that creates first impressions (Samovar and Porter, 1991a). Research in communication has revealed that as much as 90% of the social intent of a message is transmitted paralinguistically or nonverbally (Samovar and Porter). "Nonverbal communication involves all those stimuli (except verbal stimuli) within a communication setting, generated by both the individual and the individual's use of the environment, that have potential message value for the sender or receiver" (Samovar and Porter, p. 179).

Nonverbal communication serves these basic functions: to repeat, complement, or contradict what one has said; to substitute for a verbal action; to regulate a communication event; and to accentuate a message. Nonverbal messages are communicated by various means: body movements (kinesics and posture), proxemics (space and distance), dress, facial expressions, eye contact, touch, smell, and paralanguage.

French (1978) noted expectations for appropriate kinesic and proxemic behaviors. The expected kinesic behaviors include the use of gestures that match the spoken message, avoidance of adaptor behaviors that detract from the message (e.g., constantly pushing hair off one's forehead), communication of emotion through facial expression, and appropriate eye contact.

Proxemic behaviors include the maintenance of socially acceptable space or distance while conversing. One's age makes a difference in how one communicates nonverbally. For example, proxemically, children interact the closest, adolescents at an intermediary distance, and adults at the greatest distance.

Dolphin (1991) noted that there are cultural and gender differences in how children use space by age 7. Black children require less personal space than White children, and mixed-sex dyads need more space than same-sex dyads.

Paralanguage features that should be observed while assessing older students include the rate of speech, tone of voice, use of inflection, and unfilled pause time (i.e., silence) within and between utterances. Also, the presence of filled pauses (e.g., "ah," "um," "er") should be noted. Are pauses occurring so often that the message being communicated is significantly impaired? Abnormal paralanguage features impair communication as much as restricted language features do, and thus they become critical variables to evaluate during assessment. Table 9.8 lists some characteristics to assess.

How to Assess

An individual's behaviors are "relative, conditional, complex, and dynamic. Accordingly,

Table 9.8   **Assessment of Nonverbal Communication Skills**

Area	Questions to Help Assess Nonverbal Communication Skills
Kinesic and Proxemic Behaviors	Does the student: • Use facial expressions appropriately? • Have appropriate eye contact when speaking and listening? • Stand at a distance from the speaker/listener that seems appropriate and comfortable? • Use body movements to enhance communication rather than detract from it?
Paralanguage Features	Does the student: • Use an appropriate rate of speech? • Use an appropriate tone of voice? • Use a variety of vocal inflections? • Pause appropriately between utterances? Between speaker-listener turns? • Avoid overuse of filled pauses (e.g., "ah," "um," "er")?

From *Language Disorders in Older Students: Preadolescents and Adolescents* (p. 116), by V. Lord Larson and N.L. McKinley, 1995, Eau Claire, WI: Thinking Publications. © 1995 by Thinking Publications. Adapted with permission.

clinical assessment must be relative, contextual, process oriented, and dynamic" (Muma, 1978, p. 211). This type of clinical assessment can best be accomplished by using informal assessment procedures that are holistic, modifiable, and accommodating to the individual within a natural setting, rather than by conforming the individual to the test methodology. Not only is the test situation artificial, but the language of formal tests is often characteristically different from daily communicative exchanges (Lund and Duchan, 1983).

Frequently, professionals say they cannot use informal procedures because these procedures are not objective (i.e., they provide no quantitative scores). Also, they say it is too time consuming to obtain and to analyze spontaneous discourse samples across relevant situations and communication partners. We examine both of these issues next.

Objectivity is assumed when formal (i.e., standardized) tests are administered. Assume for a moment that a standardized test is more objective than an informal procedure of obtaining, observing, recording, and analyzing communication behaviors in a natural context. This objectivity should not be construed as more important than relevance (Muma, 1978). A standardized test that is supposedly objective cannot be considered worthwhile and valid if it is not assessing relevant behaviors in relevant situations.

Quantitative scores may not be as advantageous as professionals have been led to believe. Muma (1978) stated that scores may work against both the examiner and student, because when complex dynamic behaviors are reduced to numbers, essential information about the individual is lost, thus making it difficult or impossible to generate appropriate intervention goals and procedures. As Lund and Duchan (1983) noted, "Scores are of little value for the purposes of describing language and planning therapy, so clinicians must analyze performance on each item" (p. 299).

(W)hen complex dynamic behaviors are reduced to numbers, essential information about the individual is lost, thus making it difficult or impossible to generate appropriate intervention goals and procedures.

A second argument for not obtaining and analyzing spontaneous language samples is that they are too time consuming. To this, we ask, "What has allowed speech-language pathologists to conclude that assessment must be quick and easy?" Perhaps it has been large caseloads or administrative number games. Whatever the reasons, those variables that force professionals to conclude that language sampling is too time consuming should be changed and the sampling procedure should be retained. Quick and easy assessment procedures may lose more than is gained by neglecting the responsibility to assess an individual's needs appropriately (Muma, 1978). None of us would think it was acceptable for a physician or a psychologist to assess patients in a "quick and easy" fashion. The consequences may be far too severe. Why, then, should the clients served by a speech-language pathologist be any different?

At some point during the assessment procedure, the examiner must obtain from the student several discourse samples (i.e., of conversation, narration, and expository text), which in turn can be analyzed for phonological, morphological, syntactic, semantic, and pragmatic features. If such samples are not gathered and only formal tests are administered, isolated aspects of communication may be obtained. These isolated aspects do not constitute the total communication process and could lead to false conclusions. Using both selected formal tests and informal procedures, the examiner can more effectively evaluate the total communication process and thus implement a comprehensive service delivery model, which we discuss in Chapter 11.

The suggestions we provide in the remainder of this section explain how to simultaneously evaluate cognitive, language, and communication behaviors using these informal assessment procedures: a case history form, a learning style questionnaire, emotional intelligence observation, social skill checklists, oral and written discourse samples, rubrics, portfolios, and directed tasks. Although briefly mentioned in this chapter, the last procedure—directed tasks—is discussed in detail in the next chapter. All other procedures are discussed in the sections that follow.

Informal Assessment Procedures

Case History Interview Form

A case history interview form for obtaining information on the preadolescent's or adolescent's environmental, educational, vocational, health, and communication systems is provided in Appendix E. Information can be obtained by interviewing the student and parent/caregiver. Some of the information may be derived from cumulative records. In most instances, the case history interview form should not be given to the student and parent/caregiver to complete, but should be retained by the examiner, who asks the questions and records responses.

If students have the necessary skills, an alternative would be to have them write or audiotape an autobiography (Larson and McKinley, 1987, 1995; Tattershall, 2002). This option can provide insight into their perspective of the past, present, and future, and the autobiography can also double as a narrative sample.

A supplemental case history interview form is provided in Appendix H. This form can provide valuable insight into the student's perceptions of the importance of thinking, listening, speaking, reading, and writing. The student who does not value these skills, and who reports that he or she has little interest in improving skills, will approach intervention (if deemed necessary following assessment) very differently than the student who values these skills and expresses a desire to change. A questionnaire devised by Schreiber and McKinley (1995) has also been included for assessment of the student's misconceptions about listening (see Appendix F).

The completed general case history interview form should be reviewed to determine whether the student has had previous speech-language services. Also, the case history should be analyzed to determine whether there is any need to refer the student for additional professional services. If so, the examiner should determine if the student is willing to receive additional services.

The completed supplemental case history interview form should be reviewed to see if the student is aware of his or her own thinking, listening, speaking, reading, and writing abilities. The student who displays some meta-abilities may be more motivated to change these behaviors because of the awareness level and therefore may be a good candidate for speech-language services.

Learning Style Questionnaire

A learning style questionnaire has been developed by Larson and McKinley (1987, 1995) to determine when, where, what, why, and how the older student learns best. (This questionnaire is presented in Appendix I.) When using the questionnaire, the student should not be expected to read the form independently, but should be given a form to follow along with the examiner. The examiner should systematically go through the form, asking the questions and recording responses. This gives the examiner the opportunity to explain the unfamiliar terms or to ask additional questions to clarify responses.

During field testing, the form has not been useful with all students; it appears to be most useful with those who already possess a good deal of insight and self-confidence (Larson and McKinley, 1987, 1995). Students who are less secure are more likely to give answers that they think the examiner wants to hear, or that they think are correct, than they are to report how they actually learn best.

Emotional Intelligence Interview

Using Goleman's (1998) analysis, we combined the 5 dimensions of emotional intelligence and the 25 emotional competencies with assessment questions to form Appendix G: *Emotional Intelligence Protocol.* The professional should interview the student and elaborate on the answers provided. The form is not intended to be filled out by the student directly. It should be noted that the last of the 5 dimensions—social skills—has a number of competencies overlapping with other areas, such as those discussed in the next section. All the competencies within the area of emotional intelligence should be analyzed not only in terms of the impact on academic performance and personal-social interactions, but also in terms of the students reaching their vocational potential.

Social Skills Checklist

As noted by many professionals, social skills are critical to a students' academic, personal-social and vocational success (Gajewski et al., 1998a, 1998b; Goleman, 1998; Walker et al., 1994). Gajewski et al. noted these alternatives for assessing social skills:

- Naturalistic behavioral observations in which the student is observed in "real-world" situations

- Analogue observations in which the student is observed in contrived situations

- Behavioral checklists in which significant adults or the students themselves use a rating scale

- Sociometric devices through which students identify what peers are most acceptable or least acceptable

- Hypothetical situations in which the student is asked to explain what a person should do in various social-emotional situations

Walker et al. (1994) have also noted various methods to assess a student's social skills similar to those indicated above, such as Likert scales, which are used by students, teachers, and peers to rate social skills performance. They also noted that direct observation can be done using time samples, event samples, or duration recording. Whatever the method, it is critical that the students be evaluated across and within a variety of social situations in which they are likely to participate.

Students and significant adults in their lives can use rating scales and checklists like those developed by Gajewski et al. (1998a, 1998b; see Appendixes J and K) to rate a number of social-emotional skills. The adult form has 57 social-emotional skills and uses a 1-to-3 rating scale, with 1 meaning the skill is seldom used, 2 meaning the skill is sometimes used appropriately, and 3 meaning the skill is almost always used appropriately. The second rating form is that used by the students, which includes 57 behaviors stated in first person. The same 1-to-3 scale is used. It

may be advantageous to read the checklist to students if reading is a problem. Use the scales to identify problematic skills (rated 1) and those needing more practice (rated 2).

Discourse Samples for Conversations

Conversational samples are a critical part of informal assessment of older students. Such samples have been a recommended source of information for decades, and they are the preferred method of language elicitation from "toddler to adult" (Atkins and Cartwright, 1982; Retherford, 2000). We concur with this position. While a disadvantage of spontaneous conversational samples is the risk of not eliciting all the language behaviors in the individual's repertoire, a powerful advantage of conversational samples is the more realistic picture of the student's communication that is gained.

Arwood (1983), who advocates unstructured conversational sampling, commented that to rapidly determine level of functioning, professionals have only to listen to the individual talk. What can be detected about the way the student organizes ideas, expresses communicative intents, and uses a variety of structures? To the recommendation to listen, we would add, watch the student communicate. What can be noted about eye contact, gestures, body space, and facial expressions?

A partial transcript appears in the sidebar on page 258. This unstructured language sample was obtained by a speech-language

Unstructured Language Transcript of a 14-Year-Old Boy

ADOLESCENT: What do we talk on? No. Oh, I got a good one. You should see my...um, Uncle Boos had to move and they're in this really cool house. It's, it's like, it round. It's sort of li...okay, it's, it's peaked at the top and then it gets round or somethin'...no, it goes...it's...

CLINICIAN: It goes down and then (demonstrates).

ADOLESCENT: Yeah! And then inside they, they have this bedroom...They're going...Okay, there's the living room and their bedroom is...ya go up the, the st...and three stairs, and then you go up there and then they're gonna block it that off from the...so people can't see them in the living room and in the kitchen. They're gonna put a door there and plus they got this neat bar and it's real cool. They have it...um, in the living room. It's real cool. They don't have much furniture though.

CLINICIAN: They should get some.

ADOLESCENT: Uh-hum. They'll have a couch and two chairs. You should see. Oh, it's really awesome. You know, like in a restaurant. They have the table and it's like in the kitchen and it's hitched to the wall. It's real cool!

CLINICIAN: (Laughs)

ADOLESCENT: And then...okay, there's...they have about eight kids and there's one downst in the living room but two down in...Wait a minute! They have six, but counting the parents it's eight. And they...okay, upstairs they have...it's like a closet...like it's about maybe this big. About from this square and that's their bedroom. And it's, okay, from there to there. That's their bedroom. Their mom and dad's bedroom. And there's this kind of like closet thing that closes.

CLINICIAN: How can they get into it?

pathologist evaluating a 14-year-old boy. The boy successfully passed tests that measured isolated aspects of language (i.e., discrete point tests), and yet his conversational sample revealed problems in communicating messages to listeners. The excessive number of verbal mazes, lack of message cohesiveness, and high incidence of low-information words frequently left his listeners confused.

Administration

Procedures for obtaining language samples have changed very little since first recommended by McCarthy (1930). Speech-language pathologists should:

- Establish good rapport with the individual being sampled

- Keep their remarks to a minimum

- Use open-ended questions or comments that will facilitate longer responses

Usually, older students should select their own topics of conversation. The goal of obtaining a sample is that it be "representative" of the individual's communication. However, "representative" has held different meanings in the literature, including "comprehensive," "idealized," and "typical" (Gallagher, 1983).

To be comprehensive, a conversational sample has to be large enough to be reliable, but small enough to be efficient. McCarthy (1930) originally proposed a 50-utterance sample; others have recommended 100 utterances (Crystal, Fletcher, and Garman, 1991; Engler, Hannah, and Longhurst, 1973; Retherford, 2000; Tyack and Gottsleben, 1974). L. Bloom and Lahey (1978) and J. Miller (1981) recommended a minimum of 30 minutes of sampling time. Bloom and Lahey also suggested that 200 or more utterances be obtained within the recommended sampling time.

To be a representative conversational sample, the sample should evoke the best possible range of abilities (McLean and Snyder-McLean, 1978). The conversational analysis should neither underestimate nor overestimate the student's communication abilities, since "a language sample is considered unrepresentative if it leads to an analysis

that results in either one of these errors" (Gallagher, 1983, p. 3). The notion that an "idealized" sample should be collected is contradictory to the notion that it also be "typical," or representative of daily communication performances. When assessing older students, we have been most concerned with collecting samples that represent typical language performances, rather than idealized samples.

The conversational analysis should neither underestimate nor overestimate the student's communication abilities.

In addition to considering what is a representative sample, speech-language pathologists must consider how language use varies with context (Gallagher, 1983). Many clinicians have responded by obtaining language samples in more than one context, using a variety of stimuli, conversational partners, and settings (McLean and Snyder-McLean, 1978; J. Miller, 1981; Muma, 1978). The problem is that the "number of possible combinations of stimulus materials, conversational partners, and settings is infinite" (Gallagher, p. 4). The selection of combinations is either arbitrary or the result of trial-and-error sampling. Therefore, whether sampling in multiple contexts solves the assessment problems arising from language use variability is questionable (Gallagher).

There are limited data to describe how adolescents' communication varies as a function of changes in stimuli, conversational partners, or settings. Our own longitudinal study (which utilizes a school setting, and not stimulus materials, to gather data while adolescents converse with peers of their choice and with unfamiliar adults of the opposite sex) provides some of the first research that describes how language use varies in these contexts (Larson and McKinley, 1998). As noted in Chapter 3, the conversational partners (in this case, a peer of one's choice or an adult of the opposite sex) had a significant impact on the conversational features that evolved. Clearly, more information is needed.

We recommend, at the minimum, that two 10-minute conversational samples be collected, one while the student is conversing with the speech-language pathologist (usually an unfamiliar adult during initial assessment) and one with a peer of the youth's choice. Additional samples might be collected using other partners. The conversational samples should require the student to switch from an informal to a formal register. The speech-language pathologist should keep in mind that after age 15, adolescents begin to use a more formal register even with their peers, unless they are the best of friends (Wiig, 1982, 1983).

Analysis

Both partners' turns should be transcribed in order to analyze certain pragmatic features. Rather than delineating utterances, as would be done for young children, conversational units should be marked when transcribing preadolescent and adolescent language. A *conversational unit* is defined as "the utterance(s) of one conversational partner that continue(s) until the other conversational partner initiates an independent utterance" (Larson and McKinley, 1998, p. 202). A phonetic transcription may or may not be necessary. If phonological errors are evident, it may be desirable to complete a phonetic transcription. In all cases, the transcription should reflect what was actually said and include all false starts, verbal mazes, and filled pauses.

Perhaps the greatest difficulty with conversational samples is how to analyze them once they are transcribed. One reason for the difficulty is that calculation of the mean length of utterances in morphemes (MLU-M) for the purpose of comparing it with R. Brown's (1973) stages of psycholinguistic development is not appropriate for the older school-age population. Older students have far surpassed Brown's stages.

So how can professionals determine that an adolescent's language system is different from what might be expected? Loban (1976) described an analysis procedure that allows the quantification of a variety of linguistic characteristics (e.g., maze words and words per communication unit; see Tables 3.1 (on page 59), 3.2 (on page 60), and 3.3 (on page 61) in Chapter 3). This quantification begins to give a sense of the individual's functioning, but the focus is on the products of communication, rather than on processes. Adopting analysis procedures that attempt to quantify developmental changes during preadolescence and adolescence should not be the only method used, since the desired outcome is a description of the adolescent's communication, sufficiently detailed to suggest whether intervention is needed. When quantitative analysis procedures are used, they should still be combined with descriptive data that discuss how the youth's language system differs from what is typical.

J. Damico (1991) developed a procedure for gathering descriptive data called Clinical Discourse Analysis, which assesses functions of language in school-age students. It is an excellent tool for identifying students who are language impaired. The procedure is organized according to four categories described by Grice (1975) in defining his "cooperative principle." The categories and the problem behaviors pertinent to each category are described in Table 9.9. For more information about Clinical Discourse Analysis, consult J. Damico.

We have also found that the chart of competent and incompetent features of language in *Evaluating Communicative Competence–Revised* (C. Simon, 1994) provides a useful guide when analyzing the student's language. The chart, which is presented in Figure 9.2, provides a gestalt of the student's communication, not just isolated features. By noting competent features that are present, absent, or inconsistent and by describing typical utterances as evidence, the speech-language pathologist can begin to develop a sense of the total effectiveness and efficiency of a student's communication. C. Simon describes a language sample procedure that gathers observational data on 21 performance tasks that analyze a student's listening and speaking behaviors. According to C. Simon, as the student is observed performing these tasks, "it is possible to obtain a systematic description of language processing, metalinguistics, and expressive language proficiencies and deficits" (p. xi).

Drawing from a variety of sources (J. Damico, 1991; S. Duncan and Fiske, 1977; Grice, 1975; Hymes, 1972; Rhea Paul, 2001; Rees and Wollner, 1982; C. Simon, 1979; Wiig and Semel, 1980), we constructed a form called *Adolescent Conversational Analysis* (see Appendix L). This form documents the appropriateness of students' conversational skills. It is unique from other analyses in that it examines the student's role not only as a speaker during conversation, but also as a listener. In addition, the form assesses nonverbal behaviors within conversational discourse.

A personal computer can also be used for analyzing language samples. For many years now, clinicians have been using language assessment software programs such as Lingquest 1: Language Sample Analysis,

Table 9.9

Clinical Discourse Analysis

Grice's (1975) Categories	Problem Behaviors
Quantity	• Failure to provide significant information to listeners • Use of nonspecific vocabulary • Informational redundancy • Need for repetition
Quality	• Message inaccuracy
Relation	• Poor topic maintenance • Inappropriate response • Failure to ask relevant questions • Situational inappropriateness • Inappropriate speech style
Manner	• Linguistic nonfluency • Revision • Delays before responding • Failure to structure discourse • Turn-taking difficulty • Gaze inefficiency • Inappropriate intonational contour

From "Clinical Discourse Analysis: A Functional Approach to Language Assessment," by J. Damico. In *Communication Skills and Classroom Success: Assessment and Therapy Methodologists for Language and Learning Disabled Students* (p. 131), by C.S. Simon (Ed.), 1991, Eau Claire, WI: Thinking Publications. © 1991 by Thinking Publications. Adapted with permission.

by Mordecai, Palin, and Palmer (1985); Systematic Analysis of Language Transcripts (SALT), by J. Miller and Chapman (2000); Computerized Language Sample Analysis, by Weiner (1984); and Computerized Profiling (CP), by Long, Fey, and Channell (2000). These software tools assist with the sorting, calculating, and tabulating of data collected from language samples.

Lingquest 1: Language Sample Analysis (Mordecai et al., 1982) provides for an analysis of lexical items including a type-token ratio (TTR) and eight grammatical forms (i.e., nouns, verbs, modifiers, prepositions, conjunctions, negations, interjections, and *wh-* question words), mean length of utterances in words and morphemes, and an analysis of 81 subcategories of parts of speech. To accomplish this analysis, the speech-language pathologist must transcribe and code the utterances to be analyzed. This process may be difficult and time consuming,

A Clinician's Model of Expressive Communicative Competence

Figure 9.2

Competent Features			Incompetent Features		
Form	**Function**	**Style**	**Form**	**Function**	**Style**
flexible, precise vocabulary	sustains topic of conversation	considers listener's informational needs	limited vocabulary repeated often	wanders from conversationsal topic	egocentric comments
mastery of syntactic and morphological rules	selected phrasing reflects communicative intent	advance planning of content	syntactic and morphological errors	ineffective illocutionary speech acts	incoherent sequencing of details
complexity and variety of syntax	gives support for a point of view	finds words easily to express thoughts	basic syntactic patterns re-used	opinions stated as fact	word finding difficulty
mastery of irregular grammatical features	uses elaborated and restricted codes	fluency in expression	difficulty with irregular verbs, plurals, and comparatives	relies upon restricted code	false starts (mazes)
mastery of tense reference and subject/verb agreement	social and cognitive uses of language	intelligible, distinct speech	lacks consistency in tense and number reference	informal, social uses of language	slurred speech consisting of a series of "giant words"
uses clear noun referents	developed heuristic language function	comfortable speech rate	uses ambiguous pronouns	afraid to ask adults questions	rapid, jerky speech rate
uses subordinators to relate ideas	contextual adaptations of language	audible speech	unsystematic combinations of ideas	limited language flexibility	speech volume not adapted to context
	tactful deviousness used			tactless statements	
	modifies and clarifies message upon listener request			restates same information	

From *Evaluating Communicative Competence* (Rev. 2nd ed.; p. 5), by C.S. Simon, 1994, Tempe, AZ: Communi-Cog. © 1994 by Communi-Cog. Reprinted with permission.

243

with resulting summaries that are valuable but that provide no developmental information (Retherford, 2000).

SALT (J. Miller and Chapman, 2000) is based on the principles and procedures described by J. Miller (1981). SALT focuses on five major features when analyzing a language sample: transcript entry, transcript utility, standard analysis, search, and wizard word lists. The standard analysis procedures conducted by SALT are number and percentage of complete and incomplete utterances, the TTR, mean length of utterance in morphemes, a distributional analysis of the number of utterances by word or morpheme and speaker turns, the frequency of usage of structures designated by the speech-language pathologist, and an analysis of morpheme usage. This software is one of the most flexible and complicated. It allows for the examiner to have some flexibility in what features can be analyzed. Likewise, because of the sophistication, considerable practice is needed to use the programs (Retherford, 2000). However, a tutorial program is included to teach coding. A reference database has been developed up through early adolescence but is not included with the software.

Computerized Language Sample Analysis (Weiner, 1984) summarizes the frequency of occurrence and accuracy of use for 14 grammatical categories. In addition, analysis of nouns, verbs, sentence types, length of utterance, and word usage can be accomplished. A tutorial is provided that assists the examiner in learning to code utterances and to use this program. An updated version of this program is available under the title Parrot Easy Language Sample Analysis (Weiner, 1988).

Computerized Profiling, developed by Long, Fey, and Channell (2000), contains several analysis systems such as LARSP (Crystal et al., 1991), PRISM (Crystal, 1992), and "Developmental Sentence Score" found within Developmental Sentence Analysis (Lee, 1974). Pragmatic and phonological analyses are possible as well. Complex manual coding may be necessary depending on the type of analysis that is selected (Retherford, 2000).

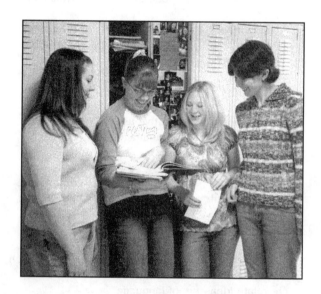

These software programs offer a range of analysis features and varying degrees of flexibility. How time consuming a particular analysis system will be is contingent upon the type of analysis chosen, the amount of information processed, and the skills of the speech-language pathologist in coding utterances (A. Schwartz, 1985). Although these software packages should ultimately allow clinicians to be more efficient, the software should also assist them to become more effective in determining the type and severity of a language disorder and in establishing appropriate intervention programs. Regardless of the software language analysis system used, the speech-language pathologist must obtain an accurate and representative language sample, transcribe the sample accurately, and code the language structures correctly.

Long and Masterson (1993) discussed what computerized language analysis software can and cannot do. They concluded that the software can:

- Conduct language analysis more quickly than when it is done by hand

- Allow for detailed analyses that, due to time constraints, would rarely be done by hand

They concluded that computerized language analysis software cannot:

- Assist in the orthographic or phonetic transcription of a student's language

- Ensure the transcript is being transcribed correctly

- Yield irrefutable truth

- Tell professionals the answers to diagnosis and intervention

This last item may be possible someday, when "expert systems" become available. The first two items have been greatly assisted

by software tools like Transcript Builder (Moore, 2001). Once the videotape or audiotape of the language sample has been digitized, Transcript Builder turns a personal computer into a video (or audio) playback unit. One side of the screen is a word processor for transcribing the language sample, and the other side of the screen is the digital audio or video file. Convenience is enhanced for clinicians, while errors are greatly reduced.

Interpretation

Quantitative data may be compared to those presented on existing developmental charts, such as Loban's (1976). Caution is advised, however, because Loban's results were obtained in a contrived conversational situation. Quantitative data in the form of a TTR should not be compared with existing data for children's utterances or with adult norms. We recommend that local normative data be obtained on the TTR of preadolescents and adolescents. With the use of the computer, this is a realistic goal.

The adolescent conversational analysis that we recommend could be interpreted with the use of the profile summary provided in Appendix L. Conversational behaviors are determined to be either appropriate or inappropriate. Determination of the appropriateness or inappropriateness of a behavior is made by judging whether it is penalizing to the student; a behavior perceived by the clinician as penalizing is marked as inappropriate (Prutting and Kirchner, 1983).

Our clinical experiences have been that the student probably has conversational deficits in need of intervention if a significant number of conversational behaviors are indicated as inappropriate (i.e., 30% or more, disregarding items marked "not observed," which approximates two standard deviations below the mean on standardized tests). Certain items (e.g., main ideas, word-retrieval skills, fluency, intelligibility, and turn-taking) should carry more weight during interpretation because they may carry more negative consequences during communication exchanges than other items do. If consistent problems are evident on any one of these items, direct or indirect intervention should be considered, even if most of the other items are judged to be appropriate.

Discourse Samples for Narrations

The use of narratives can be an excellent assessment procedure (Arwood, 1983; Strong, 1999). Narrative tasks are more structured than conversational speech, but they are less structured than the directed tasks that we discuss in Chapter 10.

Administration

The way examiners obtain a narrative language sample can result in different types of samples. For example, if preadolescents or adolescents are asked to relate a personal experience, they will reproduce a more orally structured narrative. If asked to tell a story, they will use a more literary style. However, if asked to tell a story like it is written in a book, they will use the most literary style.

When both the examiner and the student can see the stimulus picture and share in the pictorial situation, there is a tendency to resort to a more oral style and to make the narrative less explicit. Also, what is depicted in a picture may make a difference. Pictures that display an action may lead a student to describe only the action, whereas pictures that display a setting often yield a more complex story. Telling a story from a wordless picture book requires that the student recognize the scenarios depicted, whereas telling a story from a single picture requires that the student formulate and organize the story, not simply recognize it. The *Strong Narrative Assessment Procedure (SNAP;* Strong, 1999) is a comprehensive procedure using four Mercer Mayer wordless storybooks to document narrative development. *SNAP* is particularly appropriate for preadolescents and early adolescents.

Some students show minimal differences based on how the instructions are given or how the stimuli are depicted. However, others tend to switch from a more oral to a more literary mode, depending on the task. Perhaps this demonstrates that these latter individuals have a metalinguistic awareness toward story grammars.

Story reformulation has also been used as an assessment procedure (Chappell, 1980; Culatta, Page, and Ellis, 1983). In story reformulation tasks, preadolescents and adolescents have to comprehend, retain, and recall information; understand sequences; and express themselves precisely when retelling the story.

We recommend that at least two samples of narration be obtained, one formulated and the other a reformulated task. The type of story selected for the reformulation task should be sensitive to the student's social-emotional level and to memory capacity. The specific type of formulated task selected should be contingent upon whether a more oral or more literary sample is desired. Generally, we first choose a formulated task that requires the student to relate a personal experience, since the recounting of a personal story and a story reformulation task are the most distant tasks on the oral-literary style continuum. If relating a personal experience is a much stronger ability for the student

than reformulating a story, then additional formulated narration tasks requiring a more literary style may be necessary to determine where the individual falls on the continuum. The questions in the sidebar should be asked of the student to determine the ability to respond to the highest levels of the developmental hierarchy for narration.

Analysis

Once a student has formulated or reformulated a story, the speech-language pathologist should transcribe it. Recall that there are two primary ways in which narratives can be analyzed once transcribed—through a developmental hierarchy and through a story grammar taxonomy. We encourage analysis through the developmental stage progression (Applebee, 1978) because of its underlying

---

Advanced Questions on Narrations

After each narrative sample is collected, the examiner should ask questions that require the student to summarize the story, categorize it, analyze it, and generalize it. For example, these types of questions or directives might be given:

- Now tell me in one sentence what your story was about.
- What would be a good title for this story?
- In what category would you put this story (e.g., drama, mystery, comedy)?
- How else could you categorize this story (e.g., short, long, exciting, boring)?
- How did this story make you feel?
- Why do you think (main character) acted like he (she) did?
- What was the moral of this story?

From *Language Disorders in Older Students: Preadolescents and Adolescents* (p. 128), by V. Lord Larson and N.L. McKinley, 1995, Eau Claire, WI: Thinking Publications. © 1995 by Thinking Publications. Reprinted with permission.

theoretical premises (Piaget, 1959; Vygotsky, 1962). Story grammar taxonomies appear to be independent of theoretical constructs. Nonetheless, they provide a glimpse of organizational style.

Using Applebee's (1978) developmental hierarchy, we have developed a narration analysis form (see Appendix M). Applebee noted that stories do not always fit precisely into one of the first five categories. Thus, judgments will need to be made on the basis of the predominant mode of organization. Based on the student's response to the examiner's questions about summarization, categorization, analysis, and generalization, the rest of the form in Appendix M can be completed.

The myriad of choices for analyzing narratives are compiled in *Guide to Narrative Language* (Hughes, McGillivray, and Schmidek, 1997). In a very meticulous way, these authors present the range of analysis options available, matched to the manner in which the narrative sample was collected. For example, analyzing a script ("Tell me what happens at birthday parties") has different analysis options than analyzing a creative narrative ("Tell me a story about having a birthday party"). In addition to providing developmental hierarchy information, this resource guides examiners through the analysis of cohesion, clauses, and other higher-level language skills that should be in the repertoire of older students.

For another detailed analysis of storytelling skills, professionals can also consult Hedberg and Westby (1993), who provide a variety of practical ways to analyze and interpret narrative structure and content. Along with a review of the literature, their approach is illustrated using students with typical development and students with language disorders.

Likewise, Rhea Paul (2001) provides a narrative rubric to analyze the narrative skills of older students by scoring their abilities on a scale from 1 (which means not present or not developed) to 6 (which means overarching theme, dynamic characters, setting fully integrated, overarching problems, resolution supported by multiple episodes, and careful crafting of choices in a story structure) looking at parameters such as theme, characters, setting, plot, and communication. Finally, the *Strong Narrative Assessment Procedure (SNAP;* Strong, 1998) as mentioned previously, uses a story retelling method. The narrative produced by the student is analyzed for overall organization as well as for a variety of structures. The analysis procedures used have utility beyond the stories supplied by the *SNAP* resource.

Interpretation

Once the speech-language pathologist has analyzed the student's story to determine the predominant mode of organization in the developmental hierarchy, it is possible to interpret these data in terms of the underlying cognitive level and the chronological age at which most students learn various aspects of narration. Preadolescents or adolescents whose narration skills are consistently three or more years delayed, compared with their chronological age, may be candidates for language intervention.

Discourse Samples for Expository Text

As noted earlier, much of the written and spoken text that preadolescents and adolescents will encounter in the classroom is expository text (Gillam, Pena, and L. Miller, 1999; N. Nelson, 1998; Rhea Paul, 2001). The comprehension and production of this type of discourse is critical to the academic success and potentially to the vocational accomplishments of the individual.

Administration

It is important to assess both the comprehension and production of expository text across a variety of settings. Using several different procedures, the speech-language pathologist will be able to determine more readily where students are having the most difficulty and how to utilize students' strengths to help them overcome their weaknesses.

Using the student's textbooks, the speech-language pathologist can have the student read a passage silently or aloud, summarize it, and answer questions about it to demonstrate comprehension. Likewise, the speech-language pathologist might observe how well the student understands classroom lectures with and without a listening guide (i.e., a handout outlining the main points and relevant details of the lecture). By providing a listening guide, the student is

given a scaffold to focus more effectively on data pertinent to the topic. It is important to observe how using a scaffold assists (or fails to assist) the student in understanding the text.

In addition, the speech-language pathologist can give the student a topic of high interest, such as to compare and contrast rock and classical music. Ask the student to do the activity both orally and in writing to see how well he or she produces expository text using these two modalities. If the student has problems, the speech-language pathologist could provide a scaffold. For example, provide the student with an outline of the text to be written, listing main headings and space to add relevant details. After the student has an outline of the text, ask the student to summarize the information, recall details, and answer informational questions (Rhea Paul, 2001).

Analysis

Each type of expository text (both spoken and written, as well as comprehension and production) might be analyzed on the following parameters using a 1-point (least appropriate) to 6-point (most appropriate) scale as follows (Rhea Paul, 2001; Westby and Clauser, 1999):

- **Organizational text structure**—in terms of clarity; opening and closing paragraphs; topic sentences in paragraphs; cohesion devices used such as pronouns, parallel structures, and some repetitions; all ideas are presented logically using a variety of organizational techniques

- **Content and/or theme**—in terms of the content or theme being presented in an organized manner and of the main ideas being supported by appropriate details

- **Written language usage**—in terms of an appropriate variety of syntactic and semantic features being present such as simple to complex sentences and concrete to abstract vocabulary

- **Mechanics of written language**—in terms of spelling, punctuation, and correct grammar

- **Perspective**—in terms of the listener or reader being taken into account and the student assuming the perspective of the current or prospective audience

In addition, the students' behavior might be observed in the classroom regarding their ability to reason logically; predict outcomes; justify decisions; construct and explain inferences; determine and explain causes and consequences; describe objects, events, or ideas; list items relevant to a topic; compare and contrast topics; state a problem and solutions; and tell what occurred and how to do something (Rhea Paul, 2001; Westby and Clauser, 1999).

Interpretation

Each sample of spoken and written expository text should be interpreted as to whether an observed behavior was appropriate or inappropriate and where it falls on the six-point scale. Also, it is critical to determine if a behavior is inappropriate or lacking, how it is interfering with academic success. If scaffolding or mediated learning procedures are used, it is important to record how or if these procedures assisted the students. This will indicate the student's potential for learning new materials using an expository text genre.

Written Communication

Reading

The document "Roles and Responsibilities of Speech-Language Pathologists with Respect to Reading and Writing in Children and Adolescents," approved in 2001 by the American Speech-Language-Hearing Association, brought the assessment of reading into the forefront for clinicians. As children age and the lines between language disorders and learning disabilities become blurred, speech-language pathologists become a critical link to determining the extent to which oral communication deficits and reading problems overlap. Other professionals will be assessing the traditional set of reading skills if disabilities are suspect. The unique contribution that can be made by the speech-language pathologist is determining the extent to which both oral and written communication deficits co-exist.

Speech-language pathologists should choose assessment tasks that permit them to document the relationships between reading and oral communication, in particular listening. The expectations for older students with regard to these two aspects of literacy are parallel in many ways, with the exception of the modality (hearing vs. seeing). So, for example, regardless of the modality, students need to isolate main ideas and relevant details while listening or reading; they must recognize the overall organization of the speaker/author; they must identify the purpose of the communication, etc. If one looks at a list of critical listening skills, it reads nearly identically to a critical reading skills list.

Administration

Using Appendix N: *Reading Skills Profile,* the examiner is guided to provide a reading passage and a listening task. Comparable listening and reading passages should be used with regard to the density of ideas and the length. This will allow a comparison of the student's skill levels in reading as opposed to listening. Content-level material should be used for the reading passage. Likewise, a portion of grade-level content should be paraphrased and a simulated lecture delivered that spans a few minutes of time.

The content should be representative of information the student faces daily. Since most content is expository in nature in the upper grades, except for English classes which might include either narrative or instructional text, the emphasis in this assessment procedure is on the language of instruction. As the student speaks or writes

responses to the questions (whichever modality is easier), the examiner records observations on the form.

In addition to the comparison part of the profile, the examiner is asked to make judgments about the presence of other reading skills, listed earlier in this chapter in Table 9.5 (see page 228). These judgments should be made over the course of administering all the informal assessment procedures or through interviews with teachers who know the student well.

Analysis

Looking at the first part of the completed profile from Appendix N, the examiner should note what is recorded for the student's performance as a reader and as a listener. The examiner is then asked to make this comparison for each question:

- Reading was stronger.
- Listening was stronger.
- Both were about the same.

This judgment is crucial to the interpretation of performance (see next section). Moreover, it might be prudent to ask the student for his or her perceptions regarding the stronger modality and to see if the performance matches. For example, if three main ideas were part of each passage, and a student identified one in reading and two in listening, yet believes to be stronger in reading than listening, this is a mismatch that may need to be addressed during intervention.

The second part of the profile should be examined for the consistency with which skills essential for efficient reading are reported as present. If direct observation is not feasible, important informants who are well acquainted with the older student should be used. Examiners could also structure informal testing procedures that directly ask students questions germane to the second part of the profile (e.g., "How do you spell _____?" or "What purpose did the author have when he wrote this piece?").

Interpretation

If students are stronger listeners than readers, it may mean that they have comprehension skills that are obscured during reading by deficits such as decoding or fluency, and that listening skills might be used to improve reading skills. If reading comprehension skills appear to be stronger than listening skills, it may mean that students are more efficient visual learners than auditory learners, and that reading skills might be used to improve listening skills. If both skill sets are depressed, it may mean that there is a general lack of comprehension skills on the part of the student, whether the modality is spoken or written. Judgments of the presence or absence of reading skills in the second half of the profile may affect the student's overall efficiency as a reader.

Writing

N. Nelson and Van Meter (2002) emphasized the importance of gathering writing samples to determine the student's ability to engage in curriculum-based language activities. Writing samples, like conversational and narrative samples, are on a continuum from informal to more structured elicitation, resulting in different outcomes. Regardless of the stimulus, it is important to gather a sufficient number of written statements to be analyzed.

Administration

The way in which writing samples are obtained determines how the writing style is structured. For example, if asked to write a narrative, it will probably be more informal if it is autobiographical than if asked to write a story like it was written in a book. Variations will also occur in expository text writing samples. For example, a book report might be less structured than a scientific lab report, which is more rigorous in its format. Regardless of the type text—narrative or expository—each student should be provided with general directions to focus his or her writing activity (Nelson and Van Meter, 2002). These directions should include time limits, if any; whether to handwrite the document or to word-process a draft; and if there is a choice of topics. For example, you might say, "You have a half-hour to outline and draft a report on your favorite sport. During this time, you should edit and revise your report to make it the best possible. You may use the computer to type your report."

If students can choose their own topics, their samples are usually more valued by them and they take greater ownership (Roth,

2000). As the students are writing, observe how they engage in the writing process. If they are not writing at all, after 20 to 30 minutes, provide scaffolding for them in terms of planning an outline or encouraging them to write their best thoughts and not worry about mistakes.

Analysis

Once the student has provided a writing sample of at least 8–10 sentences or fragments, the sample should be analyzed both in terms of the writing process (i.e., prewriting, composing, and editing strategies used) and the writing product produced. Many times the writing process data provide more insights as to the student's writing abilities for curriculum success than does the product analysis. Appendix O provides a writing analysis profile to analyze both the student's writing process and product in terms of features that were appropriate, inappropriate, or not observed.

Interpretation

Given the analysis of the student's writing sample, the speech-language pathologist should note patterns of evidence in terms of writing process and product features appropriately or inappropriately used. It is not uncommon for students to engage minimally in prewriting and editing strategies and simply launch into the composing process. However, not to write or to need scaffolding to begin the writing process is more serious. Likewise, it is common for students to edit the writing sample for grammar, spelling, and punctuation but not for clarity of content. No notion of needing to edit or how to edit is more serious.

Rubrics

According to Benjamin (2000), rubrics are scoring guides. Rubrics or Structured-Multidimensional Assessment Profiles (S-MAPs; Wiig and Larson, in press) provide an analysis tool for both students and professionals to use to assess a given area of communication, such as story retelling, listening, writing process, and meta-abilities. The rubric or S-MAP is a 4 × 4 analysis tool in which four skill dimensions for an area are across the top and four performance levels or criteria are listed down the side. Appendix P illustrates an S-MAP or rubric for meta-abilities.

Rubrics or S-MAPs are very useful tools for evaluating authentic performance tasks derived from existing classroom work samples or by selecting a work sample from the student. These work samples and rubrics or S-MAPs can then be placed in students' portfolios to demonstrate baseline behavior; to measure student progress; and to establish appropriate goals, objectives, and/or benchmarks. Rubrics or S-MAPs allow the examiner to analyze communication tasks in a flexible manner to accomplish the following goals (Wiig and Larson, in press):

- Perform initial diagnostic testing to validate the results of norm or criterion-referenced tests

- Undertake test-retest reliability because no two work samples are the same

- Measure progress over time as a result of teaching or intervention

- Obtain a visual representation of progress, outcomes, or needed goals for parents, the student, or other professionals

Rubrics or S-MAPs have a variety of purposes. They:

- Provide qualitative as well as quantitative analysis

- Describe behavior (i.e., they do not simply state scores), allowing the IEP team to develop relevant intervention plans

- Report progress as mandated by the Individuals with Disabilities Education Act (IDEA; 1997; P.L. 105-17) and graphically demonstrate progress to students and parents

Administration

Rubrics or S-MAPs can be used effectively and efficiently as follows:

1. After listening carefully to the referral source(s), select one or two S-MAPs to extend or validate standardized test results, classroom observations, parent and student interviews, etc. The work samples to be analyzed could be provided by the classroom teacher.

2. After the student meets eligibility criteria for language services, additional work samples might be obtained from the student, using audio or videotapes, written samples, etc., and then analyzed via rubric or S-MAP to write the IEP.

3. Once the student has been provided intervention services, S-MAPs or rubrics can be used to measure and document progress.

Analysis

Once the student's work samples have been obtained, they can be evaluated using the following steps (Wiig and Larson, in press):

Step 1—Select one skill dimension (e.g., metalinguistic, metacognitive, metapragmatic, metanarrative (see Appendix P) for rating.

Step 2—Compare the observed performance to the four descriptor performance levels (expert, competent, advanced beginner, beginner) for the dimension.

Step 3—Identify the best performance descriptor and mark it on the S-MAP.

Step 4—Select each of the remaining dimensions and, one at a time, rate and record the performance level of each skill dimension.

Interpretation

Once each of the skill levels has been analyzed as to the performance level, the completed rubric or S-MAP can be used to plan the intervention process. IDEA '97 requires that present levels of performance (1) address how the disability affects classroom performance and (2) provide a baseline measure for establishing measurable goals, objectives, or benchmarks. These requirements can be accomplished with rubrics or S-MAPs. Using the descriptors within each skill dimension, one can write an objective or benchmark. Likewise, as intervention progresses, the rubric or S-MAP can be used to measure and report progress as it affects classroom performance.

Portfolios

According to Paulson, Paulson, and Meyer (1991):

> A portfolio is a purposeful collection of student work that exhibits the student's efforts, progress, and achievements in one or more areas. The collection must include student participation in selecting contents, the criteria for selection, the criteria for judging merit, and evidence of student self-reflection. (p. 60)

In portfolio assessment, the student, the classroom teacher, or both place samples of the student's work in a file or portfolio. The artifacts in the portfolio involve generalized comparisons, rather than detailed analyses of the student's work. This procedure allows for a comparison of the student's current performance with his or her past performance and helps determine the student's progress over time. For this procedure to be effective in the academic evaluation of students, the materials placed into a student's portfolio must be chosen wisely and be representative of meaningful and ecologically valid situations (J. Damico, 1993).

Paulson et al. (1991) offer the following guidelines for realizing the power of portfolio assessment:

- The portfolio should demonstrate that the student is learning about learning and engaged in self-reflection.

- The portfolio is something the student does, not something done to the student.

- The portfolio is not the same as the cumulative folder.

- The portfolio should represent the student's activities.

- The portfolio may serve a different purpose during the year than at the end of the year.

- The portfolio may have multiple purposes, but they should not conflict with each other.

- The portfolio should illustrate the student's growth.

- The portfolio should not happen by chance, but should deliberately enhance skills and techniques useful to the student.

Communication Solutions
for Older Students

The benefits of using portfolios were summarized by Wolf (1989) long before they became so popular. The sidebar focuses on the benefits when assessing written language skills.

In summary, Paulson et al. (1991) stated it best when they said:

> A portfolio, then, is a portfolio when it provides a complex and comprehensive view of student performance in context.... Above all, a portfolio is a portfolio when it provides a forum that encourages students to develop the abilities needed to become independent, self-directed learners. (p. 63)

When using portfolios, the student becomes a participant in, rather than the object of, assessment. According to Silliman, Wilkinson, and Hoffman (1993), examples of materials found in a portfolio are logs of books read, stories written, writing and dialogue journals, letters written, examples of strategies learned, reports, self-assessment scales, and video- and audiotapes showing what has been learned.

When using portfolios, the student becomes a participant in, rather than the object of, assessment.

The Benefits of Portfolios

A portfolio can be particularly helpful in assessing written language skills. Why have student portfolios?

• They help students take responsibility for their work and for evaluating their progress.

• They help students enlarge their view of what's learned, because portfolios contain a range of work (e.g., fiction, poems, essays, journal entries).

• They help students understand that learning is a process and not a product (e.g., writing is a process of planning, writing, rewriting, revising, and completing numerous drafts, not just the finished product on paper).

• They help students take a developmental point of view of how their work has progressed and to objectively evaluate their own work.

Source: Wolf (1989)

Directed Tasks

Highly structured informal procedures designed to assess a specific communication skill are directed tasks. The focus in directed tasks is on process, and not on the end product of the activities.

The next chapter outlines a number of directed tasks that we recommend for use with older students during assessment. By clustering directed tasks in their own chapter, we hope we made them more accessible for use in a clinical setting. Enough detail is provided so these tasks can be replicated by readers of this text.

Formal Assessment Instruments

To this point, we have focused on informal assessment procedures for evaluating communication behaviors of preadolescents and adolescents. But there are also many formal tests that assess a multitude of isolated variables. When selecting formal tests to use with an older school-age population, we encourage examiners to refer to the following section for a discussion on how to critique standardized assessment instruments, or to review the complete report from the American Speech-Language-Hearing Association Ad Hoc Committee on Instrument Evaluation (1986). Having done this, examiners can cautiously proceed with selecting one or more standardized tests that are relevant to the student being assessed.

Table 9.10 presents a variety of tests that the examiner might choose when assessing an older student. A number of variables have been summarized for each test, including age range, primary area(s) assessed, and norm-referenced vs. criterion-referenced measurement interpretations. The information cited in each column matches what the author(s) of the test reported in the examiner's manual. The primary areas assessed by a given test are marked in the table as to whether they assess thinking, listening, speaking, reading, and/or writing.

A standardized test has four aspects that are standardized (American Speech-Language-Hearing Association Ad Hoc Committee on Instrument Evaluation, 1986):

- The test content is fixed.

- The administrative procedures are prescribed.

- The responses are scored using predetermined criteria.

- The test scores are interpreted by reference to norms or performance criteria.

Examiners who use standardized tests need to find answers to questions found in the sidebar on page 264 for each test selected.

Worthen and Spandel (1991) cite seven common criticisms of standardized tests:

- Standardized tests do not promote learning.

- Standardized achievement and aptitude tests are poor predictors of individual students' performance.

Formal Tests for Assessing Cognitive and Communication Behaviors

Table 9.10

Test	Age Range	Primary Areas Assessed	Measurement Interpretations
Clinical Evaluation of Language Fundamentals–Revised (CELF–R) (1998), Semel, E., Wiig, E., and Secord, W., San Antonio, TX: The Psychological Corporation	5 to 16;11 years	• Listening • Speaking	Norm-referenced
Clinical Evaluation of Language Fundamentals–Fourth Edition (CELF–4) (2003), Semel, E., Wiig, E., and Secord, W., San Antonio, TX: The Psychological Corporation	5 to 21 years	• Listening • Speaking	Norm-referenced
Comprehensive Assessment of Spoken Language (CASL) (1998), Carrow-Woolfolk, E., Circle Pines, MN: American Guidance Service	7 to 21 years	• Listening • Speaking	Norm-referenced
Comprehensive Receptive and Expressive Vocabulary Test–Second Edition (CREVT–2) (1994), Wallace, G., and Hammill, D., Austin, TX: Pro-Ed	4 to 89;11 years	• Listening • Speaking	Norm-referenced
Comprehensive Receptive and Expressive Vocabulary Test–Adult (CREVT–A) (1997), Wallace, G., and Hammill, D., Austin, TX: Pro-Ed	18 to adult	• Listening • Speaking	Norm-referenced
Detroit Tests of Learning Aptitude–Fourth Edition (DTLA–4) (1998), Hammill, D., Austin, TX: Pro-Ed	6 to 17 years	• Thinking • Listening • Speaking	Norm-referenced

Table 9.10—Continued

Test	Age Range	Primary Areas Assessed	Measurement Interpretations
Expressive One Word Picture Vocabulary Test: (EOWPVT–2000) (2000), Gardner, M., Novato, CA: Academic Therapy Publications	2 to 18;11 years	• Speaking	Norm-referenced
Expressive Vocabulary Test (EVT) (1997), Williams, K., Circle Pines, MN: American Guidance Service	2 to 90 years	• Speaking	Norm-referenced
Fullerton Language Test for Adolescents (2nd Ed.) (1986), Thorum, A., Chicago, IL: Riverside Publishing	11 to 18 years	• Listening • Speaking	Norm-referenced
Gray Oral Reading Tests– Fourth Edition (GORT–4) (2001), Wiederholt, J., and Bryant, B. Austin, TX: Pro-Ed	6 to 18;11 years	• Reading	Norm-referenced
Gray Silent Reading Tests (2000), Wiederholt, J., and Blalock, G., Austin, TX: Pro-Ed	7 to 25 years	• Reading	Norm-referenced
Inventory of Essential Skills (1981), Brigance, A., North Billerica, MA: Curriculum Associates	Grade 6 to adult	• Thinking • Listening • Speaking	Criterion-referenced
Let's Talk Inventory for Adolescents (1987), Wiig, E.H., San Antonio TX: The Psychological Corporation	9 to adult	• Speaking	Norm-referenced

Continued on next page

Communication Solutions
for Older Students

Table 9.10—Continued

Test	Age Range	Primary Areas Assessed	Measurement Interpretations
Lindamood Auditory Conceptualization Test–Revised (1979), Lindamood, C.H., and Lindamood, P.C., Austin, TX: Pro-Ed	Preschool to adult	• Speaking	Norm-referenced
Oral and Written Language Scales (OWLS): Listening Comprehension and Oral Expression (1995), Carrow-Woolfolk, E., Circle Pines, MN: American Guidance Service	3 to 21 years	• Listening • Speaking	Norm-referenced
Oral and Written Language Scales (OWLS): Written Expression Scale (1996), Carrow-Woolfolk, E., Circle Pines, MN: American Guidance Service	5 to 21 years	• Writing	Norm-referenced
Peabody Picture Vocabulary Test–III (1997), Dunn, L.M., and Dunn, L.M., Circle Pines, MN: American Guidance Service	2;6 years to adult	• Listening	Norm-referenced
Receptive One-Word Vocabulary Test–2000 (ROWVT–2000) (2000), Gardner, M., and Brownell, B., Novato, CA: Academic Therapy Publications	2 to 18;11 years	• Listening	Norm-referenced
Test of Adolescent/Adult Word Finding (1990), German, D., Chicago, IL: Riverside Publishing	12 to 80 years	• Listening	Norm-referenced
Test of Adolescent and Adult Language–3 (TOAL–3) (1994), Hammill, D., Brown, V., Larsen, S., and Wiederholt, J,. Austin, TX: Pro-Ed	12 to 24;11 years	• Listening • Speaking • Reading • Writing	Norm-referenced

Table 9.10—Continued

Test	Age Range	Primary Areas Assessed	Measurement Interpretations
Test of Auditory Comprehension of Language–Third Edition (TACL–3) (1998), Carrow-Woolfolk, E., Circle Pines, MN: American Guidance Service	3 to 11 years	• Listening	Norm-referenced
Test of Language Competence–Expanded Edition (TLC–E) (1995), Wiig, E., and Secord, W., San Antonio, TX: The Psychological Corporation	9 to 18;11 years	• Thinking • Listening • Speaking	Norm-referenced
Test of Language Development–Intermediate–Third Edition (TOLD–I3) (1997), Hammill, D., and Newcomer, P., Austin, TX: Pro-Ed	8 to 12;11 years	• Listening • Speaking	Norm-referenced
Test of Nonverbal Intelligence–Third Edition (TONI–3) (1994), Brown, L., Sherbenou, R., and Johnsen, S., Austin, TX: Pro-Ed	6 to 89;11 years	• Thinking	Norm-referenced
Test of Pragmatic Language (TOPL) (1992), Phelps-Terasaki, D., and Phelps-Gunn, T., Austin, TX: Pro-Ed	5 to 13;11 years	• Speaking	Norm-referenced
Test of Problem-Solving (TOPS–Adolescent) (1991), Zachman, L., Barrett, M., Huisingh, R., Orman, J., and Blagden, C., East Moline, IL: LinguiSystems	12 to 17;11 years	• Thinking	Norm-referenced

Continued on next page

Communication Solutions
for Older Students

Table 9.10—Continued

Test	Age Range	Primary Areas Assessed	Measurement Interpretations
Test of Problem-Solving Elementary–Revised (TOPS) (1994), Bowers, L., Barrett, M., Huisingh, R., Orman, J., and LoGiudice, C., East Moline, IL: LinguiSystems	6 to 11;11 years	• Thinking	Norm-referenced
Test of Reading Comprehension– Third Edition (TORC–3) (1995), Brown, V., Hammill, D., and Wiederholt, J., Austin, TX: Pro-Ed	7 to 17;11 years	• Reading	Norm-referenced
Test of Word Finding–Second Edition (TWF–2) (2000), German, D., Chicago, IL: Riverside Publishing	4 to 12;11 years	• Listening • Speaking	Norm-referenced
Test of Word Finding in Discourse (1991), German, D., Chicago, IL: Riverside Publishing	6;6 to 12;11 years	• Speaking	Norm-referenced
Test of Word Knowledge (TOWK) (1992), Wiig, E., and Secord, W., San Antonio, TX: The Psychological Corporation	5 to 18 years	• Listening • Speaking	Norm-referenced
Test of Written Expression (1995), McGhee, R., Bryant, B., Larsen, C., and Rivera, D., Austin, TX: Pro-Ed	6;6 to 14;11 years	• Writing	Norm-referenced
Test of Written Language–Third Edition (TOWL–3) (1996), Hammill, D., and Larsen, S., Austin, TX: Pro-Ed	7;6 to 17;11 years	• Writing	Norm-referenced

Table 9.10—Continued

Test	Age Range	Primary Areas Assessed	Measurement Interpretations
Test of Written Spelling–Fourth Edition (TWS–4) (1999), Larsen, S., Hammill, D., and Moats, L., Austin, TX: Pro-Ed	Grades 1 to 12	• Writing	Norm-referenced
Woodcock-Johnson Psycho-Educational Battery–Revised (WJ–R) (1990), Woodcock, R., and Johnson, M., Chicago, IL: Riverside Publishing	2 to 90 years	• Thinking • Listening • Speaking	Norm-referenced
Woodcock Language Proficiency Battery–Revised (WLPB–R) (1991), Woodcock, R., Chicago, IL: Riverside Publishing	2 to 90 years	• Thinking • Listening • Speaking	Norm-referenced
The Word Test–Adolescent (1989), Zachman, L., Barrett, M., Huisingh, R., Orman, J., and Blagden, C., East Moline, IL: LinguiSystems	12 to 17;11 years	• Speaking	Norm-referenced
The Word Test–R (Elementary) (1990), Huisingh, R., Barrett, M., Zachman, L., Blagden, C., and Orman, J., East Moline, IL: LinguiSystems	7 to 11;11 years	• Speaking	Norm-referenced
Writing Process Test (WPT) (1992), Warden, M., and Hutchinson, T., Chicago, IL: Riverside Publishing	Grades 2 to 12	• Thinking	Norm-referenced

Questions Regarding the Use of Standardized Tests

The following questions should be answered to ensure that the test is appropriate for the preadolescent or adolescent and is a valid and reliable measure of performance.

- Is there a clearly stated purpose and definition of the population(s) with whom the test is to be used?

- Is the test content relevant to the purpose of the test?

- What stimulus presentation is used to elicit a response?

- What response mode is used to determine if a response is correct?

- Is the test valid for the population to which it will be administered? Does it have content validity?

- Is the test reliable for diagnosing a communication disorder? Does it have intra-judge and inter-judge reliability?

- What is the rationale on which the test is based? It is based on empirical data, clinical experience, theoretical constructs, or a combination of these?

- Does the test avoid cultural and sexual stereotyping and biases?

- Does it assess communication behaviors in a natural context and in a dynamic, ongoing fashion?

- Are procedures for recording and analyzing responses clearly specified?

- Are normative data available on the preadolescent or adolescent population being assessed?

- Is the sample size adequate? Has the representative sample from the population been adequately described?

- Are the manual instructions to the examiner and to the student clear and concise?

- Does the test documentation clearly list the qualifications needed (e.g., education, experience, certification) by the examiner in order to administer the test?

Sources: American Educational Research Association, American Psychological Association, and National Council on Measurement in Education (1985); American Speech-Language-Hearing Association Ad Hoc Committee on Instrument Evaluation (1986); Boyce and Larson (1983); Larson and McKinley (1987, 1995)

- Test content and curriculum content frequently are mismatched.

- Standardized tests too frequently dictate what is taught in the classroom.

- Standardized tests too frequently mislabel students in ways that are harmful to the students.

- Standardized tests are too frequently racially, culturally, and socially biased.

- Standardized tests measure only limited student knowledge and behaviors.

According to Worthen and Spandel (1991), there are some pitfalls to be avoided when using standardized tests:

- Do not use the wrong tests.

- Do not assume test scores are infallible.

- Do not use a single test score to make a decision.

- Do not forget to supplement test scores with other information.

- Do not set arbitrary minimums for performance tests.

- Do not assume that tests measure all the content, skills, or behaviors or interests.

- Do not accept uncritically all claims made by test authors and publishers.

- Do not interpret test scores inappropriately.

- Do not use test scores to draw inappropriate comparisons.

- Do not allow tests to drive the curriculum.

- Do not use poor tests.

- Do not use tests unprofessionally.

In addition to using formal tests designed to measure the communication skills of preadolescents or adolescents, speech-language pathologists should be aware of additional data that can be gleaned from tests administered by other professionals. For example, intelligence tests administered by psychologists can be a source of information.

To what extent the intelligence test may be used by the speech-language pathologist is contingent upon whether the speech-language pathologist adheres to the strong or weak cognitive hypothesis. According to Casby (1992), the strong cognitive hypothesis states that cognitive development accounts for and is a prerequisite to language development. The weak cognitive hypothesis states that cognitive abilities make certain meanings available for language (e.g., social and language-specific sources), and language has its own specific sources; more specifically, language can influence development of cognition.

Individuals such as those with developmental delays may have language skills that surpass their cognitive or mental ages (Casby, 1992). Despite this finding, the strong cognitive hypothesis or cognitive referencing model continues to influence criteria of eligibility for those who receive speech-language services in the schools (Casby; K. Cole, Mills, and Kelley, 1994). Specifically, cognitive referencing "involves the comparison of measures of language functioning and cognitive functioning to determine the amount of discrepancy between a child's *language* and *mental age*, respectively. When language functioning is significantly below cognitive functioning, the child is said to be eligible for speech-language pathology services." (Rhyner, 2000, p. 1). Casby found that 31 states use cognitive referencing as the basis for their eligibility criteria for speech-language services. Casby stated:

Certainly, cognitive and linguistic skills are highly correlated, yet it has not been established that cognition serves as a necessary or sufficient prerequisite to language development. There is now incontrovertible evidence that the strong cognitive hypothesis does not accurately reflect the relationship between cognition and language. Eligibility decisions that rely on the strong cognitive hypothesis are thus no longer appropriate. (p. 201)

K. Cole et al. (1994) conducted a study to examine the agreement of various cognitive-language profiles to confirm or refute the cognitive referencing model. Their study concluded that the use of the cognitive referencing model or strong cognitive hypothesis to establish eligibility criteria for speech-language services is questionable. Cognitive referencing was discussed in depth by the Special Interest Division 1 group's newsletter (American Speech-Language-Hearing Association, 2000a). This group of language experts have compiled excellent arguments for why speech-language pathologists should not refuse to serve children based on their language level matching their cognitive level. Nickola Wolf Nelson (2000) summed up the crux of the argument with a convincing analogy, which is printed in the sidebar that follows. Also, ASHA (2000b) has recommended the rejection of cognitive referencing in establishing eligibility for language services.

We concur with these authors and do not recommend that speech-language services for preadolescents and adolescents be based on mental age/cognitive ability being greater than language age. Many students whose language age is greater than or equivalent to their mental age can and do profit from speech-language services.

Basing Eligibility on Discrepancy Criteria:
A Bad Idea Whose Time Has Passed

Mr. Sweeney went to his physician because his blood pressure was elevated. The lab work-up also showed a problem with Mr. Sweeney's blood sugar. When it was time to discuss treatment, however, Mr. Sweeney's doctor reported that he was very sorry, but Mr. Sweeney was not eligible for treatment. In addition to the blood pressure problems and symptoms of diabetes, it seemed that Mr. Sweeney had a diagnosis of obesity. The other conditions were commensurate with the obesity, the physician explained, and because there was no discrepancy, Mr. Sweeney did not qualify for treatment.

This scenario may see far-fetched, but its equivalent is enacted regularly in school districts and clinics across America. Children who have difficulty acquiring normal communication skills on their own are denied services because their tests show commensurate levels of cognitive development.

It is ridiculous to think that a physician would deny treatment for a condition with major life implications that could respond to treatment simply because it could be correlated with another condition. In actuality, the physician might work in collaboration with a nutritionist and exercise specialist to design an individualized program that will help Mr. Sweeney improve his condition in several areas. It is equally ridiculous to think that many children are denied treatment for communication difficulties simply because their language difficulties are correlated with cognitive limitations. Yet, that is what happens when professionals apply cognitive referencing and discrepancy as the primary, or even sole, criterion to decide whether children with suspected learning disabilities or with mental retardation or pervasive developmental delay "qualify" for services.

One might argue that there are major differences between the two situations. The important variables are whether the treatment is needed and whether it can be expected to be effective, not the lack of discrepancy. I will not belabor the analogy, but I will argue that need for special services and expectation for change, in fact, are better criteria to apply in determining who needs what kinds of service than the discrepancy criterion and that neither can be adequately predicted by cognitive referencing. In other words, I will suggest that cognitive referencing should not be used as a substitute for more direct methods of determining need and expectation for change. Research evidence and dynamic assessment both show that children with flat profiles are capable of change when they receive the services they need.

From "Basing Eligibility on Discrepancy Criteria: A Bad Idea Whose Time Has Passed," by N.W. Nelson, 2000, *ASHA Special Interest Division 1, Language Learning and Education* [Newsletter], 7(1) p. 8. © 2000 by the American Speech-Language-Hearing Association. Reprinted with permission.

Points of Discussion

1. Describe several specific informal assessment tasks that would permit the examiner to gather integrated information on learning style, cognition, emotional intelligence, social skills, comprehension and production of linguistic features, discourse, written communication, meta-abilities, and/or nonverbal communication.

2. Discuss what variables you would use to critique existing standardized tests.

Suggested Readings

Damico, J. (1991). Clinical discourse analysis: A functional approach to language assessment. In C. Simon (Ed.), *Communication skills and classroom success: Assessment and therapy methodologies for language and learning disabled students.* Eau Claire, WI: Thinking Publications.

Hughes, D., McGillivray, L., and Schmidek, M. (1996). *Guide to narrative language.* Eau Claire, WI: Thinking Publications.

Chapter 10

Directed Tasks for Assessment

Goals

- Define directed tasks for assessment and describe their commonalities

- Present eight directed tasks that can be used to assess the language skills of older students

- Explain analysis procedures and provide interpretation guidelines for the eight tasks

Directed tasks are structured assessment procedures that require students to demonstrate specific communication skills. The focus of these tasks is on the process the older student uses to perform each task; a correct product is frequently irrelevant (McKinley and Larson, 1998). Also, each directed task should be followed with appropriate metacognitive, metalinguistic, and/or metacommunication questions. For example, consider questions such as:

- What did you have to think about to solve that problem? What went on in your mind?

- How did you figure out what was important to listen to?

- Was that direction difficult for you to understand? Why?

- What words were unfamiliar to you?

- What made that story (message, direction) difficult to tell?

• Do you think that was a clear message? Do you think I understood what you meant? Why didn't I understand what you meant?

These types of questions help determine what the individual knows about cognitive functions and communication. A student who has little "meta-" awareness is likely to be more impaired than one who has awareness but inconsistent application.

Directed tasks that are difficult for preadolescents and adolescents should be administered a second time, with slight variations, following metacognitive, metalinguistic, and/or metacommunication questions. This will permit the examiner to comment on the adolescent's prognosis for modification, given a structured learning experience. For example, one of the directed tasks in this chapter has the student use his or her knowledge of the organization of a grocery store (see page 272). If the adolescent fails to handle this task, the examiner could question the adolescent about knowledge of cognitive functions, such as categorization (e.g., "Do you know what some grocery store categories are?") and systematic exploration (e.g., "Do you know how you would systematically look for an item in a grocery store?"). Once these metacognitive questions are successfully discussed, the examiner might present a new problem slightly different from the first. For example, "If I sent you to a drugstore to buy aspirin, cotton balls, and toothpaste, how would you find those items?" Students who can transfer cognitive functions such as categorization and systematic exploration to this new situation would be viewed as having greater potential for learning and a more promising prognosis than those who fail to benefit from metacognitive, metalinguistic, and metacommunication discussions.

Problem Solving
Areas Assessed

The following informal assessment task for problem solving provides information primarily on cognition, but it also provides data on conversational abilities when the problem-solving task involves dialogue.

Administrative Steps

1. Say to the student, **"Let's talk about how you would handle some problem situations. Here's the first one. You try to turn on your TV with the remote control and nothing happens. You're surprised because the TV was on just a few minutes ago. Tell me about the problem."** Pause and wait at least five seconds for a response. If the student does not generate an appropriate response, repeat the situation and cue the student. If necessary, model a correct response. Once the student has satisfactorily answered or you have modeled a response, say, **"Okay. Now tell me about the**

problem by asking me a question." Pause and wait for a response. Prompt for the question form. If the student appears not to understand, model the question (e.g., "Why doesn't the TV start?"). Write the question to be answered on a piece of paper and place it in front of the student.

2. Ask the student, **"What are the ways you could answer that question?"** Pause and wait for a response. If the student says nothing, ask the question written on the paper, shrug your shoulders, and ask, **"Why?"** Usually students will say at least a generic answer like, "It's broken." That is one answer, but prompt for additional options such as "The TV is unplugged" or "The batteries in the remote control are dead." If necessary, provide these answers yourself and write them on the piece of paper below the question.

3. Ask, **"What is the best answer?"** Review the list of answers and have the student pick one. Ask, **"Why did you choose that one?"** Record the rationale.

4. Say, **"Let's make a plan to check out your best answer. What would you do next?"** (e.g., "The remote control batteries are dead"—Change the batteries and see if the TV can be switched back on.) Prompt for the student's best answer.

5. Ask, **"How will you know if your answer is the best one?"** Pause and wait for a response. Prompt as needed for a response that the TV will turn on. Ask, **"If the TV doesn't turn on, what will you try next?"** Wait for the student to choose another answer. Say, **"Let's make a plan to check out your second best answer. What would you do next?"** Prompt for an appropriate answer. Then ask, **"How will you know if that answer worked?"** Again, wait for a response like "The TV will turn on." Prompt as needed. As a last resort, supply the response.

6. Repeat Steps #1–5 with a similar problem situation: **"You just popped a movie into your DVD player. You hit the remote control's Play button, but nothing happened. What is the problem?"** Select one or two additional problem situations, or create your own based on what would be meaningful to the student (e.g., **"You have a 10-page paper due for English tomorrow and you haven't started the assignment. What is the problem?"**). Repeat Steps #1–5, adjusting questions and content to fit the new problem.

Analysis Procedures

1. On a scale of 1 to 5 (1 = independent of prompts; 5 = dependent on prompts), rate how well the student

performed during each of the problem-solving steps for situations presented. Record the student's data using a form such as Appendix Q: *Problem-Solving Recording Form.*

2. Note whether the student developed more independence as additional problem situations were presented. In particular, compare Problem #2 with Problem #1, since Problem #2 was a slight variation of Problem #1. Analyze whether performance improved toward more independence.

3. Study the student's answers during Administrative Step #3. Analyze the strength of the student's rationales and logical reasoning.

Interpretation Guidelines

- If the student does not correctly identify the problem to be solved, focus intervention on framing the problem in the form of a question to be answered.

- If the student provides only one or two alternatives (answers) and fails to generate more with prompting, focus intervention on teaching divergent thinking skills. In addition, mediate how to study a problem from many different perspectives.

- If the student fails to choose the best solution and/or to generate a logical rationale for that solution, focus

intervention on comparing and contrasting features of alternative solutions (e.g., time, money, hassle, long-term effects) and logical reasoning skills.

Organization

Areas Assessed

The informal assessment task for organization provides information primarily on cognition. However, because the task involves a dialogue between the examiner and the preadolescent or adolescent, the task may also provide discourse and "meta-" data.

Administrative Steps

1. Be prepared to record student responses on a sheet of paper throughout this step and the six that follow. Say to the student, **"Pretend I sent you to a new grocery store to buy carrots, milk, and ice cream. How would you find these items?"** Pause and wait for a response. After each idea proposed by the student, list it on a piece of paper, then ask, **"What else? How could you find these items?"** Continue prompting or, if necessary, model responses until these strategies are listed: Ask for help; look for signs; search up and down the aisles; and/or walk around the outside aisles of the store.

2. After the discussion of finding items in the grocery store, present a similar scenario for another store. Say, **"Now pretend I'm sending you to a drugstore. You need to buy aspirin and a toothbrush and cotton balls. How would you find these items?"** Pause and wait for a response. After each idea proposed by the student, list it on a piece of paper and ask, **"What else?"** The first three strategies as listed in Step #1 should be given again.

3. If the student does not need much help with the drugstore scenario, skip directly to the next step. If the student needs nearly as much help with the drugstore as the grocery store example, present a third scenario (e.g., **"Now pretend I send you to a hardware store. You need to find a garbage can, some small nails, and a screwdriver. How will you find these items?"**). Repeat the list of strategies and prompt as needed.

4. Ask the question, **"What other stores are organized?"** The student can name any store and be accurate. Once a store is named, ask, **"How is it organized?"** If the student needs prompting, use a store that is familiar in your geographical area.

5. Say to the student, **"Pretend to go to another building now. Let me send you to a school. How are schools organized?"** Pause and wait for the student to respond. Prompt for responses like grade levels, subject areas, and teachers' classrooms.

6. Ask the question **"Why is it important to organize schools?"** If necessary, model responses for the student. Then ask, **"Why do people organize grocery stores and other kinds of stores?"** Again, model responses if need be. Ask, **"Can you think of something that is not organized?"** If the student names something (e.g., a room in the house or a teacher's classroom), ask, **"How could it be organized?"** Help prompt for responses, if necessary. Then ask, **"Can everything be organized?"** Guide the student to realize the answer to that question is yes, by challenging the student to name what can't be organized, then to mediate how it could be organized.

7. Interview one or more teachers familiar with the student. Also interview one or more family members. Ask these individuals how organized or disorganized they perceive the student to be. Have them provide specific examples for both.

Analysis Procedures

1. Analyze how many different strategies for finding items in a store the student

could report. Note whether performance improved from the grocery-store to the drugstore (to the hardware store scenario) to stores named during Administrative Step #4.

2. Study the student's responses to "How are schools organized?" Judge how much support you had to give the student to generate several responses.

3. Based on responses during Administrative Step #6, determine whether the student has any awareness of the pervasiveness and the importance of organization.

4. Compare the student's performance on the organizational tasks to the examples reported by teachers and family members.

Interpretation Guidelines

• If the student has no strategies, or only one or two, for finding an item in an organized setting, and teachers or family members cite examples of disorganization that concern them, focus intervention on organizational strategies.

• If the student is disorganized and has a lack of awareness of the importance and utility of being organized, provide mediation that provides "meta-" skills related to organization (e.g., the student can eventually explain the high cost in time or money of being disorganized).

Giving and Getting Directions

Areas Assessed

The informal assessment task for giving/getting directions provides information on comprehension and production of linguistic features. It is expected that older students can give and receive multistep directions. This task can also provide data on cognition and conversation. Nonverbal communication, especially gestures, can be observed.

Administrative Steps

1. Agree on a board game or video game that is appealing and familiar to the student.

2. Have the student describe how the game is played. The board game or video game should not be present during the description. However, have paper and a pencil available in case the student wants to sketch part of the description.

3. As the student describes the game, ask scaffolding questions when the student deletes essential information or request clarification of low-information words.

4. Explain that you are now switching to a task that requires the student to follow ("get") directions. Using the school floor plan presented in Appendix R, instruct the student to

follow these directions (step-by-step direction-following is allowed for Steps a and b):

a. **"Start in 7th grade science and go out the door.** (pause) **Turn left and go to the first hallway that turns left.** (pause) **Turn left and walk to the fourth door on your right.** (pause) **Where are you?"** (6th grade office) Describe the student's performance.

b. **"Start in the art room and walk out the door.** (pause) **Turn left and go to the first hallway.** (pause) **Turn left and walk past the big open area.** (pause) **Walk past the hallway that turns left to the main entrance and enter the first door on your left.** (pause) **Where are you?"** (Special Education room) Describe the student's performance.

c. Tell the student to listen to the entire direction before taking any action. Then say, **"Start in the auxiliary gym. Go out the left door, walk straight ahead down the hall, and turn right into the third door. Where are you?"** (The janitor's closet) Describe the student's performance.

d. Tell the student to listen to the entire direction before taking any action. Then say, **"Start in the computer room. Go out the**

door and turn left, go to the end of the hallway and turn left again, then walk a few steps. Where are you?" (By the display area and the office for Special Education.) Describe the student's performance.

e. Tell the student to listen to the entire direction before taking any action. Then say, **"Start in the choral room. Take the ramp down to the Commons, walk straight ahead, turn right out of the Commons, go past two hallways, and turn into the second door on your left. Where are you?"** (7th grade-E) Describe the student's performance.

f. (NOTE: A key element has been left out of this message; to successfully complete it, the student must ask for clarification.) **"Start in the staff room for the girls' lockers. Go through the girls' lockers and out the door, then go two doors down. Where are you?"** (You can't know until you ask which door to use and if you should go left or right out of the locker room.) Describe the student's performance.

g. (NOTE: A key element has been left out of this message; to successfully complete it, the student must ask for clarification.) **"Start in 8th grade science. Go out the**

door and turn right until the first hallway, jog over and go to the second door. Where am I?" (You don't know until "jog over" is better defined.) Describe the student's performance.

Analysis Procedures

1. Analyze the student's giving of directions for organization, clarity, and precision:

    *   Could the listener follow the directions?

    *   Was the listener confused?

    *   Were essential elements consistently omitted that were necessary in the directions?

    *   Did the student include essential elements when prompted by the examiner?

    *   Were low-information words used?

    *   Did verbal mazes and/or false starts obscure the intended message?

2. Determine the student's accuracy in following (getting) directions:

    *   Were all common concept words understood (e.g., *left, right, first, second)?*

    *   Did the student retain multiple steps of the directions, or were directions needed step by step?

*   How was clarification requested when directions were incomplete?

Interpretation Guidelines

*   If the listener is confused because of low-information words, verbal mazes, and deletion of essential elements when the student is giving directions, focus intervention on vocabulary and clarity of message sending.

*   If the student does not clarify or revise directions when prompted to do so, include communication-repair strategies in intervention.

*   If the student is challenged by following directions and lacks strategies for getting them repeated or clarified, focus intervention on pragmatically appropriate ways to ask for repetition, clarification, and/or presentation in another medium (e.g., writing).

Topic Management
Areas Assessed

According to Mentis (1994), topic management is critical to coherent conversational discourse. She goes on to state that if it is an area problematic to the student, it can be severely penalizing to all aspects (i.e., social, academic and vocational) of the individual's lifestyle. One reason students may find topic management problematic is that it is multifaceted, including all areas of topic introduction and management. (NOTE: Do not do this informal assessment task unless difficulty was found in conversational discourse and topic management was assumed to be problematic.)

Administrative Steps

1. Using conversational starters and engaging students in topics of conversation of their choice, collect a 10-minute sample. Record it for later review.

2. Using Appendix S: *Topic Tally,* keep a tally of the number of topics and subtopics introduced as well as the manner and direction (types) of topics and subtopics. (This serves as baseline data to begin to evaluate more completely whether the problem exists at the linguistic level, cognitive level, and/or social level and to evaluate the influence of textual, interpersonal, situational, topical and genre conditions on topic management (Mentis, 1994)).

3. See the sidebar on page 278 for a complete assessment protocol developed by Mentis (1994) to identify and evaluate the student's ability to engage in topic management. Keep this sidebar handy for reference during administration.

4. Compare the number of topic manners and directions tallied on Appendix S. Determine if your observations fit into one of the three areas

listed under "Other Observations" on the form.

Analysis Procedures

As noted in the sidebar on page 278, topic management skills of the student should be carefully analyzed to determine if the problem is in the area of linguistic factors. That is, does the student have sufficient syntactic forms, lexical items, and semantic understanding needed to both introduce and maintain topics? For example, in the introduction of topics, does the student use adverbial conjuncts, questions, relative clauses, etc.? In terms of maintenance, does the student use appropriate pronouns, comparative adjectives, conjunctions, noun phrases, etc.? Does the student use compensatory strategies when difficulties in syntactic or semantic levels occur?

It is also important to analyze the student's performance to determine if cognitive factors are interfering with topic management skills. For example, are there problems in the student's general world knowledge, organizational knowledge structures (e.g., scripts), or attention and memory? Can the student use compensatory strategies when a cognitive factor problem occurs? Also, the examiner should evaluate the contribution of social factors to problems in topic management, as well as textual, interpersonal, situational, and genre conditions on topic management. Mentis (1994) recommended evaluating the student's topic management skills in the context of the classroom to determine the

Assessment of Topic Management

Identify whether a problem in topic management exists.

Identify which components of topic management are disrupted.
- Introduction
  - Number of topics/subtopics introduced
  - Manner of topic/subtopic introduction: change, shift, inappropriate tangential shift, noncoherent change
  - Type of topic/subtopic introduction: (a) new, related, reintroduced; (b) content (e.g. concrete/abstract)
- Maintenance
  - Length of topic/subtopic sequence
  - Type of topic maintenance contribution
    - New information: requests for novel information, requested information that is provided, unsolicited information
    - No new information: agreement/acknowledgment, repetition of old information, passes and discourse markers, clarification and confirmation requests and statements
    - Side sequences: environmentally triggered, politeness markers
    - Problematic: ambiguous, unrelated, incomplete

Evaluate contribution of linguistic factors to problems in target topic management parameters.
- Is the full range of syntactic forms, lexical items, and semantic relations needed to perform topic management functions available?
  - Introduction
    - Examples of structures that perform topic introduction functions: adverbial conjuncts, discourse particles, questions, relative clauses, conjunctions
  - Maintenance
    - Examples of structures that perform topic maintenance functions: pronouns, comparative adjectives, and determiners (reference cohesion), ellipsis, conjunctions, subordinate clauses, noun phrase postmodification through the use of prepositional phrases and appositive constructions, participial phrases, infinitive phrases, gerund phrases, modal auxiliaries, and verb tensing
- Are strategies to compensate for syntactic and/or semantic difficulties used and do they have a positive or negative effect on topic management?
- Can the required syntactic forms be acquired, or must compensatory strategies be taught?

Evaluate contribution of cognitive factors to problems in target topic management parameters.
- Are there problems in topic-related areas of cognition?
  - For example: general world knowledge, underlying organizational knowledge structures such as scripts and schemas, attention, and memory
- Are strategies used to compensate for problems in topic-related areas of cognition, and do they have a positive or negative effect on topic maintenance?
- Can the required topic-related areas of cognition be acquired, or must compensatory strategies be taught?

Evaluate the contribution of social factors to problems in target topic management parameters.

Evaluate the influence of textual, interpersonal, situational, topical, and genre conditions on topic management.

influence of the teacher, classroom interactions, and the academic curriculum on the student's abilities.

Interpretation Guidelines

- Once the data have been analyzed on the various factors mentioned above and indicated in the previous sidebar, the examiner should note if the major problems are at the cognitive, linguistic, or social levels. If serious problems exist at any of these levels that interfere with the student's ability to engage in topic management, intervention should occur. As noted by Mentis (1994), topic management is a critical skill to the student's success in being able to carry on a conversation and, in turn, develop a meaningful lifestyle across the age range.

- The nature of the intervention should take into account whether cognitive, linguistic, or social problems exist. Topic maintenance should not be treated as an isolated problem within the system.

Informational Listening

Areas Assessed

The informal assessment task for informational listening provides information on comprehension and production of linguistic features. This task may also assess narration

if the task is structured to do so (i.e., when retelling of the information is requested).

Administrative Steps

1. Obtain a 5- to 10-minute lecture (preferably videotaped) from a classroom teacher that is appropriate to the student's current grade level. Alternatively, simulate a lecture by orally presenting information from a section of one of the student's textbooks as a teacher would in a classroom. Ask the student factual questions about the content of the lecture (e.g., **"What was the main idea or main point to the lecture?"** and **"What details were presented to support the main point of the lecture?"**).

2. Obtain a second taped lecture, of equal difficulty to the first, accompanied by a printed outline that guides the student's listening. Ask the student factual questions about the content of the lecture.

3. Obtain a third taped lecture on a topic of great interest to the student but of equal difficulty to the first two lectures. Determine interest ahead of time by interviewing the student, a friend of the student, or a family member. Ask the student factual questions about the content of the lecture.

Analysis Procedures

1. Record the student's responses to factual questions regarding main ideas and relevant details on a form such as Appendix T: *Listening Skill Recording Form*.

2. Compare the student's percentage of correct answers to questions regarding the main ideas and relevant details to the actual answers for each condition.

3. Determine how the student's accuracy of answers varies based on changes in conditions.

Interpretation Guidelines

- If a student consistently answers questions incorrectly under all three lecture conditions, create listening situations such as presenting main ideas and relevant details about a given topic or asking questions about the information (see Larson and McKinley, 1995).

- If a student responds more accurately to questions when a written listening guide is present, teachers who expect classroom listening should be encouraged to prepare such guides and supply them to their students.

- If a student performs noticeably better while listening to a topic of great interest, the student might need counseling about selective listening and its negative consequences.

Critical Listening

Areas Assessed

The informal assessment task for critical listening provides information on discourse. The task also provides data on cognition, since critical listening strongly parallels critical thinking. (NOTE: Omit this directed task if all informational listening tasks indicated poor performance.)

Administrative Steps

1. Obtain taped advertisements and political speeches of relatively short length and brief content.

2. Ask the student questions about the stimulus content, such as false reasoning, prejudices, inferences, and biases. Be prepared to explain each type of content to the student.

3. Ask the student to express his or her overall impressions of what was heard in the advertisement or political speech (i.e., to summarize the message).

Analysis Procedures

1. Record the student's responses to all questions on a sheet of paper.

2. Analyze the student's responses to determine if he or she follows a consistent pattern (e.g., correct responses to factual questions but incorrect responses to opinion questions).

3. Compare the student's critical listening abilities to the student's problem-solving or other cognitive skills, since critical listening assumes a certain cognitive sophistication.

Interpretation Guidelines

• If the student consistently answers questions incorrectly across stimulus conditions, focus intervention on the student's cognitive abilities being enhanced.

• If the student inconsistently answers questions across stimulus conditions and adequately responds to problem-solving situations, focus intervention on enhancing informational listening skills.

Question Asking and Answering

Areas Assessed

The informal assessment task for question asking and answering provides information primarily on comprehension and production of linguistic features. Within a conversation, this task can also provide data on discourse. (NOTE: Do not do this directed task if a sufficient number of questions have been generated during other tasks. Skip directly to Analysis Procedures.)

Administrative Steps

1. Present one or all of the following tasks for asking questions:

    a. Use a Jeopardy quiz-game format in which the answer is supplied and the student generates the question.

    b. Direct the student to ask a question given an imaginary situation (e.g., **"How would you ask a stranger what time it is?"**)

    c. Role-play situations that require question-asking behavior (e.g., role-play an English teacher and have the student role-play someone who has missed several days of school and consequently has missing assignments).

2. Present tasks for answering questions such as the following:

    a. Role-play interviewing a student for a job.

    b. Present questions that request action (e.g., **"Would you mind moving over a seat?"**) or state information (e.g., **"Can you believe we're having another test in science?"),** and determine if the student understands what appropriate responses would be.

c. Ask questions with the same semantic intent with increasing syntactical complexity (e.g., **"Who is the president? What is the name of the president?"**).

Analysis Procedures

1. Analyze question-asking skills.

    a. Analyze the syntactic structure and semantic intent of the student's questions for appropriateness to the situation.

    b. Analyze the student's questions to determine that a variety of question forms exist and are stated clearly and concisely.

    c. Analyze to determine whether questions are asked in a pragmatically appropriate manner.

2. Analyze question-answering skills.

    a. Record answers to questions and analyze which ones are comprehended.

    b. Analyze question answers to determine if the student is answering a *why* question with a causal explanation, not a *what* description.

Interpretation Guidelines

- **Asking questions**—If a variety of question types are not asked, focus intervention on developing that variety. If all question types are not asked,

the student has restricted strategies for gaining new information and should be taught to use the missing question types appropriately.

- **Answering questions**—If a student does not answer appropriately a variety of question types, focus intervention on responding to questions in situations such as in the classroom, community, and home.

Word Retrieval

Areas Assessed

The informal assessment task for word retrieval provides information on comprehension and production of linguistic features and discourse. While the administrative steps below involve contrived situations, word-retrieval problems noted during this task are also likely to be observed within natural discourse samples. This directed task does not need to be completed if word-retrieval skills are not suspect.

Administrative Steps

1. Determine the presence or absence of a semantic deficit by obtaining a baseline measure of receptive vocabulary. Measure the student's ability to define words, to identify likenesses and differences, and/or to state synonyms and antonyms (Wiig and Becker-Caplan, 1984), or administer formal receptive vocabulary tests.

(The student's receptive vocabulary performance should be compared to either chronological or mental age to confirm or refute the presence of a semantic deficit.)

2. Once the presence or absence of a semantic deficit has been documented, measure naming accuracy and rate with a variety of tasks, such as sentence completion, naming an item upon description, rapid automatic naming, and word association (Wiig and Becker-Caplan, 1984). Snyder and Godley (1992) recommend that the examiner systematically assess those intrinsic and extrinsic variables that influence naming behavior. The following are intrinsic variables that affect naming:

   - The frequency with which words occur (i.e., the more frequently a word occurs, the easier it is to retrieve)

   - The age of acquisition (i.e., the earlier the word is acquired, the easier it is to retrieve)

   - The category type (i.e., prototypic categories such as fruits and vegetables are easier to retrieve than words from well-defined categories, such as months of the year, in which there is a small set of semantic features)

   - The degree of abstractness (i.e., the more concrete the word, the easier it is to retrieve)

   - The word class (i.e., it is easier to name concrete nouns than to name verbs, adjectives, and abstract nouns)

Similarly, the following extrinsic variables influence naming (Snyder and Godley, 1992):

   - Whether the naming is in context, such as that required in a sentence-completion task, which is easier than confrontational naming (i.e., naming a pictured object)

   - Syntactic requirements (i.e., the more difficult the sentence construction, the more difficult the word-retrieval task)

   - Whether the task requires discrete naming, which is easier than continuous instances of naming

   - Priming, which is the influence of the preceding word or words on the individual's ability to retrieve or recall a target word

3. Both intrinsic and extrinsic variables need to be taken into account when assessing a student's word-retrieval abilities. Also assess the behaviors that are indicative of word-finding difficulty, such as the nature of word substitutions (e.g., semantically related errors, phonologically related errors, visual perceptual errors, or same grammatical class errors) and performance characteristics such as accuracy (e.g.,

Is the target word retrieved on the first response? What is the speed of the response?). If the semantic deficit is determined to be present, attempt to restrict words to be retrieved to those known to be within the student's current vocabulary. If no semantic deficit is found, use words commensurate with the documented receptive vocabulary level.

Analysis Procedures

Examine data to determine the presence of a semantic deficit, a word-retrieval problem, or a combination of the two. If it is unclear which problem is more pervasive (i.e., low vocabulary or lack of word-retrieval skills), Wiig (1983) has suggested an analysis of the student's response to multiple choices. For example, if a student is pausing to find a word, supply a choice of three or four words; the individual with low vocabulary will not necessarily be assisted by multiple choice, whereas the individual with word-retrieval problems will appear to instantly recognize the desired word.

Interpretation Guidelines

- Everyone experiences word-retrieval problems some of the time. However, if word-retrieval problems are consistently present not only in naming confrontation situations but also during discourse, then a deficit area is in need of intervention.

- Students found to have deficient vocabulary, either with or without the presence of word-retrieval problems, should be considered for intervention.

Points of Discussion

1. What other directed tasks have you used with older students, or do you project could be developed?

2. Critique the eight directed tasks. Which one(s) do you think would reveal the most information about a student who is struggling with following instructions in the general curriculum and who has social skill deficits? Justify your answer.

Suggested Readings

Gillam, R., Pena, E., and Miller, L. (1999). Dynamic assessment of narrative and expository discourse. *Topics in Language Disorders, 20*(1), 33–47.

Mentis, M. (1994). Topic management in discourse: Assessment and intervention. *Topics in Language Disorders, 14*(3), 29–54.

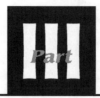

Part

Language Intervention
with Adolescents

Service Delivery Models and Issues

Goals

- Delineate reasons for serving older students with communication disorders

- Discuss service delivery options for older students with communication disorders

- Explain how to implement educational and environmental system modifications that assist older students with communication disorders

Intervention with older students who have communication disorders is paramount for their survival at school, at home, and in the community. Unfortunately, the provision of intervention by speech-language pathologists may appear inconsequential. Intervention may be considered an extra, a "frill," and certainly an expense that can be eliminated from a budget.

On the contrary, intervention for older students who have been diagnosed as having communication disorders is one of the most crucial services to provide, since the crux of students' problems often rests on their lack of adequate skills. Without intervention, the risk is great that these youth will engage in antisocial behaviors and experience school performance failure leading to personal injury, incarceration, or an unemployed or underemployed adulthood.

Rationale for Services by Speech-Language Pathologists

For speech-language pathologists who are committed to providing intervention for older students, the reasons for providing services may be challenged. Administrators or decision-makers may ask, "If students with communication disorders couldn't be 'cured' during their elementary years, why should additional services be provided by speech-language pathologists during adolescence? Why isn't the language work they receive in English and other classes enough?" To these questions, the following six counter-arguments can be offered:

1. Older students with communication disorders need continued assistance from speech-language pathologists to learn the higher level concepts and vocabulary demanded at each grade. Many of these students require special services to remain in the mainstream through the elementary grades; their need does not stop upon entrance into middle and senior-high levels. In fact, these very transitions may heighten students' needs as they move from one educational level to the next or from one educational setting to another.

2. "Turning over" language instruction to other professionals usually ensures that students will be taught communication

for academics, but not for social and vocational areas, which according to the 1997 Individuals with Disabilities Education Act (P.L. 105-17 known as IDEA '97) must be taught. IDEA '97 mandates that educators assist the student in learning the language of academics, and of nonacademic and extracurricular activities. Other professionals are concerned primarily with academic content, using communication as a vehicle to achieve their curriculum goals. Moreover, these educators are expected to teach this content in restricted time frames to large groups of students with varied needs. The speech-language pathologist may be the only professional who is concerned primarily with communication, using content (academic, social, and vocational) to achieve speaking, listening, reading, writing, and thinking goals. It is also the speech-language pathologist who has been specifically educated to break down the complexities of the communication process. A speech-language pathologist has the expertise to determine the finite steps that provide a language scaffold for students to learn and achieve communication goals for school, home, and community settings.

3. Students generally make the transition from the concrete period into the formal period of cognitive development at the adolescent level (Piaget and Inhelder, 1969). The formal

level of thinking permits students to consider new realms of possibilities; students are no longer tied to the present. Learning abstract concepts that require formal operational thought is required at the secondary level for most courses. Students who have not reached this level of cognitive growth will require supportive services to help master curriculum concepts.

4. Strong programs for adolescents with communication disorders, in combination with other special programs (e.g., those for learning disabilities and vocational education), have been effective in reducing dropout rates to well below the national average (C. Flores, personal communication, July 8, 2002). Nationwide, the percentage of 16- through 24-year-olds who are not enrolled in a high school program and have not completed high school is 11.8%, an estimate consistent over the past decade (Kaufman, Kwan, Klein, and Chapman, 2000). Studies have also documented that weekly earnings are substantially increased when workers have completed high school, and they are greatest for those who have a 2- or 4-year degree and for those who possess higher literacy skills (e.g., $355 per week for those with Level 1 literacy skills, vs. $531 for Level 3 literacy skills and $910 for Level 5 skills; Sum, 1999).

5. Speech-language pathologists need to document precisely the growth in language development that occurs over time with adolescents who are receiving intervention. This documentation of language growth is convincing evidence that intervention does make a difference for these students and that significant progress can be made in oral and written communication skills.

6. Taxpayers will ultimately pay for older students with communication disorders at some point—if not in high school, then during their later years in the form of adult literacy programs, basic job training, unemployment compensation, incarceration, or in the form of other attempts to reverse the pattern of failure. Wouldn't it be prudent to hire more full-time speech-language pathologists in the middle and high schools to help lessen the often predictable burden to society as these youth mature into adults?

Appropriate intervention that teaches older students communication skills for academic, social, and vocational situations is the key to their ability to "fit" into society— to function as family members, lifelong learners, citizens, participants in leisure, and as consumers and producers of goods and services (Apel, 1999b; Larson and McKinley, 1995; Rhea Paul, 2001; Valletutti and Bender, 1982). These are not just nice intervention goals or accomplishments to adhere to, but simply stated, it is the law! IDEA '97 mandates that the curriculum taught must result in the student being able to compete and achieve in today's society.

This chapter addresses how speech-language pathologists can best intervene with older students to help them function as effective communicators—so that they succeed at school, at home, and in the community.

Service Delivery Models

Historically, service delivery to all students with communication disorders has undergone change, with the focus of the speech-language pathologist's role changing from specialist in the 1970s, to expert in the 1980s, to a collaborative consultant in the 1990s (Blosser and Kratcoski, 1997). The focus of treatment in 2000 was outcome-based, with the speech-language pathologist functioning as a facilitator of service delivery.

A number of service delivery models have been discussed by the American Speech-Language-Hearing Association (1999) regarding the facilitation and selection of an appropriate model for an individual student with a communication disorder. These models are described in the sidebar that follows.

This range of options allows the speech-language pathologist to select and a student to experience more than one option depending on the student's needs. Moore-Brown and Montgomery (2001) and ASHA (1996)

noted that three important concepts should drive all service delivery model decisions:

1. Service delivery is a dynamic process that must change depending on the needs of students.

2. A variety of service delivery models should be used, and no one model should be used exclusively.

3. Regardless of the model chosen, time must be set aside for collaboration/ consultation with parents, other educators, and service providers.

Appropriate service delivery for older students must be carefully selected or their cooperation with intervention will be minimal. Primary choices for service delivery options for older students are suggested in Figure 11.1, and they are discussed next.

Traditional Delivery Model

Traditionally, services by speech-language pathologists have been delivered through pull-out models (i.e., removing students from classrooms in which they are struggling and providing services in an isolated therapy room). While younger children are excited to be singled out for such attention, older children often react negatively. At an age during which students' desire to conform—not to appear different than their peers—is greatest, the undesired "visibility" of leaving an existing class or study period may sabotage intervention. Furthermore, removing older students

Service Delivery Options

Monitor: The speech-language pathologist sees the student for a specified amount of time per grading period to monitor or "check" on the student's speech and language skills. Often this model immediately precedes dismissal.

Collaborative Consultation: The speech-language pathologist, regular and/or special education teacher(s), and parents/families work together to facilitate a student's communication and learning in educational environments. This is an indirect model in which the speech-language pathologist does not provide direct service to the student.

Classroom-Based: This model is also known as integrated services, curriculum-based, transdisciplinary, interdisciplinary, or inclusive programming. There is an emphasis on the speech-language pathologist providing direct services to students within the classroom and other natural environments. Team teaching by the speech-language pathologist and the regular and/or special education teacher(s) is frequent with this model.

Pullout: Services are provided to students individually and/or in small groups within the speech-language resource room setting. Some speech-language pathologists may prefer to provide individual or small group services within the physical space of the classroom.

Self-Contained Program: The speech-language pathologist is the classroom teacher responsible for providing both academic/curriculum instruction and speech-language remediation.

Community-Based: Communication services are provided to students within the home or community setting. Goals and objectives focus primarily on functional communication skills.

Combination: The speech-language pathologist provides two or more service delivery options (e.g., provides individual or small group on a pullout basis twice a week to develop skills or preteach concepts and also works with the student within the classroom).

From *Guidelines for the Roles and Responsibilities of the School-Based Speech-Language Pathologist* (p. 273), by the American Speech-Language-Hearing Association (ASHA), 1999, Rockville, MD: Author. © 1999 by ASHA. Reprinted with permission.

from study periods for intervention is equivalent to removing younger students from recess in earlier grades. Another disadvantage of the pull-out model is the discontinuity of intervention and classroom instruction. Students are still expected to know the information presented during class while they are out of the room for intervention.

Collaborative Consultation Delivery Model

To coordinate speech-language goals and academic content, a model of choice has increasingly been collaborative consultation. Collaboration and consultation are independent concepts: "collaboration defines

Figure 11.1

Service Delivery Model Options

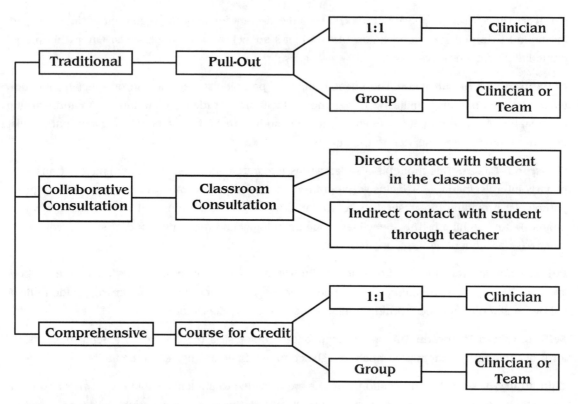

From *Language Disorders in Older Students: Preadolescents and Adolescents* (p. 154), by V. Lord Larson and N.L. McKinley, 1995, Eau Claire, WI: Thinking Publications. © 1995 by Thinking Publications. Adapted with permission.

how we interact" and "consultation defines the process" (Coufal, 1993, p. 4). Collaborative consultation may take one of three basic forms, as shown in the sidebar that follows.

While classroom consultation is a viable, practical intervention model for preschool and elementary students, the educational system is structured counterproductively with respect to consultation at upper grade levels. With whom might a speech-language pathologist collaborate? Once students reach middle grades and beyond, classroom teachers focus on curricular content, almost to the exclusion of basic skills. Since oral language skills are assumed to be intact within older students by most classroom teachers, few will appreciate the benefit of taking class time to focus on such skills. And if a professional were to pull a small group aside within a classroom, it is frequently more embarrassing to a pre-teen or teen than resorting to the traditional pull-out model.

Forms of Collaborative Consultation

1. **The formula model**—The speech-language pathologist and collaborative partner plan lessons weekly. Each then teaches a lesson to a different group of students in the classroom.

2. **The communication enhancement model**—The speech-language pathologist guest-teaches a demonstration lesson for all students while the classroom teacher assists.

3. **The curriculum-based model**—The speech-language pathologist notes the language of instruction in the classroom, then provides complementary lesson components and advises how language can be taught to students in an effective and efficient manner.

Source: C. Simon and Myrold-Gunyuz (1990)

Since oral language skills are assumed to be intact within older students by most classroom teachers, few will appreciate the benefit of taking class time to focus on such skills.

There are some unique challenges to collaborative consultation at the secondary level, and these challenges are listed in Table 11.1. As seen in the table, six characteristics and challenges must be resolved if the older student with a communication disorder is to benefit from a classroom inclusion model of intervention. These challenges help illustrate why this is often not the best choice for older students.

At the same time, speech-language pathologists need to be cognizant of analyzing general education curricular goals, designing goals and objectives that focus on the student's success in meeting general education requirements, and interacting in partnership with other educators so that the student can be successful in the classroom setting.

Consultation at the secondary level is most feasible when it occurs between the speech-language pathologist and another specialist (e.g., a learning disabilities specialist, or a school-work transition liaison). These educators, like the speech-language pathologist, have a vested interest in the communication skills of students. Team-teaching situations involving the speech-language pathologist and another specialist can also be very powerful for effecting changes in preadolescents and adolescents.

Silliman et al. (1999) presented an inclusion model for intervention, basing

Unique Challenges to Overcome during Collaborative Consultation at the Secondary Level

Table 11.1

Characteristic	Challenge
Many secondary-level students demonstrate basic skills that plateau at the 4th to 5th grade level when they reach the 10th grade.	The amount of time needed to teach the required number of complex skills exceeds the amount of time that can reasonably be allocated to instruction in the mainstream classroom.
The existing structure at the secondary level tends to be large-group instruction.	The student with a language disorder often needs intensive, small-group teaching to make progress.
The existing curriculum at the secondary level assumes higher order skills.	The student with a language disorder has strategy deficits that are not present in students experiencing success in the mainstream.
Teachers have significant autonomy within their subject areas.	Teachers often need to be convinced that a consultation model is important for some of their students. Once that is accomplished, they need to be further convinced that consultation with the speech-language pathologist is an intricate link with their content area.
Secondary-level teachers see their students only 50 minutes per day, approximately.	Since the secondary teacher spends very little time with a given student compared to the elementary teacher, his or her understanding and addressing the student's strengths and areas of need are more difficult through a consultation model.
Secondary-level students (especially early adolescents) want to "blend into the peer group."	Doing something that calls attention to the special needs of a student in front of his or her peer group may be more devastating than working with students "out of sight" from others (e.g., using a comprehensive model or classroom setting).

their discussion on the premise that "the question is no longer if intervention will involve curricula or be classroom based but rather how intervention will be provided in this context" (p. 1). They noted that the discussion should center around whether the intervention will involve full inclusion or optional inclusion. Full inclusion advocates contend that all students should be provided with an equal opportunity to have their educational needs met in the regular education classroom. Whereas those who advocate optional inclusion, which is a more middle ground choice, recommend that while access to regular education should be a priority for all students, more critical is that the placement be selected on the basis of the student's needs. This position coincides with the 1997 provision of IDEA.

Many professional groups, such as the American Speech-Language-Hearing Association (1996) and the Learning Disabilities Association (LDA; 1993), as well as parent organizations, argue that the full inclusion model does not meet the educational and communicative needs of every student with a language disorder or learning disability. It should be noted that with the approval of IDEA '97, a number of market-driven changes in school practice have taken place (Huffman, 2000). They are delineated in the sidebar.

Comprehensive Delivery Model

The most effective intervention model, advocated by us since 1983, is the prototype service delivery model (Boyce and Larson, 1983; Larson and McKinley, 1987, 1995; Larson, McKinley, and Boley, 1993; McKinley and Larson, 1985), which we have since

---

Market-Driven Changes in School Practice

- Analyzing the general education curricular goals and designing individualized education programs (IEPs) focusing on student success in meeting general education requirements

- Conducting student assessment in the context of classroom performance and expectations, resulting in using dynamic and authentic assessment procedures and curriculum-based assessment

- Interacting in partnership with general educators so that the student can be successful in the classroom setting

- Delivering services where the student can learn most effectively, which might be in the classroom using materials such as the textbook, software, and so on

Source: Huffman (2000)

renamed the comprehensive delivery model for secondary-level students (Larson and McKinley, 2002). The essence of this model is that services are provided by the speech-language pathologist through a class that has the same requirements as any other course the student takes (i.e., it meets for so many minutes each week, a grade is given, and credit is granted toward high school graduation). This model is uniquely different from the traditional pullout model and the much advocated collaborative consultation model, which grew out of the Regular Education Initiative (REI) several decades ago.

The comprehensive delivery model consists of six major components:

1. Information dissemination
2. Identification
3. Assessment
4. Program planning
5. Intervention
6. Follow-up

Table 11.2 presents details of the model. All six components must be intact to ensure that appropriate services are provided to older students with communication disorders. Mutual interdependency exists among components. A missing component, or lack of coordination, will result in disparate services.

Each of the six components of the delivery model includes direct and indirect services. *Direct services* refer to activities in which the speech-language pathologist has actual contact time with adolescents who are, or may be, viable candidates for intervention. For example, selectively screening adolescents with suspected communication disorders, assessing adolescents, and providing remediation are direct services in the sense that the interactions are between the speech-language pathologist and the adolescent.

Indirect services refer to activities in which the speech-language pathologist does not have actual contact time with adolescents. Rather, the clinician assists, trains, and consults with other persons important to adolescents (e.g., a teacher, a parent, or a friend) for the benefit of the adolescent with a communication disorder. For example, teaching other professionals to utilize a referral form to identify adolescents with suspected communication disorders and organizing parent support meetings are indirect services. Table 11.2 shows what are considered direct and indirect services for older students.

Whenever indirect services are discussed hereafter, reference will be to the adolescent's educational and environmental systems. The *educational system* encompasses the adolescent's structured learning situations and the speech-language pathologist's interactions with professionals and paraprofessionals in those settings. Learning situations may be traditional (e.g., a senior high school) or nontraditional (e.g.,

Comprehensive Delivery Model
for Secondary-Level Students

Table 11.2

	Who?	Information Dissemination		Identification		Assessment	
		What?	**How?**	**What?**	**How?**	**What?**	**How?**
Direct	**Adolescents** **Early** **Middle** **Late**	Expectations and problems Normal developmental data Benefits of adequate communication Self-referral process Prevention	Publications Career days, job fairs Classroom lectures Intake screening	Match-mismatch with expectations for communication	Self-referral Selective screening	History Learning style Emotional intelligence Social skills Cognition Linguistic features Discourse Written communication Meta-abilities Nonverbal communication	Informal assessment procedures Interviews Questionnaires Checklists Profiles Oral and written samples Rubrics Portfolios Directed tasks Formal assessment instruments
Indirect	**Educational system members**	Expectations and problems Normal developmental data Benefits of adequate communication Referral process How related professionals can help the adolescent Prevention	Inservice Media Telecommunications	Match-mismatch with expectations for communication	Observational checklist referral form	Structure of educational system Teacher language and classroom routines Curriculum variables	Structure of educational system checklist Self-evaluation technique Curriculum analysis form
	Environmental system members	Expectations and problems Normal developmental data Benefits of adequate communication Referral process How family and friends can help the adolescent Prevention	Media Telecommunications Informational and support meetings	Match-mismatch with expectations for communication	Observational checklist referral form	Family members Peer group Employment setting	Interviews Observations Checklists

Continued on next page

Communication Solutions for Older Students

Table 11.2—Continued

Who?	Program Planning		Intervention		Follow-Up	
	What?	How?	What?	How?	What?	How?

Direct — **Adolescents** Early Middle Late	Adolescent's involvement
	
	Adolescent's motivation
	
	Program selection
		Writing goals and objectives
		
		Motivational procedures
		
		Selecting programs
			Thinking
			
			Listening
			
			Speaking
			
			Reading
			
			Writing
			
			Meta skills
			
			Nonverbal communication
			
			Paralinguistic skills
				General procedures
				  Learning strategies
				  Mediation
				  Bridging
				  Enhancing skills
				    Speaking
				    Listening
				    Reading
				    Writing
				  Specific intervention methods
				    Referential communication
				    Narrative activities
				    Expository activities
				    Word-finding activities
				    Emotional intelligence activities
				    Social skills activities
					Baseline data
					
					Benefits of program
						Study design
						
						Survey methodology
						  Interviews
						  Questionnaires

Indirect — **Educational system members**	Educational policies and procedures
	
	Consultation
	
	Peer involvement and attitude modification
		Administrator's involvement
		
		Collaborative approach
		
		Peer tutoring
			Modifications of the system	Consultation
				  Organization of curriculum materials
				  Classroom discourse
				  Oral language/ written language of textbooks
				  Peer tutoring
					Benefits of services for adolescents
					
					Benefits of consultation model
					
					Benefits of counseling
						Survey methodology
						  Interviews
						  Questionnaires

Environmental system members	Alteration or maintenance of parent's attitudes and behaviors
	
	Awareness of referral agencies
	
	Sibling acceptance and involvement
		Informational and support meetings
		
		Newsletters, phone campaigns, home visits
		
		Sibling tutoring
			Modifications of the system	Oral language
				
				Learning environment
				
				Attitudes and feelings
					Benefits of services for adolescents
					
					Benefits of consultation model
					
					Benefits of counseling
						Survey methodology
						  Interviews
						  Questionnaires

From *Communication Assessment and Intervention Strategies for Adolescents* (inside back cover), by V. Lord Larson and N.L. McKinley, 1987, Eau Claire, WI: Thinking Publications. © 1987 by Thinking Publications. Adapted with permission.

homebound instruction for hospitalized youth; instruction at a juvenile delinquency center for incarcerated adolescents). The professionals who may be involved within the educational system are classroom teachers, administrators, special educators, social workers, psychologists, guidance counselors, nurses, and probation officers. The paraprofessionals who may be involved are teacher aides, communication aides, and peer tutors.

The *environmental system* refers to family members and peers who interact with the adolescent with a communication disorder. Obviously, the educational system is a part of the environmental system. Since the educational system plays a major role during adolescence, that system is presented as a separate area within indirect services.

While an individual adolescent might receive only direct services or only indirect services, it is more common that a combination of direct and indirect services is needed.

Information Dissemination

The first component, information dissemination, refers to educating people about adolescents' communication disorders and varied characteristics. Information dissemination is synonymous with what business calls "marketing the product." The average person—and sometimes even those within the discipline of communication sciences and disorders—

does not know what can be done for adolescents with communication disorders or how best to proceed.

Normally, a speech-language pathologist's position is already in existence in a school district, but a position to work specifically with the adolescent population frequently needs to be created. Professionals must express with clarity and conviction why a school board should add a new speech-language pathologist position at the secondary level. Without such information dissemination, professionals are vulnerable to being considered an expendable service, thus putting at risk any guarantee of appropriate services to adolescents with communication disorders.

Visibility of speech-language pathology services must also be heightened for adolescents themselves (direct services) as well as for persons important to the adolescent (indirect services). The identification component is activated once adolescents and the people around them become aware of what constitutes a communication disorder and how they might benefit from intervention. Until people know what constitutes a communication disorder during adolescence, what impact such a problem can have on the individual, and what intervention services can be provided, referral for a suspected disorder will not occur.

Communication Solutions
for Older Students

Until people know

what constitutes a

communication disorder

during adolescence, what

impact such a problem can

have on the individual,

and what intervention

services can be provided,

referral for a suspected

disorder will not occur.

Identification

The second component in the comprehensive delivery model is identification, the process of defining which adolescents have a suspected communication disorder that warrants further evaluation by a speech-language pathologist. Many agencies rely on screening for identification. The term *screening* refers to "the use of a systematic procedure to identify provisionally those (individuals) from a population who manifest, or are likely to manifest, an attribute which is judged to require special attention" (Hill, 1970, p. 1). While screening may be viable for young populations, it is inappropriate for adolescents. First, the time it would take to screen is not warranted.

Second, no screener exists that would be sensitive enough to pick up the range of communication problems that might be contributing to a student's poor performance.

As an alternative to screening, we recommend using Table 6.1 (see page 133) as a reference for educating key people in the lives of students with suspected communication disorders. Once others—such as administrators, school psychologists, and classroom teachers—recognize the characteristic problems of older students with communication disorders, appropriate referrals can be made for investigating the suspected disability, following all the IDEA '97 regulations for this activity. Table 6.1: Characteristic Expectations and Problems of Older School-Age Students with Language Disorders allows speech-language pathologists and colleagues to use a match-mismatch model, which detects students who fail to match the expectations of others within a particular environment (e.g., a high school).

A referral form based on Table 6.1 is available in Appendix A. We recommend that speech-language pathologists serving older students use this form and or create a variation (e.g., one that captures unique features of a given student population or community).

Assessment

Assessment, the third component in the comprehensive delivery model, is the thorough documentation of communication performance. This component of the comprehensive delivery model was addressed in depth in Part II of this text; consequently that information will not be repeated here. Simply recall that assessment should confirm or reject initial impressions of a communication disorder observed during identification and should determine if it constitutes a disability that adversely affects academic performance and warrants special services. In addition, assessment should document the awareness that adolescents have about their disorder, and their motivation to modify their communication behaviors. Adolescents with documented communication disorders who acknowledge their problems and are willing to work to improve their communication may be better candidates for program planning than adolescents without these traits.

Program Planning

The fourth component, program planning, is the connecting link between assessment and intervention. Before effective intervention can occur, an appropriate individualized education program (IEP) must be drafted; IDEA '97 specifies that this program must tie to the general education curriculum. In addition, IDEA (§ 602 [30]) mandates that older students with disabilities must also begin preparing for transition by age 14. A plan must be in place for the student's movement from school to post-school activities (e.g., vocational training, post-secondary education, or integrated employment). Note that the IEP teams must specifically address the development of skills that students need to master to hold a job.

Program planning occurs both before an adolescent's entrance into intervention, as well as during the adolescent's involvement. Ongoing and direct program planning might involve contracting with the adolescent to learn specific behaviors, or earning points toward a quarterly grade for communication improvement. Indirect services related to program planning might include planning with teachers how to modify curricula or how to modify the learning environment for the benefit of the adolescent.

Planning should directly involve the adolescent whenever possible. For example, adolescents may offer suggestions for their own goals and objectives. In fact, it is desirable for them to do so to have them "buy into" the intervention process. Unlike younger clients who willingly cooperate and who are often thrilled with the speech-language pathologist's stickers or other reinforcers, adolescents are often reticent to take advantage of intervention. Thus, careful program planning is needed to ensure appropriate cooperation. Motivation can usually be enhanced by a variety of techniques, such as those that follow.

Course for Credit

Developing successful intervention programs in which older students are willing to participate is paramount. Recognition of the student's efforts by offering communication intervention as a course at the middle-school or junior-high level and as a course for credit (e.g., one-half credit per semester) at the senior-high level is probably the single most important factor in the development of these programs. In these courses, students invest at least as much time and energy working on their communication skills as they do on other skills taught in courses for credit.

Our idea of a course for credit can be traced back to a high school student in Wisconsin who wondered if he could get credit for intervention after observing he spent as much time and effort on his communication disorder as on singing in choir or building something in industrial arts. His school board ultimately agreed, and he was granted credit. Thus, the course or course-for-credit model can be applied to one student at a time, or to groups that might grow to 10 or 12 students. The course may meet several times a week or daily, depending on the structure of the school schedule and the amount of credit being granted for the intervention time.

If a decision is made to offer communication intervention as a course for credit, it should be determined whether this is to be an elective course or whether a required course can be waived (i.e., credit for the communication course can substitute for a required course credit, such as that for English). The speech-language pathologist and the student need to determine which option is most suitable (i.e., elective or substitute). Questions to consider when making this decision are listed in the sidebar.

Should Intervention Be a Required Course or an Elective?

- Is the student attempting to function in required mainstream courses but failing, or nearly failing, one or more? If so, is the failure resulting from poor comprehension of vocabulary and concepts, or from the high cognitive demands of the curriculum? When one or both factors are contributing significantly to failure in a required course, a rationale can be built for the student to receive a waiver from that course on the grounds that insufficient language and cognitive skills inevitably prevent success in the course. When the communication course replaces the class being failed, prerequisite language and cognitive abilities become goals and objectives in the student's IEP.

- What other electives are in competition with the communication course? Students with language disorders, especially those who need intervention at the secondary level, frequently wish to take vocationally oriented classes, which usually are offered as electives. These students need flexibility to take these electives because the courses are important for their future vocational success. Also, these students are often more motivated to participate in elective courses than in required courses. Since these same students may be at risk for dropping out of school, they must be kept in courses that spark their interest. If there are many electives in which the student is interested, it might be best to build a rationale for communication intervention being offered as substitute credit.

Grading

Offering communication intervention courses entails giving grades for student performance. Giving a letter grade or using a satisfactory/fail system, as other courses would, is appropriate. If the communication course is substituting for a required course, a letter grade may be mandatory if this is the grading policy for other required courses. Another option is to grade by progress, resulting in a description of performance and not a letter grade. Grading by progress most accurately reflects performance on individual goals and objectives and could possibly be combined with other mandatory grades.

Even when communication intervention is not organized as a course for credit, grading should be explored as an option. As much as grades appear to be aversive to students, they are inherent in the student's educational experience. Grades are a way to give credibility to intervention. Several options exist regarding their use. They are captured in the sidebar.

Keep in mind that IDEA '97 mandates that progress of students with IEPs needs to be reported to parents as often as reports are made to parents of students without disabilities. Students need to understand that grading will occur and realize when and how grades will be reported. Appendix U illustrates an example progress grading report that contains essential elements to consider for older students.

Grading Options

- Assign a percentage of the grade to each course requirement (e.g., 25 percent for class discussion, 25 percent for projects, 25 percent for examinations, and 25 percent for daily assignments).

- Assign points for participation and work completed and remove points for inappropriate behaviors. At the end of a grading period, have a minimum number of points needed for each letter grade.

- Have the student's performance in communication intervention contribute to a percentage of the student's grade in another course. For example, if the student is being removed from part of English class for intervention, propose to the English teacher that a portion of the student's grade be determined by his or her communication performance.

- Request a space on the student's regular report card for communication performance, and record a letter grade or satisfactory/fail notation.

- Include a communication progress report with the student's regular report card.

Communication Solutions
for Older Students

A word of warning about grading should be given here. In school districts honoring communication intervention as a course for credit and permitting letter grades, other teachers and parents may raise validity questions: "Is an A or a B given for communication intervention of less value than an A or a B earned for algebra?" "Should an A or a B in communication intervention contribute the same to class rank as an A or a B in English?" Since class rank affects scholarship and college admission decisions, to name just a few issues, the impact of grading for communication intervention may have broad implications. At least one school district we know of resolved the dilemma by disallowing grades for special courses, such as the communication intervention course, in class-rank calculations. This was not a supportive decision for the adolescents with disabilities in that school system, but it was the best compromise that could be struck among the speech-language pathologist, parents, teachers, and school board members.

Scheduling

Another motivational issue to consider is scheduling the communication course so the student receives appropriate intervention, rather than token services. Meeting twice a week for 20 or 30 minutes using a pullout model is almost never sufficient to help older students make significant progress in communication behaviors. What may happen during these short time blocks is that the student may experience some

success but become frustrated further when the intervention time cannot be extended.

A more viable means to schedule intervention is to use existing time modules and to have the administrator who sets the class schedule incorporate the course like all other subject areas. Meeting for full-time modules will allow more time for intervention and will eliminate the problems in middle, junior high, and senior high schools caused by students entering a class after 20 minutes of intervention or leaving a class midway to go to intervention. This obvious entering and leaving causes disruptions and is one more way youth with communication disorders seem different from their peers.

While an obvious solution to scheduling might appear to be removing students from resource rooms or media center time, caution is advised. Some students offer such extreme resistance to intervention during their individual study time, if it even exists in their schedules, that they refuse to participate. Others disrupt sessions so severely that they need to be removed. From the perspective of the professional, these youth may be using their time inefficiently for academic activities, but students may insist on personal nonclass time for social reasons or for relaxation.

Other students, particularly those in early adolescence, often willingly accept being removed from study time for intervention. They may have few friends with whom to relate socially during study time, and they may possess few acceptable relaxation outlets (e.g., reading a book or writing a letter). They would rather work on structured objectives and activities with the speech-language pathologist than work on homework assignments for which they lack basic skills. These homework assignments can be used as the medium for achieving communication goals, but with extreme caution, lest your colleagues begin to view you as a tutor. When homework is used, it should become the medium for teaching new strategies or providing application opportunities for strategies previously taught.

Acceptable Course Titles

The speech-language pathologist must consider and select titles for courses that students feel comfortable using. "Speech Therapy" or "Language Therapy" may be unacceptable titles for students with communication disorders trying to appear similar to their peers. Better titles might be "Individualized Communication Class" or "Communication Strategies." The title selected is also important because it will appear on the student's report card and transcript, which may be seen by future employers. The confidentiality of the student's past history of intervention should be protected by choosing transcript wording carefully.

Areas of the School

Providing intervention services out of the mainstream areas of the school is frequently viewed negatively by older students. A room located in a part of the school that is perceived as part of the mainstream is less likely to carry a negative image.

Many times, because of overcrowded conditions, the speech-language pathologist cannot have a private classroom throughout the day that is large enough for groups of students to meet. However, a classroom somewhere in the building is generally open because secondary-level teachers have staggered preparation periods.

Providing speech-language services out of the mainstream areas of the school is frequently viewed negatively by older students

Given a willingness to be flexible and to tote their materials from classroom to classroom, speech-language pathologists can meet in areas of the school viewed positively by older students. As a toehold is gained for the profession of communication sciences and disorders at the middle and secondary levels, buildings being constructed or remodeled should take the speech-language pathologist's space needs into account.

Communication Solutions
for Older Students

Intervention

Intervention, the fifth component in the comprehensive delivery model, refers to any method of ameliorating or reducing the communication disorder within the adolescent. One of the primary goals of intervention during the period of adolescence is acquisition of functional communication for academic, personal-social, and vocational settings. As such, intervention will involve a coordination of efforts among a variety of professionals who may be working with the adolescent in different environments.

- The Stage I early adolescent will tend to have intervention goals and activities directed toward functional communication for academic and personal-social settings.

- The Stage II middle adolescent will often have functional communication goals for all three settings: academic, personal-social, and vocational.

- The Stage III late adolescent will have goals of intervention focused most often on personal-social and vocational settings.

Intervention for a given adolescent may include direct or indirect services, or a combination of the two. Intervention will vary in intensity and content, depending on the individual needs of the adolescent. Ongoing assessment and program planning during intervention, whether it be direct or indirect, are necessary to remain most responsive to the changing needs and abilities of youth with communication disorders. The last part of this chapter, as well as the remaining chapters within Part III, continues to address the intervention component.

Follow-Up

The last component in the comprehensive delivery model is follow-up. *Follow-up* refers to any activity designed to measure the real and perceived benefits of services delivered by a speech-language pathologist. The activity may occur while the older student is still in the secondary school system, or post high school. We believe that the discipline of communication sciences and disorders has not validated its intervention approaches. For a given communication disorder, little evidence exists that approach X is more successful than approach Y.

Research shows a "continuum of failure" as children grow older (i.e., young children with language deficits often have residual problems during adolescence; C.J. Johnson et al., 1999). If they do receive intervention during the secondary level, what model is being used and how much progress is occurring? Will these youth continue to experience significant communication problems during their post high school years? Only valid follow-up studies can begin to answer these questions.

Research shows a

"continuum of failure" as

children grow older.

Adolescents who receive services from speech-language pathologists might be involved in follow-up activities, or other adults might be used as informants. If follow-up activities are used, they should occur both during and after services are terminated. We have created a follow-up survey procedure that can be easily adapted and implemented in individual programs. It is found in Appendix V. The data from these surveys can be used to demonstrate the effectiveness of the program delivered by the speech-language pathologist, which can be a major factor when budget cuts threaten the future of services for secondary-level students with communication disorders. In addition, students should make journal entries to get filed in their portfolios that address topics like those shown in the sidebar.

Choosing to implement a comprehensive delivery model does not negate other service delivery options. Many professionals organize their schedules so that part of the day is spent delivering services through each of the major models. The main goal is to match the student's needs with the most appropriate delivery model. Failure to do so will sabotage even the most brilliant lesson plan.

Portfolio Questions

The following are questions that might be used as follow-up documentation for progress made in communication intervention.

- How have your communication skills improved?

- How has the communication program helped you be a better student?

- What language skills have you learned that will help you be a better worker?

Comparing responses to the same questions over several years helps document the growth in communication skills brought about through the intervention program. These qualitative data can also carry weight when decisions are being made about the amount of staff time to make available for older students.

The remainder of this chapter revisits the intervention component within the comprehensive delivery model. The focus is on indirect intervention with older students. Then Chapters 12 and 13 are dedicated to direct intervention ideas for older students.

Indirect Intervention

Indirect intervention involves people from the student's educational and environmental support systems in activities that assist the youth to communicate more effectively. Of most concern are those students who have communication disorders accompanied by problems within their support systems at school, at home, or in the community (e.g., they are having difficulty understanding the language that teachers use in the classroom, that parents use at home, or that supervisors use at work).

During indirect intervention, the speech-language pathologist attempts to effect positive modifications for the student without face-to-face contact with that student. More often, direct and indirect intervention occur simultaneously, and three-way interchanges occur (e.g., a work supervisor, the student, and the speech-language pathologist are concurrently involved).

When the student's deficits revolve around language, two main choices can be made: Either the educational and environmental systems need to be modified to meet the existing performance of the student, or the student's performance must be changed to cope with the systems. Again, in reality, both activities may occur simultaneously. Of the two choices, we strongly advocate for the second (i.e., change the student's performance). This approach is addressed in detail in the Chapters 12 and 13. Time is running out for the student to receive intervention during secondary school, so the more independent the student can become at recognizing and voicing the modifications needed in his or her environment to cope with the language demands, the better the chances are for adjustment in school, home, and community settings.

Modifications of the Educational System

When the educational system is modified to meet the language needs of older students, changes might occur in these areas:

- The organization of curriculum materials
- The oral language of the educator during classroom discourse
- The written language of textbooks and other printed materials
- The use of peer tutors

When approaching modifications of the educational system, professionals need to remember that deficiencies could exist in the system itself, which compound the older student's communication disorder. For example, the curriculum materials may be sequenced inappropriately, demand cognitive abilities that exceed the student's present capacity, or require written responses that surpass the student's ability level. (See Appendix D for how to analyze the curriculum.) The oral language of the teacher may be too rapid, complex, or disorganized for the older student to comprehend. Perhaps the teacher is using too many unfamiliar vocabulary terms or lengthy sentences. (See "Teacher Language and Classroom Routines" on page 188 in Chapter 8 for how to analyze the teacher's language). Likewise, the written language of the textbook and other materials may be too complex or many contain an abundance of novel terminology.

When approaching modifications of the educational system, professionals need to remember that deficiencies could exist in the system itself, which compound the older student's communication disorder.

Organization of Curriculum Materials

The overall organization of the curriculum is typically generated by a curriculum committee that formally reviews specific content areas every few years. Often this process is linked with new textbook selection. Speech-language pathologists should make known to administrators, department heads of specific academic areas, and classroom teachers that they are uniquely qualified to appraise the language and cognitive demands of the curriculum, as they affect students with language disorders and learning disabilities. We urge speech-language pathologists to volunteer for curriculum committees in their local communities.

In some schools, volunteering to serve on a curriculum committee meets with quick

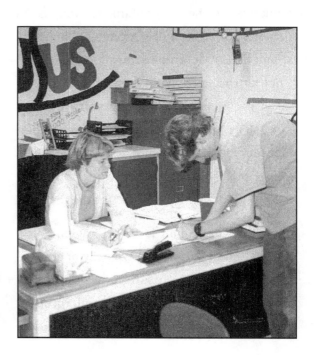

approval. In other places, the voluntary request will be suspect and the speech-language pathologist may have to launch a campaign to educate others as to how the discipline of communication sciences and disorders may contribute positively to the outcome of the curriculum committee.

Often, professionals can make inroads on elementary-level curriculum committees before they can at the middle and high school levels. A phone call from the elementary principal to the secondary principal may remove roadblocks more quickly than other approaches, assuming the elementary principal speaks positively about the benefit of input from speech-language pathologists.

Once appointed to serve on a curriculum committee, the speech-language pathologist should analyze the language and cognitive demands of the curriculum as well as its organization from a developmental language standpoint. A determination should be made whether the curriculum is sequential or spiral in nature. Recall that in a spiral curriculum, skills gradually build upon each other; in a sequential curriculum, content and skills are relatively independent and each new topic provides a "fresh start" for the student.

If the curriculum is to be implemented with students performing typically and those with disabilities, a cross-section of performance may be needed from both groups. Through these types of efforts, some schools develop alternative curricula or "schools within schools" to serve at-risk students and those with marginal academic skills. The pendulum swings back and forth in education as to whether such tracking of students is "good" or "bad" policy. In the 1990s, one of the passwords was "inclusion," and a modified curriculum occurred in response to every individual's unique needs. The reality of implementing this concept in a classroom with dozens of students has remained challenging. In the 2000s, the passwords have shifted to "benchmarks" and "standards" and "access to the general education curriculum." Literacy is paramount, as is standardized test performance. Students with marginal academic skills have remained a challenge in mainstream classrooms, and achieving the standards required in the general education curriculum continue to elude these students.

Speech-language pathologists should also be involved when committees are formed to review and modify the curriculum in special education areas. The special education curriculum naturally includes language and communication as areas to teach. However, the scope and sequence of objectives may be organized inappropriately, or important objectives may be missing. Relevant objectives may not be considered, especially if special education aligns itself in a parallel fashion with general education and teaches the same curriculum, only at a slower rate. For example, social communication objectives might be overlooked because they are not part of the curriculum for general education students.

Speech-language

pathologists should also be

involved when committees

are formed to review and

modify the curriculum in

special education areas.

In some cases, language goals might be buried in other areas of the curriculum. For example, the concept of "left-right" might be a goal tucked in the "adaptive physical education" area of the curriculum. Teachers may fail to grasp the strong language component contained within such goals. Speech-language pathologists can assist other special educators in seeing the pervasiveness of language within their curricula.

Oral Language of the Educator during Classroom Discourse

Good teaching involves adjustment of the form and content of messages to reflect an awareness of the needs and feelings of students. When selecting discourse style for the classroom,

> Teachers use a combination of prior knowledge about the expected linguistic and cognitive abilities of their students along with immediate verbal and nonverbal feedback. In this way, they adjust their speaking styles to fit the presumed capabilities of the children they teach. (N. Nelson, 1984, p. 175)

Students outside the educator's expected group norm for language ability will have difficulty succeeding in that teacher's classroom. Occasionally, educators will overshoot the majority of the group, as reflected by such student comments as, "Nobody understands what's going on! I think Mr. B. talks to himself most of the time." Teachers may also undershoot, as reflected by student comments such as, "This class is so easy, it's boring! She must think we're babies." The teacher language evaluation forms in Appendixes B and C were developed so that teachers can gain their students' perceptions and compare them against their own.

Once the speech-language pathologist has established a firm relationship with the classroom teacher, that teacher can be encouraged to use several speaking styles for his or her students. For example, the rate of delivery may need to be slowed down, the information may need to be repeated, or perhaps the content may need to be handed out in a study guide too. When students look perplexed, a re-explanation using more concrete language should follow. If the teacher's spoken language is excessively cluttered by verbal mazes, false starts, and revisions, the use of clearer messages and questions should be encouraged. These teachers in particular might be encouraged to use listening guides that capture main ideas and relevant details that students are expected to comprehend. If teachers are resistant to developing listening guides (often those who are in need of the most change are the ones least likely to accept help or are the most defensive), then speech-language pathologists can develop study guides by using notes from students who are performing well in the class. Politically, relationships remain more amicable in school settings when teachers are not forced to make modifications, even when those changes are desirable for students.

How the teacher responds to student requests for clarification, even those that seem unnecessary at the time, will set the learning tone in the classroom. Perhaps most of us can remember a teacher in our past who ridiculed or embarrassed students for asking a question or for confessing to a lack of understanding. Students attempting to survive in these classrooms quickly learned that it was safer to say nothing at all and to suffer the consequences (e.g., completing an assignment incorrectly) than to risk the ire of the teacher.

How the teacher responds to student requests for clarification, even those that seem unnecessary at the time, will set the learning tone in the classroom.

Speech-language pathologists should encourage teachers to remain receptive to student questions, to share that receptive attitude with students, and to resist making the assumption that the students' questions are irrelevant. For example, directions may appear clear to educators because of their familiarity with the material but be ambiguous to students. Rather than reacting negatively to a question, educators might pursue a student's perspective by countering with a question like, "What is confusing you about the directions?"

When student requests for clarification are global (e.g., "I don't get it! Say it again"), teachers should help these students isolate the information that was not understood and then restate the question more precisely. Often, students do understand some of the directions, but they lack the necessary skill to ask a specific question about what was not understood.

Sometimes discourse rule differences between regular classrooms and resource programs may complicate school language for students with communication disorders. For example, if the resource room is informal and students can ask questions whenever they arise, students may have difficulty adjusting to teachers who expect questions for clarification to be asked only at particular times, such as before or after class. The student who blurts out questions informally may be judged by the classroom teacher as "bumbling" or rude (Donahue, 1985). A signal system might be devised between the teacher and the student so that the student knows when the behavior is appropriate. Also, during direct intervention, judging when to ask questions and when to hold them could be emphasized with the student.

Teachers should also realize that indirect requests (e.g., saying, "Don't you know you're supposed to begin reading Chapter 6 as soon as the bell rings?" to stop a student from engaging in a conversation) are frequently misunderstood by students with language disorders. Frequently, they miss the illocutionary force of indirect requests.

Rather than assuming that indirect requests for action are understood, the teacher could ask students to explain what is expected. Perhaps better yet, for some students, is for the teacher to make direct requests until comprehension of indirect requests is taught as a specific communication skill.

Written Language of Textbooks and Other Printed Materials

For many older students with language disorders and learning disabilities, the reading level of classroom textbooks is too high for them to comprehend without modifications. One such modification is to color-code textbooks for students with some reading skills but for whom the amount of print is overwhelming. When color-coding textbooks, one color or several might be used. For example, a yellow highlighter might be used for main ideas, a blue highlighter for relevant details, and a green highlighter for new vocabulary words. If multiple colors prove to be confusing to students, then the system should revert to a simple one-color approach. The challenge is to leave more words that are not highlighted than are highlighted. When multiple books from different subject areas are being coded, an identical system of colors should be used, which will require agreement among professionals.

For many older students with language disorders and learning disabilities, the reading level of classroom textbooks is too high for them to comprehend without modifications.

Communication Solutions
for Older Students

Initially, classroom teachers should do the color-coding, since they are most familiar with the material and with their expectations for students' performance. However, during consultation, a plan should be devised whereby the students are gradually taught to color-code the textbooks themselves. The plan should also include who will be responsible for teaching the skill of color-coding to students.

Sometimes, the greatest resistance to color-coding comes from administrators who fear color-coding will damage textbooks. One solution is to start with older textbooks that will be phased out in the next few years and which may already be worn. Professionals should assure administrators that there will always be a group of older students who need the assistance of color-coded textbooks. Once books are coded, they will still be very useful to future students. Another solution is to obtain permission to photocopy chapters from the chosen textbooks and to teach color-coding skills through the use of those copies. Ideally, students should learn how to color-code for themselves, and they can practice only when they have their own copies. Color-coding may become increasingly more important as students enter postsecondary learning experiences and are expected to learn independently.

Another viable modification when it comes to the written language of textbooks is to make available audiotape recordings of the material. This permits students to listen and relisten to the printed information for specific content areas. A number of states, as well as the Library of Congress, have books on tape already recorded for students with visual handicaps, and these tapes are often available to students with reading difficulties. A phone call to your state department of education can verify whether textbooks on tape are available and the procedures for obtaining them.

If textbooks on tape must be created, contact youth groups interested in service projects (e.g., the Honor Society, 4-H clubs, Boy Scouts, Girl Scouts, and Thespians). At the same time, find someone in your agency familiar with audio equipment who can guide the volunteers to produce quality recordings. A local radio or television studio committed to youth might even let you use a professional recording studio free of charge during off hours.

Another modification that could be considered is to provide a summary of key ideas that students should glean from written material. As mentioned previously, teachers could also provide listening guides to summarize main ideas and relevant details of information delivered through a lecture. Additional notes in class could be obtained through a "buddy" system. A "buddy" who takes concise, well-organized notes shares them with students struggling to grasp the information presented through lectures. The sharing may be accomplished through photocopies or hand-copying of notes by students with language disorders and learning disabilities. With the burgeoning use of computers in schools, these data can also be transferred electronically from student to student.

While another option is tape-recording teacher lecture information, it is a less desirable option because of the time it takes to re-listen to the information. Frequently, the students who might need to tape-record lectures are the same students who fall behind in their schoolwork. Often, time is not available to re-listen to lectures. However, tape-recording of instructions for completing an assignment might be prudent and requires little time for re-listening.

Some teachers might perceive infringement of academic freedom when tape-recording is done. These teachers may refuse to allow taping in their classes, despite the best possible advocacy on the part of the speech-language pathologist. Professionals need to be aware that Section 504 of the Rehabilitation Act of 1973 and the 1990 Americans with Disabilities Act both state that reasonable accommodations must be made for individuals with disabilities. Reasonable accommodations might well include tape-recording of information so it can be listened to again. Perhaps if other professionals were made aware of legal requirements for accommodations, they would be less likely to resist audio-taping (D. Vetter, personal communication, 1986).

The Use of Peer Tutors

One of the major mechanisms for involving peers and changing their attitudes toward adolescents with communication disorders is through a system of peer tutoring. Professionals typically think that the major advantage of peer tutoring is to the recipient. However, peer tutoring may be as important to the tutor (i.e., for changing attitudes). Also, helping another person learn usually results in all people having a greater understanding of the behaviors being modified.

The peer tutoring system planned by the speech-language pathologist should emphasize teaching tutors how to assist adolescents who have communication disorders to improve performance. When using a peer tutoring system, the speech-language pathologist must spend a considerable amount of time and energy planning the tutorial program. If a peer tutorial system already exists in the educational agency, speech-language pathologists should collaborate with those persons implementing that system to determine if it meets existing needs of adolescents with communication disorders. If a peer tutorial system does not exist, some of the issues to consider when planning such a program include the following:

1. **Gaining Educators' Support—** Administrators can "make or break" tutoring programs. To gain the administrators' supportive enthusiasm, it is necessary to explain the program to them, the benefits derived from such

Communication Solutions
for Older Students

a program, and the resources needed for the establishment and maintenance of the program. Teachers should be consulted about the program to determine if they are willing to have their students participate and which students might be best in the role of the tutor.

2. **Recruiting and Selecting Tutors—**Obviously, supportive teachers can be instrumental in recruiting and selecting tutors for the program. In addition to the teachers' assistance, the program can be advertised through posters, brochures, newsletters, media, and personal solicitations. Once the tutors have been identified, a structured selection process must be followed. This entails interviewing the tutors and having them complete an application form (see Appendix W) that reveals their strengths and weaknesses. Using the data submitted on the form and gleaned from the interview, it should be feasible to select good tutors. Some of the characteristics of a good tutor include: Ability to relate to adolescents with communication disorders; knowledge of the behaviors to be taught; patience; ability to teach someone else; positive attitude toward education; available time to participate; and ability to prepare, to implement, and to evaluate lesson plans and activities.

3. **Training, Supervising, and Supporting Tutors—**It is essential to orient tutors about the tutoring program. Tutors should be trained to engage in interesting activities; to implement time-management techniques; to help tutees feel good about themselves; to respect confidential information about students; and to establish and to maintain tutoring logs. Answers to questions such as the following should be provided to the tutor during the training session: Who am I going to tutor? What will I be doing during the session? When will I tutor the tutee? How do I encourage effort and reinforce success? Where am I going to do the tutoring? What type of records must I keep?

During the training session, it is important to discuss tutoring strategies that make a difference. Some tutoring strategies that have been found to be successful include: (1) focusing on the student's strengths, (2) working with the student's interests, (3) listening to students, (4) accepting students at their level, (5) helping students learn how to pay attention, (6) helping students complete assignments independently, (7) creating a challenging situation for students, (8) encouraging appropriate risk-taking, and (9) developing and maintaining a learning environment in which the tutee feels comfortable to ask questions (Koskinen and R. Wilson, 1982). In addition, we would recommend that each tutor be required to read about tutoring. For example, the *Allyn and Bacon Guide to Peer Tutoring* (Gillespie and Lerner, 1999) would be appropriate reading for tutors who are late adolescents or young adults, such as those who are in vocational-technical institutes or colleges and universities. *Caring and Sharing: Becoming a Peer Facilitator* (Myrick and Erneg, 2000) and *TLC: Tutoring, Leading, Cooperating* (McLaughlin and Hazouri, 1992) would be appropriate resources for those who are in early or middle adolescence. These are pertinent resources for helping the tutor to better understand peer tutoring, and the role, responsibilities, and guidelines for being a peer tutor.

Once the tutor has been trained, it is critical to have weekly or biweekly contacts to evaluate progress and to detect and to prevent problems. The tutor should be supervised and should be encouraged to discuss all issues with the speech-language pathologist as they occur.

4. **Selecting the Tutee**—Not all adolescents with communication disorders will benefit from having a tutor. Therefore, it is equally important that careful planning be given to the selection of the tutee. The tutee should be someone who needs to learn tasks that can be taught by a tutor, who is not embarrassed to work with a peer; and who has time available to participate in the program. The peer tutoring program is conducted independent of the time spent in communication intervention and other courses, and therefore must be incorporated into the students' schedules. Quite frequently, peer tutoring is feasible during resource hours when both tutors and tutees are available.

Modifications of the Environmental System

When the environmental system is modified to meet the language needs of older students, changes might occur in these areas:

- The oral language used within the environmental system

- The structure of the learning environment away from the student's school program

- The attitudes and feelings toward the student with the disorder

Oral Language

Through information sharing, the speech-language pathologist can advise parents, siblings, employers, and others when their language is too rapid or too complex for the

Communication Solutions
for Older Students

student with a language disorder to comprehend. Through changing rate of speech, repeating information, and reducing the length of sentences, the level of frustration when communicating with preadolescents and adolescents with disorders can be greatly reduced. At the time, during direct intervention, older students can be coached to request repetition of information and to ask others to slow down their rate of speech.

When students have strong reading skills, they could ask for written messages that summarize the oral language. This strategy would be particularly appropriate for employment settings (e.g., when a supervisor gives a string of oral directions, it could be reinforced with a printed list). Initially, the involved professionals could work with employers to implement this modification; ultimately, older students should self-advocate for the modification.

Learning Environment

The learning environment at home should match as closely as possible the variables involved in how the youth learns best. For example, if the student learns best when there are few distracting noises, the family should be encouraged to provide that environment at home. Realistically, not all households can accommodate the student's learning style, but other options exist, such as community libraries. Nonetheless, it is valuable information for many families to develop an appreciation for the learning style of the individual with the language disorder

and to recognize that a modified setting can frequently make learning a less frustrating experience.

Students pursuing postsecondary education would be particularly wise to know their learning style and to adapt their environmental accommodations (and they are typically willing to do so), because increased productivity is likely to be the result. Employers also need to comply with the 1990 Americans with Disabilities Act, which states that reasonable accommodations must be made for people with disabilities.

Attitudes and Feelings

The most challenging modifications probably reside in the realm of attitudes and feelings. As children become older, there are more opportunities and years during which others can build up negative attitudes and feelings toward students with communication disorders. Parents, siblings, peers, and employers are increasingly realizing that a communication disorder is not something that will be outgrown if it persists during adolescence. As language demands and expectations increase, many students with disorders do not keep pace. Their feelings of failure in school and their frequent lack of a strong support group of friends contribute to the likelihood of developing at-risk behaviors.

Even once armed with information about disorders and disabilities, parents and siblings cannot usually just "decide" to change attitudes and feelings about the family member with the communication disorder without the benefit of some type of counseling or support group. Sue (1981) cautions, however, that counseling is "a white, middle-class activity that holds many values and characteristics different from those of... (other cultural) groups" (p. 28). During counseling, there is typically an emphasis on verbal communication using standard English, and imposition of class-bound values (e.g., strict adherence to time schedules; an ambiguous or unstructured approach to problems; or the seeking of long-range solutions and goals), and an assumption of culture-bound values by the counselor (e.g., using an analytic cause-effect approach; distinguishing between mental and physical well-being; or encouraging verbal/emotional/behavioral expressions). These characteristics of counseling may be sources of conflict and misinterpretation by family members and peers who are not White middle-class members unless adjustments are made by the counselor to accommodate other language systems, different class-bound values, and alternative culture-bound values.

Employers may also be slow to change attitudes toward individuals with disabilities. Often a supported employment arrangement involving a job coach or a school-to-business partnership is the best way to begin changing attitudes and feelings. Speech-language pathologists should form alliances with school-to-work transition specialists, offer to analyze the language required in various employment settings, and then provide intervention ideas for students struggling with oral and written directions at work. Also, social communication skill resources (e.g., *Social Skill Strategies*, by Gajewski, Mayo, and Hirn, 1998a, 1998b, and *Job-Related Social Skills*, by Montague and Lund, 1991) should be shared with school-to-work transition staff members. The transition from school to work is discussed further in Chapter 14.

Points of Discussion

1. Critique the comprehensive delivery model. If you worked in a high school with only a traditional pull-out model in existence, what would you do to develop other service delivery options?

2. How would you help the older student become aware of the modifications being made in his or her educational and environmental systems? And how would you teach self-advocacy for these changes?

Suggested Readings

American Speech-Language-Hearing Association. (1999). *Guidelines for the roles and responsibilities of the school-based speech-language pathologist.* Rockville, MD: Author.

Larson, V. Lord, and McKinley, N. (in press). Service delivery options for secondary students with language disorders. *Seminars in Speech-Language Pathology.*

Overview of Intervention with Older Students

Goals

- Present six intervention guidelines that should be considered when serving older students

- Explain the importance of class meetings during intervention

- Delineate what skills to teach older students in these areas: thinking, listening, speaking, reading, writing, meta-abilities, nonverbal communication, and paralinguistics

- Discuss how to intervene using techniques that result in students learning strategies for acquiring skills

Figure 12.1 provides an overview of the who, the what, and the how involved in direct intervention with older students. As indicated in the Who? column, all intervention tasks should be designed by keeping in mind the stage of adolescence in which the older student presents: early, middle, or late. What is relevant at each stage is kept at the forefront of intervention (this concept is elaborated upon later in this chapter in considerable detail).

General skill areas of what to teach older students are listed in the What? column of Figure 12.1. Each of these skill areas has subskills that are itemized later in this chapter and provide the nucleus for developing individualized education programs (IEPs).

Figure 12.1   # Direct Intervention of Older Students

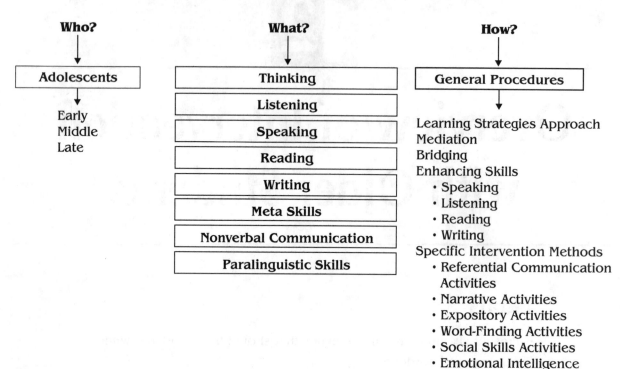

Who?	What?	How?
Adolescents	**Thinking**	**General Procedures**
Early Middle Late	**Listening**	Learning Strategies Approach
	Speaking	Mediation
	Reading	Bridging
	Writing	Enhancing Skills
	Meta Skills	• Speaking
	Nonverbal Communication	• Listening
	Paralinguistic Skills	• Reading
		• Writing

Specific Intervention Methods
• Referential Communication Activities
• Narrative Activities
• Expository Activities
• Word-Finding Activities
• Social Skills Activities
• Emotional Intelligence Activities

The How? column of Figure 12.1 summarizes the general procedures recommended for intervention with older students. In addition, the six specific intervention methods presented in Chapter 13 are foreshadowed.

Before delving into the what and how of intervention, six intervention guidelines are discussed. These guidelines are critical to consider regardless of the content of a student's IEP.

Intervention Guidelines

Basic intervention guidelines pervade speech-language services for older students.

The guidelines we believe are important are as follows:.

1. Determine the purpose of intervention.

2. Establish responsibility for the communication disorder.

3. Be prepared to counsel.

4. Adjust to the social-cognitive development of students.

5. Be cognizant of adult learning theory.

6. Establish ground rules for intervention sessions.

These guidelines are explained in the sections that follow.

Determine the Purpose of Intervention

A profile of relative strengths and weaknesses should have emerged from the assessment results. Moreover, this information should have been explained to the student in such a way that awareness of the communication disorder was established and the need for intervention was made clear. Mutual planning of goals and objectives by the student and the involved professionals should occur at the outset of intervention and periodically throughout the process so that the adolescent is always certain about the purpose of intervention. There needs to be no "hidden agenda" when providing intervention services for adolescents. Preschoolers and early elementary students frequently do not know what the terminal objectives are during their remediation, and this is developmentally appropriate. With older students, however, professionals should communicate openly and honestly about what needs to be accomplished and why it is to be done.

There needs to be no "hidden agenda" when providing intervention services for adolescents.

Many older students with communication disorders have multiple problems, so it is crucial to prioritize what should receive attention first. After goals and objectives that address these problems are identified, the student should assist in ranking them by importance. Certainly, professionals can provide guidance by pointing out when prerequisite objectives are necessary to reach top-ranked goals. Unlike younger children, however, who have no investment in the goal-setting process, older children must fully participate if they are to be active and cooperative learners during intervention. Otherwise, goals may be self-defeating. In essence, students determine what is most critical for their particular lives; they are not told what to do.

Recall from the last chapter that the developmental stage of the student affects the selection of goals and objectives to be emphasized. The following general guidelines may be helpful:

- **Pre-teens and youth in early adolescence**—Goals should focus on developing the language necessary for academic progress and personal-social growth (i.e., peer-group acceptance).

- **Students in late adolescence**—Goals should focus on developing the language necessary for enhancing vocational potential and personal-social growth (i.e., one-to-one, long-term relationships).

- **Students in middle adolescence**—Goals may focus on any or all of the three areas (i.e., academic progress, personal-social growth and/or vocational potential). The corresponding objectives and activities need to be authentic, meaningful, and relevant from the student's perspective, not just the professional's viewpoint.

Establish Responsibility for the Communication Disorder

With adolescents, it is important to establish that they—and not the involved professionals—are responsible for taking care of their disability, and that they are the ones who stand to lose if they do not develop appropriate communication skills. If an adolescent does not want responsibility, denies the existence of a problem, and/or remains unmotivated to change, we recommend that services be discontinued. Until students recognize their communication disorders, and take ownership of them, they will not be motivated to make behavioral changes.

Until students recognize

their communication disor-

ders, and take ownership of

them, they will not be

motivated to make

behavioral changes.

Contracts between students with communication disorders and professionals have often been helpful in establishing this sense of responsibility. Some students seem to be motivated to learn when they sign a contract that specifies goals for communication performance and the time frame within which the goals are to be accomplished. When using contingency contracts with preadolescents and adolescents, make the contracts appear adultlike and official (Larson and McKinley, 1985b). Develop the contract jointly with the student, allowing sufficient time for the student to help shape its content. The contract should specify the consequences for positive performance or lack of performance. A sample contract is shown in Appendix X.

Be Prepared to Counsel

The focus of counseling during speech-language intervention is to give information to students about the impact of their communication disorders on academic progress, personal-social growth, and vocational potential. During counseling, it is critical to obtain information from students about their perceptions of the disorders and to provide release and support for associated feelings. Counseling should be specific to problems associated with the communication disorders. It should not address topics in which speech-language pathologists are unqualified to intervene (e.g., domestic violence or suicide proneness). Preadolescents and adolescents with problems that extend beyond their communication disorders need more help than empathic responses from speech-language pathologists; they need referrals to trained counselors. It is unethical and impossible to try to handle all of the problems associated with preadolescence and adolescence within the confines of a communication intervention program.

Intervention with certain adolescents may involve 50% communication work and 50% counseling (C. Simon, 1981). During sessions, try to use behaviors that communicate understanding to teenagers. The sidebar suggests behaviors that are likely to communicate understanding and those that may not.

Counseling about the communication disorder should not be a segregated part of intervention, but an integral part of the process. Opening each session with a "class meeting" is a recommended way to integrate counseling, and is discussed a little later in this chapter (see page 331).

Adjust to the Social-Cognitive Development of Students

As indicated in Chapter 1, adolescence is a time of major transition in social-cognitive skills. Materials, methods, and procedures that are geared for younger children are not

Behaviors Most Likely to Communicate Understanding

- Suggesting ways to solve the problem
- Taking time to sit down and talk
- Spending time to discuss the problem
- Listening to what the student has to say
- Asking the student questions about the problem
- Sticking to the problem about which the student wants to talk

Behaviors Least Likely to Communicate Understanding

- Jumping to conclusions before the student finishes giving the facts
- Changing the topic immediately after the student introduces concern
- Hurrying the student through the telling of an experience
- Avoiding talking with the student about the problem
- Sitting there "like a bump on a log"
- Looking at something else while the student is talking

Source: Baggett (1969)

Communication Solutions
for Older Students

appropriate for older students. As a group, early adolescents are intellectually and socially different from middle adolescents, who are different from late adolescents. These differences have implications for how professionals intervene. Major implications are outlined in the sidebar.

Part of adjusting to the social-cognitive level of older students involves recognition by the professional that students are too old to show up for communication intervention simply for a trivial reinforcer, and too young to show up because they realize the lifelong importance of developing adequate communication skills. As we have told many workshop

Adjusting Intervention to Social-Cognitive Levels

- Design curricula to stimulate development toward formal operational thinking rather than assuming students have already reached that period. Most early adolescents and many adolescents at the middle and late stages have not yet attained formal operational thought; others are inexperienced in this mode of thinking; and yet others fail to apply it to their communicative behavior.

- Design intervention activities to emphasize "doing" communication in an instrumental sense since most early adolescents and many adolescents at the middle and late stages are at a concrete operational level. Introducing formal operational aspects, such as persuasive tactics, are not usually productive for opening activities; introduce formal operational aspects with concrete activities.

- Design intervention to involve a group process, rather than individual work, at all stages of adolescence. Group activities allow adolescents to interact and learn from one another, a consistent theme that is emphasized in cognitive developmental literature. Discussion is particularly appropriate.

- Design activities that are sensitive to the peer pressure felt during adolescence. Peer influence and conformity reach greatest intensity by ages 11 to 13 and decline slowly thereafter. Classes emphasizing speech are "risky" for adolescents because of their public nature. For example, an early adolescent who is required to "pick something that interests you to talk about" may be devastated to discover that the peer group finds the topic choice peculiar.

- Design activities that encourage students to become increasingly responsive to each other. Early adolescents are primarily concerned with themselves and are convinced that others are also preoccupied with their appearance and behavior. The adolescent is continually constructing or reacting to an imaginary audience; this probably accounts for such behaviors as extreme self-consciousness, constant preening, and adolescent boorishness. In the 14- to 17-year age range, adolescents are better able to consider different perspectives and to engage in appropriate interpersonal communication behaviors based on another's needs.

Source: Ritter (1981)

audiences over the past several decades, "The power of your stickers has worn off!" As much as professionals wish that students would develop an intrinsic motivation to improve communication skills, it is often not forthcoming until late adolescence or young adulthood. Thus, we recommend using token economy systems to motivate students to participate in communication intervention. When such systems are used, they should be implemented in very different ways than for younger children. The sidebar on page 330 captures the primary recommendations we make when using token economy systems with older students. These concepts are explained in even greater depth in *Daily Communication* (Schreiber and McKinley, 1995). Of course, if students do not need such systems, valuable time should be saved for other activities. Based on our clinical observations, students seem to "self-wean" between eighth and ninth grade.

Be Cognizant of Adult Learning Theory

There is a body of information available on the topic of adult learning (Knowles, 1973; Knowles, Holton III, and Swanson, 1998). We do not mean to imply that adolescents are adults, but neither are they small children. Older adolescents may be developing learning patterns that are more typical of adults than of children. Educators providing intervention services for this age group should be aware that adult learning theory exists and that it could have ramifications for certain students on the caseload.

One of the basic tenets of adult learning theory is that adults learn what they want and when they want (i.e., they feel control over the learning situation). Hence the "required inservice" or workshop, which is scheduled at a set time, is often viewed more negatively by adults than a workshop that they can freely choose to attend at their convenience. Late adolescents are similar to adults in their approach to learning; they need to feel like they are learning what they want to learn. The "no hidden agenda" plan cited earlier becomes especially important during late adolescence.

Establish Ground Rules for Intervention Sessions

Enforce basic social communication rules at all times (and teach them when they are outside the students' current repertoire of behaviors). Character traits, such as respect for others in the group and their property, are essential to emphasize. Intervention time needs to be safe for older students—both physically and mentally.

Having said that, ground rules (e.g., talking respectfully to others in an intervention group) may be nearly impossible to enforce when groups have members of gangs or clubs that do not interact with each other outside of school. Professionals need to be aware of the dynamics of who is being grouped together and determine when it is worth the risk and the effort to put youth who dislike each other together, and when it should be avoided. This is particularly

Characteristics of Token Economy Systems for Older Students

- Give "big" points. Don't give 1 or 5 or 10 points; give 100, 500, and 1,000. Let the student leave the communication intervention sessions with 50,000 points in a day. (What difference does it make to you, since giving points costs you nothing?) A number like 50,000 is so much more exciting than 50 to an older student.

- Make each student "bank" his or her points. Go to your local bank or credit union, and get all the paperwork for an account—a deposit book, a savings deposit record book, and check blanks. Have the student make deposits, transfer points between checking and savings accounts, etc. (You might be amazed at the organizational challenges. The student has to record large numbers and keep an accurate running amount in the record books.)

- Have students determine what privileges or goods the points can buy. Don't second guess what is motivating to them; have them tell you. It might be the opportunity to drink a can of soda during the communication session—and they bring it! You just have to work out the privilege with your administrator. One eighth grade boy worked for gum. Obviously steering students toward items that are low cost to the communication program is preferable to high-ticket items.

- Help set the response cost system, and make it relate to behavioral management issues. Do certain students always need to get a drink of water when they see you? If so, make it cost dearly to get that drink, and then have the student write out a check for that amount before getting the drink. Suddenly, thirst is not taking so much precious intervention time. Are students worried about a test later in the day because they failed to study for it the night before? Do they want study time during the intervention session? Don't just give in to a study day—make it hurt "financially," and allow students to buy a study day at a level that nearly bankrupts them.

- Teach all the functional language of banking. To write out a check, the student has to monitor whether all the correct information has been entered. Of course, the mechanics of writing are very laborious for some students with language disorders, and it deters them from spending points. They often become your "savers" and they should get much experience transferring to their savings accounts and keeping their columns of numbers organized.

- Have a plan in place for spending saved points. One program with whom we have consulted had an auction day, and the students learned how to follow the auctioneer call—a unique language skill that is assumed to be intact by adulthood. Another had an end-of-the-school-year pizza party, and they practiced their social skills while eating together.

- Adapt the token system to paperless banking, if you wish. Students still need a system for verifying that their records match the "electronic" version. (Be certain to make some recording errors to give students practice in comparing their system with the bank's.) Discuss predictable errors that could happen (e.g., recording an entry that has the decimal point shifted over one place).

Sources: Larson and McKinley (2002); Schreiber and McKinley (1995)

important for speech-language pathologists who work with incarcerated youth. Finding and "winning over" the kingpin(s) in the groups is often imperative before ground rules can be enforced, since their help is usually needed to win over others to follow the rules and cooperate.

Professionals need to be aware of the dynamics of who is being grouped together and determine when it is worth the risk and the effort to put youth who dislike each other together, and when it should be avoided.

Speech-language pathologists should also establish rules of confidentiality with students, particularly since counseling is sometimes necessary. Students need to feel secure that what they say and do will remain a private matter between themselves and the educator. Naturally, they also need to know when adults are legally obligated to report illegal activities and child abuse/neglect. If you sense it would be better that students not share certain information within a group session, arrange a private meeting time with the individual student. Few events cause more mistrust in you and in the services provided than a breech in confidentiality.

Ground rules are best established and maintained through a class meeting. We recommend that every intervention session with older students begin with a class meeting. This starting point for every intervention session is explained in the next section.

Class Meeting

Opening each intervention session with a "class meeting" can be a prime vehicle for keeping the six intervention guidelines in the forefront. The class meeting contains three parts:

1. Self-reports on how successfully students have transferred two or three communication behaviors outside of the intervention setting

2. Issues or problems that are of primary concern to the students, particularly as they relate to communication disorders

3. Opportunities for participants to reinforce themselves or to compliment one another

Self-Reports

The self-report part of the class meeting targets two or three behaviors that the student is trying to incorporate into daily living situations (e.g., using mnemonic strategies to remember information). The speech-language pathologist and the student mutually select these behaviors. Once appropriate use of the behavior is reported for 10 consecutive sessions (or arbitrarily select another number if the student is being seen only a few times a week), the behavior is replaced with a different behavior. Reporting relies on the honesty of the student. While teens and pre-teens might occasionally misrepresent the truth, their peers in the intervention session tend to challenge these misrepresentations. Honesty is certainly desirable, but dishonesty does not destroy the value of self-reporting on communication behaviors outside the intervention setting. Whether honesty or dishonesty prevails, the value of students' thinking about their communication (i.e., metacommunication) is retained. Taking the time to self-report reinforces the message that use of newly learned communication behaviors outside of the intervention time is the goal. Generalization cannot be expected without time spent on having students reflect on where and when they used the behavior apart from the speech-language pathologist.

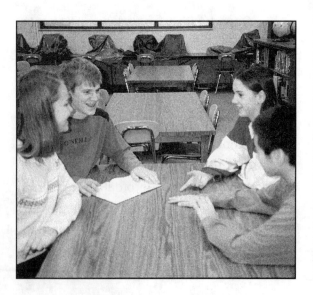

Issues or Problems

The issues or problems part of the class meeting affords a routine mechanism for uncovering significant problems in the lives of youth. Once professionals become trusted adults in the lives of older students, they will hear about students' issues whether they want to or not. Students will burst through the door upset about something a peer, teacher, or parent said or did. When the cause of the anger or frustration is rooted in a communication breakdown, the issue is often worth discussing at length.

When professionals are open recipients to students' feelings and attitudes, they often absorb the brunt of listening to significant problems and helping students determine possible solutions. These problems tend to be paramount to the students at that moment in time. Failure to address the problems would be detrimental to the remainder of the session. The best-planned lesson is doomed if students arrive at a session preoccupied with a burning issue or problem and it is dismissed as irrelevant. The best lessons with preadolescents and adolescents use topics of deep interest to them—such as those that surface during the issues or problems section of the class meeting—and weave these topics into existing goals for communication intervention.

When problems are addressed during this portion of the class meeting, it is often helpful to have students refer to a problem-solving chart (Schreiber and McKinley,

1995). Figure 12.2 is an example of such a chart. Whether this particular chart or an adaptation is used, the logical flow of the steps within the model tends to guide the discussion of the problem effectively. The professional monitoring the discussion should also mediate how a problem-solving model can assist in analyzing and resolving other difficult issues throughout the student's daily life.

Some days there are no issues, and the class meeting proceeds quickly to the third part. On other days, problems surface that require referral to other professionals. If the speech-language pathologist is team teaching with other specialists (e.g., a social worker or learning disabilities specialist), a wider range of problems can be addressed as they surface. At no point should the speech-language pathologist assist a student with an issue that goes beyond the discipline's professional training. And remember, some issues (e.g., abuse, probation violations) must be reported legally to others.

Reinforcement or Compliments

The third part of the class meeting is a time for students to reinforce themselves and to compliment one another. Professionals should be prepared to model compliments, since the individuals receiving intervention often have received few of them. As much as possible, compliments should focus on actions (e.g., "I like the way you said 'Good morning' to me") rather than on physical

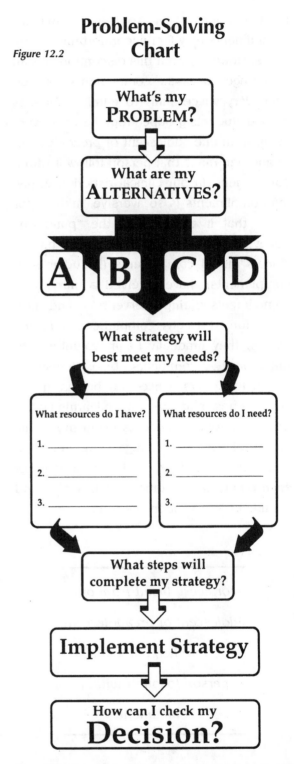

Figure 12.2

Problem-Solving Chart

From *Daily Communication: Strategies for Adolescents with Language Disorders* (p. 38), by L. Schreiber and N. McKinley, 1995, Eau Claire, WI: Thinking Publications. © 1995 by Thinking Publications. Reprinted with permission.

ags et's write properly.

**Communication Solutions
for Older Students**

attributes (e.g., "I like your shirt"). Initially, compliments may feel uncomfortable to students. However, even this discomfort has an advantage, because compliments can be used very successfully to eliminate insults among students grouped together. For every insult from one adolescent or preadolescent to another, make that person follow it with a compliment. In our clinical experience, giving compliments is so aversive, initially, for youth that it extinguishes the "put-down" behaviors. Once students have seen professionals model compliments (including self-compliments), have received a number of compliments during intervention, and have been "forced" to give compliments following insults, they gradually begin voluntarily to make positive comments about themselves and fellow peers. Once that begins, group cohesiveness and cooperative learning often become stronger, students seem more willing to take risks to change communication behaviors, and their emotional support of each other may become evident inside and outside of intervention sessions.

For every insult from one adolescent or preadolescent to another, make that person follow it with a compliment.

The class meeting takes approximately the first 5 to 10 minutes of the session if there are no issues and the meeting consists only of self-reports and compliments. The meeting may last the entire session if the issues or problems are weighty, are appropriate for group discussion, and are intertwined with intervention goals and objectives.

What to Teach

Given the mutual planning of goals and objectives discussed in the previous section, it is important to use terms familiar to preadolescents and adolescents. We recommend that terms like *thinking, listening, speaking, reading,* and *writing skills* be used, since those are common words and ones that likely surfaced during the assessment process. Table 12.1 lists important thinking, listening, speaking, reading, and writing skills, plus meta-abilities, nonverbal communication, and paralinguistic skills to consider during intervention. Note that certain skills were "forced" into a category for the sake of simplifying the list (e.g., the skill "understands and produces complex stories with multiple embedded narratives" is listed only as a "speaking skill," even though it also makes reference to listening skills.)

Many of the goals for intervention presented in Table 12.1 correlate directly with benchmarks in the general education curriculum. The 1997 Individuals with Disabilities Education Act (P.L. 105-17, known as IDEA '97) requires that student IEPs target goals that provide access to the general curriculum. Table 12.1 is in concert with this requirement.

Table 12.1

Skills to Teach during Intervention

Thinking Skills	Goals for Intervention
Input	The student: • Uses senses (e.g., hearing and seeing) to gather clear and complete information • Uses a plan so that important information is not being skipped or missed • Consistently names objects and events so that they can be remembered and talked about clearly • Describes events and objects in terms of where and when they occur • Describes characteristics of objects and events as the same even when changes take place (e.g., a square tilted onto its corner is still recognized as a square) • Organizes information by several characteristics simultaneously (e.g., by date and by time of day; by size and by shape) • Knows when and how to be precise and accurate (e.g., when reporting data about an emergency to the appropriate authorities)
Elaboration	The student: • Defines problems and determines what needs to be done • Uses only the information that is relevant to the problem and ignores the rest • Forms "good pictures in the mind" about what must be done to solve a problem • Makes a plan that includes steps needed to reach a goal • Remembers the various pieces of information needed to solve a problem • Looks for relationships by which separate objects, events, and experiences can be tied together (e.g., a flat tire, a sick child, and an overdrawn checkbook have made my mother very upset today; therefore, this is not the time to ask for a new jacket) • Compares objects and experiences to others to determine what is similar and what is different • Finds the class or set to which new objects or experiences belong • Thinks about different alternatives and what would happen if one or another were chosen • Uses logic to prove answers and to defend opinions

Continued on next page

Table 12.1—Continued

Thinking Skills	Goals for Intervention
Output	The student: • Is clear and precise in language so that the listener understands the message • Thinks through the response instead of immediately trying to answer and making a mistake • Uses restraint before saying or doing something that will be regretted later • Uses a strategy to help find answers rather than panicking when stuck on a problem

Listening Skills	Goals for Intervention
Comprehension of Linguistic Features	The student: • Differentiates grammatical phrases, clauses, and sentences as incorrect or incomplete • Comprehends various sentence transformations • Comprehends sentences of various lengths and complexity • Comprehends various semantic features (e.g., multiple-meaning words, verbal analogies, inclusion-exclusion, and idioms)
Informational Listening	The student: • Comprehends factual information (e.g., directions and dates) • Concentrates attention on the speaker • Uses advantageously the time differential between thinking and speaking speed (i.e., people think two times faster than they listen) • Understands and differentiates between main ideas and supportive details • Formulates questions of clarification
Critical Listening	The student: • Identifies and recognizes the credibility of the source or speaker • Recognizes and uses inductive and deductive reasoning • Detects false reasoning (e.g., discriminates between fact and opinion) • Recognizes propaganda devices (e.g., loaded words) • Draws inferences and judges statements heard

Table 12.1—Continued

Speaking Skills	Goals for Intervention
Production of Linguistic Features	The student: • Uses simple and complex sentences • Uses appropriate sentence fragments (e.g., a response of "eleven o'clock" to the question, "What time will you be home tonight?") • Avoids an excessive number of run-on sentences that are strung together with *and* or *and then* • Uses a variety of question forms, such as *wh-* questions, tag questions, interrogative reversals, and questions marked by rising intonation • Uses figurative language, such as slang, jargon, idioms, metaphors, similes, and language for the purpose of entertainment or humor • Avoids overuse of nonspecific language, such as low-information words (e.g., *things, stuff,* and *everybody);* when requested to do so, the student rephrases, using more specific language • Displays few, if any, word-retrieval problems • Uses cohesion devices that contribute to the continuity of meaning in the conversation or narration • Uses cohesion devices in a way that avoids the disruption of continuity
Functions of Communication	The student: • Gives an appropriate amount of information • Gets information (i.e., asks questions) • Describes an ongoing event with sufficient detail for the listeners • Gets the listener to do, believe, or feel something (i.e., persuade) • Expresses his or her own intentions, beliefs, and feelings (i.e., practices self-disclosure) • Indicates a readiness for further communication • Uses language to solve problems • Uses language to entertain
Fluency	The student: • Avoids an excessive amount of verbal mazes that interfere with communication • Avoids an excessive amount of false starts that interfere with communication

Continued on next page

Table 12.1—Continued

Speaking Skills	Goals for Intervention
Conversations	The student: • Applies the rules of conversation • Initiates conversations in a variety of situations • Selects appropriate topics • Maintains a topic over a number of speaker-listener exchanges • Switches topics in an appropriate and orderly manner • Terminates conversations in a timely manner

Narrations	The student:
	
	• Summarizes stories
	
	• Categorizes stories both subjectively and objectively
	
	• Understands and produces complex stories with multiple embedded narratives
	
	• Analyzes stories (13–15 years of age)
	
	• Generalizes from the meaning of the story, formulating abstract statements about the theme or message, and focusing on reactions to the story (16 years–adulthood)
	
	• Uses a story grammar taxonomy as evidenced by the following:
	
	  • A setting is provided.
	
	  • The characters are identified and described.
	
	  • The events of the story are presented sequentially.
	
	  • A goal is present.
	
	  • There is an initiating event.
	
	  • There is a causal relationship between events.
	
	  • An internal response is present.
	
	  • There is an attempt to attain the goal.
	
	  • There is a consequence.
	
	  • Multiple plans are used to meet the goal.
	
	  • A partial or complete episode is embedded in the episode.
	
	  • There are two characters with separate goals and actions that influence each other's actions.

Table 12.1—Continued

Speaking Skills	Goals for Intervention
Expository	The student: • Shifts focus of attention from one question to another • Shifts from one perspective to another • Integrates verbal and visual information • Integrates old and new information • Reasons logically • Predicts outcomes • Constructs and explains inferences • Uses abstract vocabulary • Uses grammatical complexity to reflect conceptual complexity • Justifies a decision or position • Determines and explains causes and consequences • Describes what something is • Lists items relevant to a topic • Compares and contrasts topics • States a problem and solutions • Tells what occurred and how to do something
Reading Skills	**Goals for Intervention**
Early	The student: • Has phonological awareness skills as demonstrated by such tasks as rhyming, syllable and phoneme segmentation, and syllable and phoneme blending • Has rapid automatic naming of visually presented symbols, such as letters, digits, and common objects • Has phonological memory skills to repeat strings of digits, words, or letters presented auditorily • Has letter identification skills, such as naming the alphabet • Has the skill of "speech to print letters" in terms of spelling • Has single-word decoding skills • Has oral reading fluency • Has reading comprehension as measured through questions, paraphrasing, and story retelling tasks • Has knowledge of derivational morphology and orthographic patterns of irregularly spelled words

Continued on next page

Communication Solutions
for Older Students

Table 12.1—Continued

Reading Skills	Goals for Intervention
Late	The student: • Has knowledge of different text structures and genres, such as narratives and expository passages • Has knowledge of the different purposes of text, such as to persuade, negotiate, inform, and entertain • Has strategies for different styles of reading, such as skimming, overview, analytic, and critical • Has strategies for facilitating comprehension, storage, and retrieval of information, such as using headings and subheadings, tables of contents, indexes, summaries, and end-of-chapter questions

Writing Skills	Goals for Intervention
Prewriting	The student: • Develops ideas • Gathers information about a topic • Organizes content • Takes the reader (audience) into consideration • Has considered the purpose for writing (e.g., to tell a story, to explain a process, or to give directions)
Composing	The student: • Uses appropriate syntax and semantics to write a passage • Spells and punctuates appropriately
Editing	The student: • Edits the written product • Finds errors (e.g., spelling and grammatical) and makes revisions

Table 12.1—Continued

Meta- Skills	Goals for Intervention
	The student: • Shows evidence of metalinguistic skills (e.g., the ability to assess communication breakdowns and revise them) • Shows metacognitive skills (i.e., the ability to assess one's own thinking or to think about thinking) • Shows metapragmatic skills (i.e., the awareness and application of cultural rules for using language appropriately across and within various social contexts) • Shows metanarrative skills (i.e., the awareness of story elements and structure so as to manipulate intentionally the various story elements)
Nonverbal Communication Skills	**Goals for Intervention**
	The student: • Uses facial expressions appropriately • Has appropriate eye contact when speaking and listening • Stands at a distance from the speaker/listener that seems appropriate and comfortable • Uses body movements to enhance communication rather than detract from it
Paralinguistic Skills	**Goals for Intervention**
	The student: • Uses an appropriate rate of speech • Uses an appropriate tone of voice • Uses a variety of vocal inflections • Pauses appropriately between utterances and between speaker-listener turns • Avoids overuse of filled pauses (e.g., "ah," "um," or "er")

Sources: Applebee (1978); ASHA (2001b); Creaghead and Tattershall (1991); Reuven Feuerstein (1979); Isaacson (1991); Larson and McKinley (1995); McKinley and Larson (1990); Stein and Glenn (1979)

Note that Table 12.1 does not include all potential reading and writing skills, but rather a selective list that relies heavily on language and cognitive skills. The content for those portions of Table 12.1 was extrapolated from the American Speech-Language-Hearing Association (ASHA; 2001b), Creaghead and Tattershall (1991), and Isaacson (1991). Reading and writing are integrated processes and are highly interactive in the general education curriculum. As Scott (1999) stated, "High school students read to find out what to write and write to demonstrate that they understand what they read" (p. 224). Reading and writing have become an essential part of the speech-language intervention process, especially when they support the acquisition of oral communication skills.

At about third grade (i.e., 8–9 years of age), children increasingly use their sentence-level knowledge and narrative discourse processing skills in reading (Snyder and Downey, 1991). Before that age, children appear to focus much of their processing efforts on reading at the word level (Chall, 1983). Between 8 and 9 years, the decoding process is sufficiently mastered to the point where it can be automatically applied to print (Chall, 1983). It is at this same time that expository text becomes an important part of the general education curriculum and a major medium for acquiring content knowledge about the various academic subjects that the student will encounter (ASHA, 2001b). It should be noted that printed language is not just speech written down; rather, it differs from speech in complexity, style, and level of decontextualization. Reading is usually an individual activity, unlike speaking, which has a social context. As a result of these differences, reading involves higher-level thinking processes (ASHA, 2001b; Catts and Kamhi, 1999).

"Helping students gain explicit knowledge of text structures and linguistic cohesion devices may help them to improve their reading comprehension and written discourse structures, and vice versa" (ASHA, 2001b, p. 36). At this level, students expend less effort on the phonological and lexical processing required for decoding and word recognition and begin to allocate more attention and processing resources to the syntactic and discourse operations required for the higher order processing of text (connected discourse). Thus, it is at this stage that children are thought to move into fluent reading (Synder and Downey, 1991.

Youth with language disorders do not attain decoding automatically and are thought to become "stuck" at the early stages of reading, thus preventing progress to the more advanced stages of reading for meaning (Chall, 1983). The different dimensions of language processing appear to have an impact on reading at the word and text levels (Kamhi and Catts, 1989).

Some researchers (Catts and Kamhi, 1999; Kamhi and Catts, 1986, 1989; Wallach and L. Miller, 1988) have suggested that reading-related oral language skills develop as school-age children interact with formal instruction and written texts. Fawcett (1994) cited the intricate interconnections among language processes and noted "that growth in oral language supports growth in written language and vice versa" (p. 39). Thus, there appears to be reciprocity in the oral-written language relationship (Snyder and Downey, 1991), and intervention must include thinking, listening, speaking, reading, and writing goals and activities, as well as meta-, nonverbal, and paralinguistic skills.

How to Intervene

Use a Learning Strategies Approach

Four primary program approaches exist for communication intervention:

1. Basic skills approach
2. Tutorial approach
3. Functional curriculum approach
4. Learning strategies approach

The one we recommend for older students the majority of the time is the learning strategies approach.

Each of these approaches will be explained briefly, since the outcome of intervention hinges on the choice(s) made by the speech-language pathologist. However, approaches are not exclusive. For example, a learning strategies approach can be combined with a functional curriculum approach. Also, in any given day, the speech-language pathologist may switch from one approach to another for individual students.

In a *basic skills approach*, skills are taught that approximate the student's achievement level. For example, if an adolescent has third-grade comprehension skills, intervention tasks are designed to teach the next comprehension skills at that grade level. This approach makes the assumptions that identifying and sequencing of prerequisite skills are possible; that past instruction has been inappropriately or incompletely delivered, or the elementary child was not ready for the instruction when it occurred; and that the secondary student will benefit, in spite of a history of not benefiting, from similar intervention to that used in the elementary grades. While the proposition of increased competence in basic skills is attractive, the reality is that limited time is available to older students, thus making it unlikely that enough progress can be made to reduce the gap between grade level and functioning level.

A *tutorial approach* concerns itself with instruction in academic content areas. We urge speech-language pathologists to resist the temptation to make classroom assignments a primary goal of intervention. While providing tutorial assistance meets the immediate needs of students, it is a short-term solution. Little time is left to intervene with the actual, underlying problems when so much time is spent on assisting students with academic assignments and using them as a medium during intervention. The focus should be on teaching strategies for learning the academic content, not merely tutoring that content. Using classroom assignments as the vehicle for teaching learning strategies helps students gain independence, whereas a simple tutoring approach keeps students dependent on adults for academic success.

In a *functional curriculum approach,* the focus is on equipping students to function in society (i.e., teaching them survival skills). This approach has merit in that, at least over the short term, students are equipped to function independently in society. A better approach would be to combine a functional curriculum approach with a learning strategies approach. With the combined approach, intervention could focus on survival language for a specific situation (e.g., for using a microwave oven) and at the same time teach strategies for learning the language to use for the next household appliance being invented (e.g., to ask questions for clarification or to highlight key ideas in the instruction manual).

For the majority of older students, the *learning strategies approach* is the most appropriate. Emphasis is on *how* to learn (i.e., process) rather than *what* to learn (i.e., product). "Learning strategies are defined as techniques, principles, or rules that will facilitate the acquisition, manipulation, integration, storage, and retrieval of information across situations and settings" (Alley and Deshler, 1979, p. 13). Youth who attain competence in learning strategies maximize their

learning efficiency; they apply their metacognitive abilities successfully in both academic and nonacademic settings (Ehren, 2002b).

Learning strategies allow students to make changes in response to immediate concerns and to generalize to other situations. The emphasis on *how* to learn is better suited than other approaches to the ongoing adaptation that students will be facing in their lifetimes.

Provide Mediation

How students learn new skills and strategies is the topic of an ongoing theoretical debate. Traditional behaviorists would have educators believe that learning involves a stimulus-response (S-R) situation (Skinner, 1957). Piaget (1959) revolutionized how professionals think about learning by interspersing an "O" between the "S-R"—in effect, reminding them that the stimulus-response is affected by the cognitive level of the organism ("O") receiving the stimulus and generating the response.

Learning of the S-R or S-O-R type is direct exposure learning. The organism (student) interacts with the stimulus, derives meaning, and formulates a response. Direct exposure learning does not explain, however, the vast amount of learning that takes place, according to Reuven Feuerstein (1979). He posits that mediated learning experiences account for much of human learning, especially by children who cannot have direct exposure experiences. For example, most of what people know about history is acquired through mediation, not through direct exposure. Mediation is different from direct exposure in that some human (H)—a teacher, a parent, a sibling, a friend—comes between the stimulus and the organism and/or between the organism and the response. Figure 12.3 illustrates how mediation compares to other theoretical explanations for learning.

The "human" involved in mediation frames, filters, and schedules the stimuli. He or she may cause certain aspects of the stimuli to be salient and other aspects to be suppressed. For example, in teaching the social significance of World War II, the mediator might focus on the shifts in attitude that occurred and deliberately not focus on the details of the war itself. When teaching writing, the mediator might provide a critique of the content and deliberately ignore spelling and punctuation errors.

There is an intention to transcend the immediate teaching situation during mediation (Feuerstein, 1980; Reuven Feuerstein, Rafi Feuerstein, and Schur, 1997). Even something as simple as asking a student to close the door can be mediated. Simply saying, "Close the door" does not mediate. But if you say, "Please close the door because there's a strong draft in the hallway, and I'm afraid the wind might ruin our art projects," then you have established a reason for closing the door that goes beyond the immediate situation. You have established a relationship between closing the door and preventing a problem (destruction of art projects) and have modeled how to anticipate predictable mistakes.

Mediation occurs from birth onward. "Good" parents mediate without having the label for it. They are constantly scheduling stimuli for their children such as when and where to eat, and how much. "Do's" and "don't's" are followed by explanations that go beyond the immediate needs. "Don't touch the stove. You'll get burned," "Pet the dog. He likes you," or "Put your shoes on. The sidewalk is very hot." The immediate

Figure 12.3 **Theoretical Explanations for Learning**

S-R
Stimulus-Response
Learning

S-O-R
Organism's
Cognitive Level
Considered

S ⇒ H ⇐ O ⇒ H ⇐ R
Mediated
Learning
Experience

Sources: Reuven Feuerstein (1979); Piaget (1959); Skinner (1957)

needs are to avoid touching the stove, to pet the dog, or to put on shoes, but the "good" parent adds information that goes beyond the immediate need and draws connections between actions and results. "Good" educators do the same.

The more mediation a child has, the more capable he or she becomes to learn independently through direct exposure to stimuli. So states Reuven Feuerstein's (1980) theory of cognitive modifiability. When a young child arrives at school with a history of appropriate mediated learning experiences, his or her cognitive functioning is typically adequate. When mediated learning experiences have been lacking, deficient cognitive functioning is the result.

The more mediation a child

has, the more capable he or

she becomes to learn inde-

pendently through direct

exposure to stimuli.

When children past the age of 10 experience concomitant cognitive deficiencies and language disorders, a lack of mediated learning experiences can almost always be traced in their development (Reuven Feuerstein, 1980; Reuven Feuerstein et al., 1997). In some youth, cognitive ability is greater than their language age; in others, the pattern is reversed. In either case, intervention can be very effective, for as language skills increase, the student's cognitive functioning often improves. And as students think better, they communicate better.

One of the greatest travesties in the provision of speech-language services is denying students intervention simply on the basis that they are currently communicating better than their cognitive levels would indicate. When both language and cognition are lagging years behind chronological-age expectations, intervention is warranted regardless of any discrepancy that might exist between the two measures (Casby, 1992). Provision of the mediated learning experience that has been lacking is a prime focus of intervention, whether language exceeds cognition, cognition exceeds language, or both are equally impaired.

Granted, some individuals are so neurologically impaired that mediation is generally unsuccessful. Mediation is not a panacea. There are individuals who require such an investment of the professional's time to make minor cognitive and language gains that one questions the efficacy of such intervention. This is not the population being addressed in this text. Rather, the older school-age child with inclusion into regular education all or part of the day is modifiable, and mediation is paramount for the development of adequate cognitive functioning. Readers will see continual reinforcement of the need to mediate for older students in parts of this chapter and in Chapter 13.

Structure Bridging Opportunities

Bridging is another essential aspect of intervention that should occur concurrently with mediation (Reuven Feuerstein, 1983). While the professional mediates, the student bridges. Bridging involves the application of an idea, concept, or skill being used in one situation to a different situation. For example, if the student has just learned how to interrupt politely, he or she describes a situation when this skill might need to be used in a community setting. Or the student is given an assignment to interrupt someone politely the next day and then to report back on the experience. Bridging might also be thought of as "transferring" or "generalizing." We prefer the term *bridging* because it provides a visual image for students.

Bridging involves the application of an idea, concept, or skill being used in one situation to a different situation.

You cannot bridge for your students. Rather, you guide students to do the *bridging* through the questions asked and the time allowed. Without the consistent inclusion of bridging in intervention, students will make minimal gains in using their new communication behaviors in other settings.

During bridging, students apply new behaviors and strategies learned within intervention sessions to novel academic, personal-social, or vocational situations. Professionals structure intervention so students engage in bridging, but only the students themselves can make a meaningful application. The application should be specific enough to demonstrate the understanding of how to apply the new behavior or strategy in other relevant situations. Table 12.2 provides examples of strong bridges, in contrast with weak bridges, for a variety of behaviors and strategies.

Within Table 12.2, only one guide question for each new behavior or strategy is indicated. This is not to imply that only one probing question would be used. Rather, the professional should generate many ongoing questions about each behavior or strategy that will trigger bridging responses from students throughout the intervention process. When weak bridges are given (e.g., the first response in Table 12.2, "In math class"), professionals should ask follow-up questions that encourage expansion (e.g., "When, in math class, might you switch topics of conversations with the teacher?").

A common pattern is for older students to generate no bridges, or weak bridges, initially. The realization of an application for what is being learned in an educational situation appears foreign to many students. However, with guidance from the adult

Table 12.2 **Strong and Weak Bridging by Students**

New Behavior or Strategy	Professional's Guide Question	Strong Bridge	Weak Bridge
Switching topics (of conversation) appropriately	When might you have to switch topics when talking with a teacher at school? (academic bridge)	When I have two things to ask, like what assignments I'm missing and what's on the test.	In math class.
Formulating questions for clarification	Are there times when you want to ask questions for clarification, but it's not appropriate? (personal-social bridge)	When I want to ask my mom something but she's on the telephone.	At home.
Making a plan to reach a goal	Who earns a living by making plans? (vocational bridge)	City planners.	Adults.

mediator(s), preadolescents and adolescents gradually improve the quantity and quality of their bridges. Improvement is facilitated by providing a partial bridge and by encouraging its completion. The transcript in the sidebar that follows, taken from a group session, illustrates this facilitation of bridging.

From the transcript, notice how the professional assisted the young adolescents to think about a particular communication behavior as it affected their lives. Sometimes this process is facilitated by the use of a hands-on activity, rather than relying on students answering questions (e.g., bringing in a telegraph key and practicing formulating actual telegrams). Additional specific ideas for bridging will be provided throughout Chapter 13. With frequent exposure to the general procedure of bridging, students gradually begin to generate spontaneous responses that result in positive transfers in daily communication.

Apply Mediation and Bridging Consistently

No matter what the focus of intervention or the objectives, mediation and bridging become general principles that guide the process. Common questions and statements

Sample Transcript of a Bridging Dialogue

PROFESSIONAL: We have been practicing giving clear messages. We made it a rule to use the fewest words possible, but still to communicate the message. Think for a minute. Where else is it important to give clear messages using the fewest words possible?

YOUNG ADOLESCENTS: (No response after waiting 5 to 10 seconds)

PROFESSIONAL: Suppose you are at a pay phone. You need a ride home. You put your money in the phone and discover it is a long-distance call to your home. The voice message tells you to deposit another coin. You now have no more money. When you call from a pay phone, you can only talk for a few minutes long distance before depositing more money. How would giving a clear message be important in this situation?

YOUNG ADOLESCENT 1: Better tell Mom to pick you up. Tell her to get there fast.

PROFESSIONAL: Good idea! You'd really want to get right to the point of your message when you're stranded at a pay phone. Now think for a minute about telegrams, like a Western Union message. You've been studying about telegrams and the Morse code in history. Why is it important to send short messages when wiring a telegram?

YOUNG ADOLESCENTS: (No response after waiting 5 to 10 seconds)

PROFESSIONAL: Does anyone know...Is it free to send a telegram or does it cost money?

YOUNG ADOLESCENT 2: No, people gotta pay.

PROFESSIONAL: All right. When people send a telegram, they have to pay so much for each word. So why would it be important to send a telegram using the fewest words possible?

YOUNG ADOLESCENT 2: So it don't cost much.

PROFESSIONAL: Good thinking! So it doesn't cost as much. Sometimes sending a clear message may save us money. Let's think of another situation. You are in the middle of study hall and you need to tell your friend something. How will clear messages help now?

YOUNG ADOLESCENT 3: You better tell your friend fast. Or else the teacher may catch you and put your name on the board.

PROFESSIONAL: In our school, that's true. In this case, sending a clear message could help you avoid trouble. You've done a good job of bridging some examples of when and why it is important to give clear messages using the fewest words possible.

From *Language Disorders in Older Students: Preadolescents and Adolescents* (pp. 177–178), by V. Lord Larson and N.L. McKinley, 1995, Eau Claire, WI: Thinking Publications. © 1995 by Thinking Publications. Adapted with permission.

that emerge time and time again appear in the sidebar.

The level of questioning may seem high. However, comparable questions appear in textbooks and in teacher-student exchanges in the middle grades and beyond. Students are expected to handle thought-provoking questions. Mediation will help them handle higher level questions across a variety of settings.

The prevalence of metacognition and metalinguistics in these questions is apparent. Students are repeatedly being asked to think about their thinking and to communicate about their communication. This is intentional and sets intervention with older students apart from intervention with younger children (i.e., children younger than age 10). Bliss (1993) stressed the importance of not explaining the communication act or commenting on its importance to children or

---

Mediation and Bridging Questions

Mediation (Focusing Questions)

- What do you see on this page?

- What do you think we're supposed to do on this page? (Or, what do you think the problem to be solved is?)

- What were the cues that helped you figure out what we're supposed to do?

- What strategy(ies) do you think you could use to complete the tasks on this page?

Bridging Questions

- Where else have you seen _____? (Or, where else have you ever had to _____?)

- You used this strategy: _____. When else have you used that strategy in school? At home? In the community?

- Who might use this strategy at his or her place of work? Give an example.

- What mistakes might you make if you didn't use a strategy (plan)?

A word of caution: Expect dead silence when first asking these kinds of questions of older students. On average, they have not been asked to apply what they are learning. Be prepared to assist them in composing relevant answers as long as necessary—probably 6 to 9 months. Once they are well versed in mediation and bridging experiences, you can transition some of the thinking and talking time to written assignments.

Source: Larson and McKinley (2001)

adolescents. We believe, however, that as young children mature, especially those who lack mediated learning experiences, explaining the significance of learning various communication skills (and having them bridge the significance of the skills to meaningful academic, personal-social, and vocational settings) is an essential component of intervention that promotes the intrinsic motivation of the student to improve communication skills.

A difference between intervening with children past age 10 and with those younger than age 10 is that older students are capable of "meta-" activities like

- Thinking about their thinking
- Thinking about their talking
- Talking about their thinking
- Talking about their talking

Note that "talking" should be interpreted as speaking and listening. Extending this to written communication, they can also:

- Think about their writing
- Write about their thinking
- Write about their writing

This ability to engage in higher-level cognitive discussions and tasks should be routinely incorporated into intervention as students learn how to learn. The "good" mediator helps students select meaningful skills to learn, structures questions and activities so students understand why the skills are important, and provides opportunities to bridge the skills to relevant academic, personal-social, and/or vocational situations. Put another way, professionals need to help students "think meta-, plan meta-, do meta-" across all goals and activities (Larson and McKinley, 2002). Mediation of these meta-skills requires using and teaching the vocabulary of critical thinking.

B. Bloom, Engelhart, Furst, Hill, and Krathwohl (1956) provide an organized schema for professionals to use with older students. The sidebar on page 352 lists critical thinking terms within each cognitive domain. These words are essential for older students to learn in order to develop higher level cognition and meta-abilities, thus improving their success in the general curriculum.

Enhance Speaking

Traditional intervention procedures have systematically taught phonology (articulation), syntax (grammar), semantics (concepts), and pragmatics (social communication, functional language) as isolated skill areas. Of these, pragmatics has often been ignored in deference to the other three areas. In contrast, emphasis with older students should be on teaching the natural interactions among the skill areas and making pragmatics the "umbrella" that encompasses the other skills. Figure 12.4 compares the two approaches.

Communication Solutions
for Older Students

Key Words in Academic Assignments (Organized by Bloom et al.'s [1956] Taxonomy)					
Knowledge →	Comprehension →	Application →	Analysis →	Synthesis →	Evaluation
count	repeat	add	analyze	categorize	appraise
define	reproduce	apply	arrange	combine	assess
describe	associate	calculate	break down	compile	compare
draw	compute	change	combine	compose	conclude
identify	convert	classify	design	create	contrast
label	defend	complete	detect	derive	criticize
list	discuss	compute	develop	design	critique
match	distinguish	demonstrate	diagram	devise	determine
name	estimate	discover	differentiate	explain	grade
outline	explain	divide	discriminate	generate	interpret
point	extend	examine	illustrate	group	judge
quote	extrapolate	graph	infer	integrate	justify
read	generalize	interpolate	outline	modify	measure
recall	give examples	interpret	point out	order	rank
recite	infer	manipulate	relate	organize	rate
recognize	paraphrase	modify	select	plan	support
record	predict	operate	separate	prescribe	test
	rewrite	prepare	subdivide	propose	
	summarize	produce	utilize	rearrange	

Most older students have some type of oral language system, albeit an ineffective or inefficient one. The challenge during intervention is to help students use the system they do have in the most appropriate way possible. How can they use their current language to communicate better in daily living situations?

This is not to imply professionals will avoid working on articulation problems or grammatical errors of older students. However, when phonology or syntax or semantics are addressed in intervention, the mediation will relate to a pragmatic base. For example, the student will be assisted to see that his or her articulation errors are causing intelligibility problems in academic situations (e.g., when making a report) and rejection or ridicule in personal situations and consequently realize that there are strong pragmatic and social communication reasons for taking responsibility for correcting the articulation errors.

When pragmatic and social communication skills are the primary deficit area, there is a growing call for speech-language

Figure 12.4 ## Oral Communication Intervention Approaches

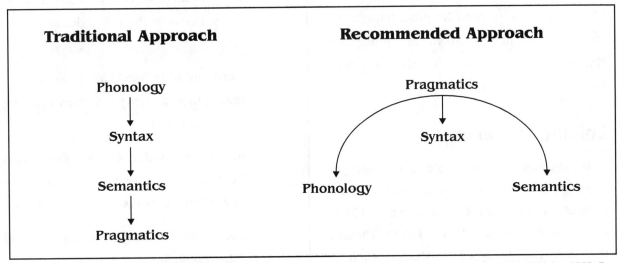

From *Language Disorders in Older Students: Preadolescents and Adolescents* (p. 181), by V. Lord Larson and N.L. McKinley, 1995, Eau Claire, WI: Thinking Publications. © 1995 by Thinking Publications. Adapted with permission.

intervention (Walker, Schwarz, Nippold, Irvin, and Noell, 1994). Children who have weak social skills and problematic peer relations in the early years of their school careers risk a host of negative outcomes (e.g., low self-esteem, underachievement, juvenile delinquency, dropping out of school; Strain, Guralnick, and Walker, 1986). Preventing these negative developmental outcomes hinges on proactive, systematic social skills training (Walker et al., 1994). (Specific intervention ideas for social skills are presented in Chapter 13.)

Intervention activities should be relevant and contextually based with a focus on the communication process, not the end product. Activities (e.g., referential communication

tasks or barrier games that are slightly higher than the student's skill level) can produce great learning moments when a "safe" environment—one allowing youth to experiment and make mistakes—is set. (Referential communication activities are further explained in Chapter 13.) Discussion should center on why the speaking or listening task succeeded or failed. Was the success or failure due to actions of the speaker or the listener or both? The purpose of this discussion is not to focus blame but to determine how to send and/or receive successful oral messages.

This type of discussion assumes basic conversational rules are intact or can be taught to the students in the group. Basic rules of conversation based on Grice's (1975) fundamentals are summarized in Figure 12.5 and should be provided graphically for students as shown. Schreiber and McKinley (1995) provide specific activities for how to teach these rules.

Enhance Listening

Listening has been the least taught and yet most used in the educational and environmental system (Boyce and Larson, 1983; Larson and McKinley, 1987, 1995). Though there are different types of listening, such as informational and critical, classroom listening or listening to lectures is crucial to the older students' success in the educational system because:

- Curriculum demands at the secondary level place a heavy emphasis on the ability to listen.

- In some secondary classes, listening is the main activity (e.g., 97% of the time in English may be spent listening).

- Social and job situations require good listening skills.

Figure 12.5   **Rules of Conversation Poster**

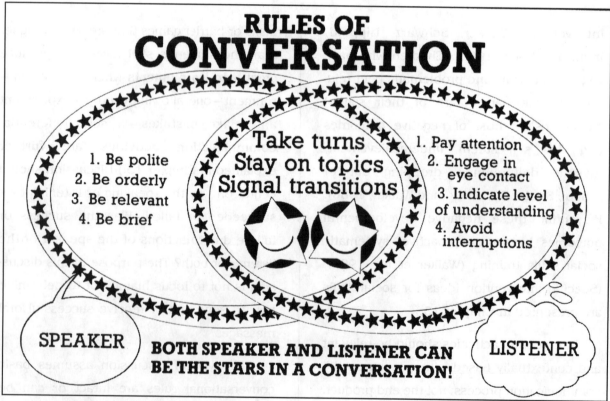

Sources: Grice (1975); Schreiber and McKinley (1995)

• Listening performance can be improved through instruction.

Listening instruction begins with prelistening strategies.

Prelistening Strategies

Prelistening strategies are those applied before the act of listening begins. The strategies include several factors:

1. **Having knowledge of barriers to listening and how to avoid poor listening habits**—Students should be made aware of the difference between their good and bad listening habits. This can be accomplished by having the students view a 15-minute videotaped lecture in their typical manner and then providing them with some good listening habits to see if they can glean more information from the lecture.

2. **Being mentally prepared to listen**—Have students review materials from a previous class, read the current day's materials, relate the current day's lecture topic to other topics they are knowledgeable about, or review and understand the vocabulary of the current day's lecture.

3. **Being physically prepared to listen**—Encourage students to sit near the teacher when lecturing and bring the appropriate materials to each class. This latter behavior can be accomplished by writing a checklist of materials needed for each class on 3 × 5" cards and keeping them in a pocket or purse.

Following prelistening strategy development, students should learn listening strategies.

Listening Strategies

Listening strategies include the following factors:

1. **Listening for organizing cues**—Guide students to notice if the teacher outlines the lecture, provides key points on the blackboard or in a handout, or uses verbal cues such as, "Today we will discuss three main points."

2. **Listening for verbal and nonverbal cues**—Using videotaped lectures, note verbal phrases like "in summary" and "last but not least"; observe vocal inflections and emphasis; and identify nonverbal cues like eye contact, gestures, body positions, facial expressions, and pauses.

3. **Listening for main ideas and relevant supporting ideas**—Critical for being a successful learner of classroom lecture materials, this strategy can be learned by having students hear a short selection or lecture and then suggest a title; tell a short story and then summarize it in a sentence; listen to a lecture and then pick out the main ideas and supporting details.

4. **Questioning for clarification**—This is a strategy that will help students glean the most information from classroom lectures. Students need to be taught how (politely and in an inoffensive manner) and when (during pauses or discussion points) to ask questions during a lecture.

5. **Seeking and using feedback**—Many times students do not realize that, as a listener, they can have a powerful influence over the speaker/teacher. The listener can use verbal cues (e.g., groans) and nonverbal cues (e.g., facial expressions). Students need to learn how to give positive or constructive feedback to teachers.

6. **Applying memory strategies**—This tactic helps students retain information presented in lectures. Three strategies proven to be helpful are (1) rehearsal—which allows one to review material presented because of the differential between speaking and thinking speed; (2) visual imagery—which allows the student to visualize each topic; and (3) clustering and coding—which allows the student to organize material, such as a list of main points, using mnemonic devices, which helps one to remember the list.

7. **Taking notes**—This strategy might be taught to students so that they are efficient (e.g., outlining, key words or concepts) and effective (e.g., meaningful to the situation).

Postlistening Strategies

Finally, listening skills can be enhanced with postlistening strategies. Postlistening strategies engage the student after the lecture is over. They include:

1. Reviewing the lecture material immediately or soon after the lecture for key ideas.

2. Adding any information needed to complete ideas.

3. Asking themselves questions about the lecture.

4. Writing a set of summary statements or conclusions from the lecture.

5. Skimming notes before the next lecture and preparing via prelistening strategies for the next lecture.

Using these prelistening, listening, and postlistening strategies will result in more effective listening to classroom lecturers.

Enhance Reading

Interest in and concern over enhancement of reading skills with older students is relatively new as educators have realized that instruction in early grades is not enough to create strategic readers in upper grades (Ehren, 2002a; Vacca, 2002). In 2002, the National Institute of Child Health and Human Development (NICHD) held workshops on adolescent literacy and set a national research agenda focused on how older students can learn to become competent readers (National Institutes of Health, 2002).

Reading should be taught using a strategy approach so that students develop content-area reading skills (D'Arcangelo, 2002; Minskoff and Allsopp, 2003; Vacca, 2002). Reading intervention for older students needs to be a careful balance between learning skills that should have been developed at an earlier age, like phonological awareness and alphabetic principles, while simultaneously teaching higher-level language skills needed to survive in the educational curriculum, such as metacognitive skills, to interpret lectures and textbooks.

A report by ASHA (2001b) contained suggestions for providing a balanced approach to reading intervention at the word, sentence, discourse, and metacognitive levels. ASHA's suggestions are summarized in the sidebar on page 358. In general, intervention with younger students typically focuses first on sound-symbol relationships and decoding, then on fluency; intervention with older students is concerned with comprehension, and then constructing knowledge from text.

Professionals should assist older students with readiness activities. For expository text, prepare students for reading by having them identify what prior knowledge (e.g., knowledge of the topic or vocabulary) they have. Alternatively, if the reading passage is narrative text, what knowledge does the student have about the setting? The characters? The author? The title? For both types of text, if students have little or no prior knowledge, an oral discussion leading into the reading can provide a critical orientation to the content of the text. To enhance comprehension of the text during or after reading, the use of Bloom et al.'s (1956) taxonomy (Kindsvatter, Wilen, and Ishler, 1988; Wiig and C. Wilson, 2002) and graphic organizers is effective (Minskoff and Allsopp, 2003; Vacca, 2002; Wiig and Wilson, 2001).

Providing students with opportunities to answer higher level questions, based on Bloom et al.'s (1956) taxonomy, has been effective with students who have comprehension difficulties. Table 2.3 (on page 45) suggests higher level questions that could be asked.

If using graphic organizers, the graphic should show the overarching organization of ideas (or story) presented by the writer(s), the main ideas and relevant details, and their relationship to one another. (This approach is similar to the classroom listening strategies crucial to teach to older students. Parallels between the two skill sets should be drawn.) Once the graphic is developed, have students practice discussing the main ideas of the author(s) by referring to the visual they have created. This will be an indication of the level at which they have comprehended the text and used it to construct knowledge. Such knowledge, built over time, adds to readiness for reading in the future.

A variety of acrostic devices can also be used effectively to enhance reading strategies (Minskoff and Allsopp, 2003). Several

357

Suggestions for Enhancing Reading Skills

At the word level:

• Teach strategies to learn the vocabulary of the school curriculum, such as the vocabulary of math, science, history.

• Teach prefixes and suffixes of words and how they affect the root or base word.

• Teach multiple-meaning words.

At the sentence level:

• Teach comprehension of the meaning of complex syntactic structures.

• Teach the impact of various clauses (noun, verb, adverbial clauses) on the meaning of the sentence.

At the discourse level:

• Teach awareness that reading is more of a monologue than a dialogue.

• Teach understanding of the macrostructure of the composition (e.g., problem/solution) as well as the microstructure (e.g., headings and subheadings; paragraphs).

• In expository discourse, teach recognition that information can be organized in various ways depending on the overall scheme (e.g., description, compare-contrast, cause-effect).

• Teach how to state the main idea of the text; provide a summary of the material; generate a title for the text.

At the metacognitive level:

• Teach self-monitoring skills to determine when there is a failure to comprehend the text.

• Teach knowledge of why a passage is being read (i.e., reading a passage with a purpose in mind, such as for entertainment, for information, or for instructions), which alters the strategy for how the reader reads it (e.g., skimming, analyzing).

• Teach the abstract interpretation of literate language.

• Teach higher-level language skills (e.g., awareness of derived words, sensitivity to high and low frequency words) along with strategic behaviors (i.e., learning to think with text).

Sources: ASHA (2001b); Westby (1999)

that are particularly helpful for older students faced with reading challenging expository text are in the sidebar that follows.

Before completing a lesson centered on a chosen reading passage, make certain that students understand the purpose of the writing by the author(s). Discuss any emotive reactions the students had and analyze how the writer(s) achieved that communication with their readers. Have the students think

Reading Strategies

IF IT FITS (for remembering new vocabulary)

- **I**dentify the word that is unfamiliar.
- **F**ind the definition.
- **I**solate the word by writing it on a card.
- **T**ell the definition aloud and write it on the card.
- **F**ind a keyword you already know that's like the new word.
- **I**magine an interaction (e.g., create an unusual visualization).
- **T**hink about the strategy (i.e., think of the keyword and make sure it triggers the definition of the new word).
- **S**tudy the strategy by testing yourself (and find stronger interactions if your strategy fails).

ABCDE (for getting the overall idea of a passage)

- **A**cclimate—determine what you know about the topic.
- **B**efore reading—survey the headings, pictures, graphics.
- **C**reate questions—ask yourself "teacher-like" questions.
- **D**uring reading—answer the questions.
- **E**nd of reading—summarize.

RAP-Q (for understanding main ideas of what was read)

- **R**ead a paragraph/passage.
- **A**sk myself, "What was the main idea?"
- **P**ut the idea in words and tell someone else (i.e., paraphrase).
- **Q**uestion myself about what I've just read.

ASK 5 Ws & 1 H & Answer (for comprehending details of what was read)

- While taking notes or in a graphic organizer, ask detailed questions about each main idea by using these questions as headings:

  Who?
  What?
  Where?
  When?
  Why?
  How?
- **Answer** the questions using the notes taken, or using the graphic organizer made while reading.

Source: Minskoff and Allsopp (2003)

about what skills they used, and have them bridge the lesson in one or several ways (i.e., generalize where else they will use or have used the skills just learned or practiced). Questions such as these might be asked:

- The purpose of the author was to inform. What else do you read that informs you?

- The author succeeded in helping you feel angry about someone being treated unfairly. What else have you read that made you feel similar?

- As you read this passage, you had to figure out the meanings of many words with multiple meanings. How did you figure them out? Name another time you will need to use a similar strategy(ies).

Enhance Writing

Traditionally, teachers have asked students to complete assignments that include a page or less of writing and that stress subject-area concepts (Applebee, Auten, and Lehr, 1981). These same teachers have emphasized mechanical aspects of writing (spelling, punctuation) over text-formatting aspects and have usually asked students to write about information already known to them so they are not looking for novel ideas.

Increasingly, teachers in individual schools across the country are now using writing as the means for learning (e.g., "journaling"). For students to become better writers, they need to write more and to do so by completing meaningful, authentic activities. This may be accomplished by having students write for at least 20 minutes every day (ASHA, 2001b). Scott (1999) noted that writing includes writing a particular type of text and/or in a particular genre. For example, just because one can write in one genre (e.g., narrative), it does not mean one can write in another (e.g., argumentation or persuasion; Scott, 1999). Our schools require that students be able to write a variety of types of text, both personal and impersonal, to succeed in the curriculum. Classification schemes of typical school writing genres are presented in Table 12.3 (Catts and Kamhi, 1999).

Writing needs to serve as a tool for learning rather than as a means to display acquired knowledge (Applebee et al., 1981). Like oral communication, written language needs to be seen as a process with a number of distinct aspects. One simple formulation is to use an instruction sequence of prewriting, writing, and editing (Applebee, 1981). Westby and Clauser (1999) explicitly pointed out that writing strategies should not be linear, but rather be recursive; that is, planning and revising should be in all phases of the process. Likewise, they advocated the use of self-verbalization at all phases of the process to think aloud about what they are doing and why. They stated, "as with strategies for effective reading comprehension, strategies for effective writing must consider declarative, procedural and conditional knowledge" (p. 304). They defined each of these types of knowledge as follows:

- Declarative knowledge is what is expected at each stage of the process

Classification Schemes
of Typical School Writing Genres

Table 12.3

Type of Text	Chronological	Nonchronological (logical)

Personal	Narratives
	    Personal experience
	    Biographical
	    Fictional
	    Historical
	Personal journals
	Letters
	Procedures
		Persuasion
		Reports
		Composition
		    Generalization
		    Speculation
		    Argument

Impersonal	Narrative (what happened) Recount	Factual (the way things are) Procedural (how something is done) Descriptions (what some particular thing is like) Reports (what an entire class of things are like) Explanation (a reason why a judgment has been made) Exposition (arguments why a thesis has been proposed) Persuading *that* (analytic) Persuading *to* (oratory)

From *Language and Reading Disabilities* (p. 238), by H.W. Catts and A.G. Kamhi, 1999, Needham Heights, MA: Allyn and Bacon. © 1999 by Allyn and Bacon. Adapted with permission.

- Procedural knowledge is knowing how to employ various strategies

- Conditional knowledge is knowing when and where to employ these strategies

Prewriting Strategies

Prewriting involves thinking about a topic, gathering information, talking, and reading. In authentic writing situations, this period may extend for weeks or even months. In classroom situations, some teachers only allow students just over three minutes (Applebee et al., 1981)! Most writing assignments in school begin with the expectation that the student already knows what to write and can rapidly start.

Discussion of a topic is an excellent technique that can be used to enhance both written and oral communication. One way to collaborate within the classroom is for the classroom teacher or learning disabilities specialist to formulate a writing assignment and then allow time for the speech-language pathologist to have students discuss the topic, formulate strategies for gathering and organizing the information to complete the assignment, and outline or map the amassed data. The outline or map might be accomplished through a program such as Inspiration (Inspiration Software, 1997), through word-processing software, or with traditional recording methods. The advantage of using a software program, such as Inspiration, is that it allows the student to create a visual map or organizational scheme that quickly converts to a traditional outline, or vice versa. A plan-think sheet might be generated that the student uses to note the following:

- "The Topic
- Who: Who am I writing for?
- Why: Why am I writing?
- What: What do I know? (Brainstorm a list of what is known about the topic).
- How: How can I group my ideas?" (Westby and Clauser, 1999).

Discussion of a topic is an excellent technique that can be used to enhance both written and oral communication.

It is effective when older students use such methods as the STOP strategy (Westby and Clauser, 1999) as part of their planning for certain genre (e.g., persuasive writing), which involves the following:

- **S**uspend judgment.
- **T**ake a side.
- **O**rganize ideas.
- **P**lan more as you write.

Composing Strategies

Writing involves the composing process. The topic is developed on paper (or computer screen). Concern should be on expressing ideas, not on formulating sentences. Westby and Clauser (1999) recommend that during the writing process, the student be taught to use self-regulating behaviors, such as (1) focusing attention and planning by thinking, "I need a topic sentence and supporting details"; (2) self-evaluating and error correcting by thinking, "I didn't say that clearly; I know I can do better"; (3) coping and self-control by thinking, "I'm not going to start all over until I think more about this topic"; and (4) self-reinforcement by thinking, "This is one of my best sentences."

Multiple drafts may be needed before the various sections of writing support each other. In contrast, some teachers require only one draft and do little to mediate the notion that cohesive writing almost always requires a successive refinement process. Unless the written piece is very short, students should anticipate and be required to produce more than one draft. Word-processing the document for use in sequel revisions is strongly recommended. Mediation should be used to help students focus on sections needing greater clarity or stronger arguments. Students should also bridge to situations when various writing expectations will be demanded of them (e.g., writing a letter or a paper to persuade vs. writing to tell a story).

Editing Strategies

Editing involves "polishing"—attending to spelling, punctuation, usage, and other mechanics. Westby and Clauser (1999) noted that students do not like to engage in revising their writing, and if they do, they confine it to proofreading for the mechanics of writing and not to revising to improve the meaning, clarity, and organization of their writing. K. Harris and Graham (1996) have a very straightforward procedure for revising or editing text. They suggest students SCAN each sentence as follows:

- Does it make Sense?
- Is it Connected to my central idea?
- Can I Add more detail?
- Note errors.

Another concept put forth by Westby and Clauser (1999) is that of an author's chair, where the student comes forth and reads their written work aloud and peers react to the writing by carefully listening to the text, commenting on what they like about the text and why, and commenting on something they believe could be improved and how to revise it. This can be most helpful if students are taught to give constructive feedback.

When teachers have a "first-and-final draft" mentality (and some do), that copy is also surrounded by demands for accuracy and neatness—a rather unrealistic expectation even for the best writers among us. While word processing helps greatly to omit the "messiness" factor, the writing and the editing phases should still be approached as separate, albeit related, factors.

When teachers comment on student papers, they function in much the same way as an editor's evaluation. In authentic writing situations, the editing would be acted upon and students would write another draft, using the editorial suggestions and revisions to produce a better manuscript. Unfortunately, in many school situations, the editorial comments simply become private criticism for the author that may or may not prove beneficial. After all, educators cannot assume that students' reading of their critiques (if indeed they're read at all) results in learning how to correct their errors.

Writing should be motivated by a need to communicate to a reader who does not already know what is going to be said (Applebee et al., 1981). The best lessons for older students view writing as a vehicle for learning, which emerges naturally from other activities. When oral and written communication skills are interwoven in clinical activities, the power of language to create meaning is maximized, and "meaning-making is the general purpose of all forms of language text or all skills" (J. Damico, 1992, p. 10).

Points of Discussion

1. Do you agree with the intervention guidelines presented for working with older students? Why or why not? Would you add others?

2. Think of three relevant intervention activities that you might do with an older student. Mediate the importance of learning the skills taught within the activities.

Suggested Readings

Ehren, B. (2002). Getting into the adolescent literacy game. *The ASHA Leader, 7*(7), 4–5, 10.

Ehren, B. (2002). Speech-language pathologists contributing significantly to the academic success of high school students: A vision for professional growth. *Topics in Language Disorders, 22*(2), 60–80.

Feuerstein, Reuven, Feuerstein, Rafi, and Schur, Y. (1997). Process as content in education of exceptional children. In A.L. Costa and R.M. Liebman (Eds.), *Supporting the spirit of learning: When process is content* (pp. 1–22). Thousand Oaks, CA: Corwin Press.

13
Chapter

Specific Intervention Methods

Goals

- Outline specific intervention methods for referential communication activities, narrative storytelling activities, expository discourse activities, word-finding activities, emotional intelligence activities, and social skill activities

- Demonstrate the kinds of questions to ask to mediate strategies

- Provide bridging questions that focus students on how to transfer communication skills learned during intervention to other places at school, in the home, and in the community

Volumes would be needed to delineate the many specific methods (i.e., procedures and materials) that could be used for teaching thinking, listening, speaking, reading, writing, meta-abilities, nonverbal communication, and paralinguistic skills. Methods abound and vary with the theoretical underpinnings selected for intervention. Instead of attempting to present several methods superficially, we present a few representative methods in depth in this chapter:

- Referential communication activities
- Narrative storytelling activities
- Expository discourse activities
- Word-finding activities
- Emotional intelligence activities
- Social skill activities

These methods have been selected because they are ones we advocate for older students with language disorders. They are consonant with our theoretical constructs presented in

Chapter 1 and with the recommended general program approach of learning strategies.

For each method, we describe the procedure, discuss materials, highlight areas of emphasis, list sample bridging questions that could be asked by the adult providing intervention, and summarize potential strategies that could be mediated for the student. (For an explanation of bridging and mediation, see Chapter 12, pages 344–351.)

Referential Communication Activities

Referential communication activities, also known as *barrier activities*, emphasize the communication functions of giving and getting information. To perform these functions, adequate speaking and listening skills are required when exchanging information orally, and reading and writing skills when using a written medium. This ability to express and to comprehend informative messages is a function repeated many times by competent communicators throughout a typical day. However, students with language disorders often have difficulty engaging in precise message formulation and reception. Referential communication activities improve this precision.

Referential communication activities are appropriate for preadolescents and youth in all stages of adolescence. By altering the content

and the level of difficulty, the activities become adaptable to any age and ability level.

Procedure

Referential communication activities require a minimum of one speaker and one listener (or one writer and one reader). They are seated near each other with a physical barrier (i.e., a screen of some type) between them. The speaker and the listener have identical sets of materials that are concealed from each other by the screen. The speaker explains to the listener how to use the materials to construct or reconstruct an identical two- or three-dimensional model that only the speaker can see.

Barrier activities may involve more than one speaker (or writer) and one listener (or reader) simultaneously. One speaker may give directions to many listeners. Numerous speakers could collaborate on sending one clear message to one or many listeners; this is a common communication experience (e.g., a committee deciding how to word a statement; two parents agreeing on what to say after their child has misbehaved).

Another option for including more than one speaker and one listener during referential communication activities is to appoint one or more observers (or an editor(s) for written messages). The observer is free to study the model that the speaker is describing and to observe the responses of the listener. The observer can often see firsthand when and why any communication breakdowns are occurring. The format of assigning "speaker-listener-observer" roles is based on the idea that people can more easily focus on the relation between speaker (message) and listener (response) when not enmeshed in one of those roles (Shantz, 1981). It may be that "vicarious" role reversal occurs by the observer, thus making it an effective experience.

Whatever combination of participants is used during barrier activities, the outcome is natural communication. There is a reason for the speaker (writer) to formulate a message and a reason for the listener (reader) to attempt to understand it. All participants, including any observers (editors), are afforded the opportunity to observe the effects of adequate and inadequate communication.

The professional providing intervention should use a number of variations during referential communication activities (Schreiber and McKinley, 1995). A few are listed in the sidebar. They provide opportunities for the professional to mediate when these variations occur in daily communication and how message sending and receiving need to be adjusted to accommodate for them (e.g., if the speaker (writer) knows no questions for clarification are allowed, the message should be delivered after more planning and perhaps with a slower rate of speech (or with a step-by-step list in writing)).

Materials

Materials for referential communication activities may be either two- or three-dimensional. In both cases, the materials should be sophisticated enough so they do not cause embarrassment to the older student (e.g.,

Referential Communication Variations

• **Clarification questions vs. no questions.** Asking questions for clarification could be allowed initially during the message exchange. They should not only be encouraged, but also modeled by the adult providing intervention. If the student's message is too general, saying, "I've got [4, 2, or however many] items like that. I'm not sure which one you mean. Can you help?" is more effective than asking "Which one?" or simply guessing which referent the speaker (writer) intends (e.g., "Is it this one?"; Robinson, 1981).

As participants become more proficient in producing and comprehending messages, occasional sessions might be held during which questions for clarification are not allowed. During and after these sessions, students should discuss and bridge their experience (e.g., "How did the rule of 'no questions' affect your understanding of the message?"; "Was the activity more or less difficult when questions were not allowed?"; "What questions(s) would you have asked if you could have?"; and "In what other situations have you been where you were not allowed to ask questions for clarification?").

Continued on next page

Communication Solutions
for Older Students

Continued

- **State vs. state-restate.** The usual sequence of events during barrier activities is for the speaker and the listener to compare models after the message has been given and questions for clarification, if allowed, have been asked. Another option is for the listener to restate the entire message to the speaker before the comparison of models is shared. The restatement may also be accomplished sequentially (i.e., after the speaker gives one part of a step-by-step message, the listener then restates the information). Restatement may allow for identification of the sources of any communication breakdowns and permit repair.

- **Gestures vs. no gestures.** Gestures that help clarify the spoken message may initially be allowed, especially for students who need the activity to be as concrete as possible. Gestures might be particularly tempting to use when spatial orientation is an important attribute to describe. Disallowance of gestures that substitute for description (e.g., pointing to a piece of the model rather than describing it) should be enforced most of the time. Alternate use and nonuse (e.g., seat people back to back during the exchange) of gestures will allow the opportunity for discussion concerning how the oral message becomes modified with and without accompanying gestures and facial expressions.

- **Partial message vs. complete message.** When students begin referential communication activities, they are more likely to be successful if partial messages are sent and received in sequential order. Later on, the speaker (writer) could be required to send the entire message at once, and listeners (readers) might be required to receive the whole message before beginning a response. This requires memory strategies, thus making the level of the task more difficult.

- **Information questions vs. clarification questions.** This variation requires the listener (reader) to ask questions for information rather than questions for clarification. The speaker (writer), in turn, supplies responses to these questions rather than initiating the content of the message. For example, if *wh-* questions are allowed, questions might include "What shapes are used?"; "What size is the triangle?"; or "Where is it placed?" The activities could also be structured to require the listener to ask yes-no questions. The speaker remains in control of the model to be duplicated. However, the listener must employ careful questioning strategies to obtain all the necessary information to complete the activity successfully.

- **Time limit vs. no time limit.** This variation introduces the impact of time pressure on the fluency and efficiency of the message. When students are given a structured time limit (e.g., one minute) to send a message, more planning must occur than when messages have no restrictions. Discussion should focus on how speakers (writers) and listeners (readers) alter their behaviors when time is of the essence.

Source: Schreiber and McKinley (1995)

colored building blocks will usually be viewed negatively). Regardless of the material selected, two or more identical sets will be needed.

The adult providing intervention should explain to the student that the model constructed or reconstructed with the materials is secondary to the communication process occurring. Also explain that referential communication is not successful until the speaker and the listener share a common meaning for the message. When communication breakdowns occur, they should be analyzed and repaired. Depending on the focus of the referential communication activity, the materials may be natural or contrived. For example, actual objects may be used (i.e., natural materials), and the speaker must describe to the listener how to orient them to one another. On the other end of the spectrum, materials may be contrived, such as drawing two-dimensional representations of objects.

A commercial material that provides 100 drawings that become gradually more challenging to explain is a great timesaver for the professional (i.e., *Make-It-Yourself Barrier Activities* [L. Schwartz and McKinley, 1987]). Such a material allows professionals to easily find patterns that are challenging but not frustrating for students.

An additional material that is sometimes desirable during referential communication activities between speakers and listeners is a tape recorder. With a tape recorder, the speaker's message can be recorded and replayed to prevent discrepancies between what the speaker perceived to have communicated and what he or she actually said.

Areas of Emphasis

The most common areas of emphasis during referential communication activities are speaking and listening. The role of the student engaged in the activities may alternate between speaker and listener, or one role may be assigned throughout. Regardless of the specific content of an activity, ongoing opportunities are available for producing and comprehending clear messages. The roles of speaker-listener are easily replaced by writer-reader when a focus on written language is desired.

If the content of the referential communication activities is carefully planned, then areas of emphasis may also include thinking behaviors and nonverbal communication. Thinking may be emphasized more specifically if the materials selected require application of spatial, quantitative, and qualitative concepts. Nonverbal communication may be emphasized if messages that could be more easily communicated with gestures, or a combination of gestures and oral language, are utilized. For example, giving each student a group of pictures illustrating such actions as someone waving a flag, starting a lawn mower with a pull rope, and bouncing a ball. Through gestures, the student can communicate to the receiver(s) what picture is to be matched. Also, using the technique of gestures vs. no gestures (discussed in the sidebar on pages 367–368) provides a means for focusing on nonverbal communication. When imposing a time limit, paralinguistics (especially rate of speech) can be emphasized.

Bridging Questions

Consider asking these bridging questions during or after referential communication activities:

- "In what other situations has it been important to communicate a message clearly?"

- "Tell me about a time when you were talking and a breakdown in communication occurred (i.e., when you, as a speaker, were the cause of the breakdown). What were the consequences?"

- "Tell me about a time when you were listening and a breakdown in communication occurred (i.e., when you, as the listener, were the cause of the breakdown). What were the consequences?"

- "Give an example of when you asked a question for clarification. Did it prevent a communication breakdown?"

- "You have just been restricted from using gestures and eye contact when saying your message. When else might you be prevented from using nonverbal communication?"

Strategies to Mediate

A partial list of strategies to mediate for youth during referential communication activities includes these:

- Visualizing the information being spoken or listened to (i.e., seeing the model "in your mind")

- Using a plan to organize the information (i.e., what is most important to say (write) first, next, last?)

- Concentrating attention on the speaker when in the role of a listener (i.e., blocking out distractions)

- Knowing how and when to ask a question for clarification

- Using appropriate concepts (e.g., spatial, quantity, quality) to make messages concise

- Taking the listener's (reader's) perspective when producing a message

Narrative Storytelling Activities

A wide array of discourse-level skills are needed for successful participation in social and academic pursuits. One essential narrative skill is storytelling. As children reach adolescence, the ability to comprehend and to produce larger units of language becomes increasingly important for peer acceptance and academic survival. Whereas younger children often receive help from teachers and parents to fill in narrations, adolescents are expected to be more independent. Both oral and written narrative skills must be part of their repertoire.

Narration activities can be used during preadolescence and during early, middle, and late stages of adolescence. They should be chosen with the student's social-emotional level and interests in mind.

Procedure

Westby (1991a) has suggested three levels of activities for enhancing narrative skills. Goals for each level have been summarized as follows:

- **Early Stage**—Provide exposure to literate language. Structure interactions to facilitate reporting.

- **Middle Stage**—Facilitate understanding of relationships among character traits, emotions, and events. Require the child to structure the narrative.

- **Advanced Stage**—Facilitate comprehension of more complex embedded narratives. Facilitate metanarrative skills. (Westby, 1991a, p. 351)

Although it is desirable for older students to be performing at the advanced stage, they may need to acquire more concrete behaviors before abstract abilities (e.g., metanarrative skills) develop. Obviously, activities at the early, more concrete, level (Westby,

1984), which provide exposure to literate language for young children (e.g., "show and tell" time), are not appropriate at the preadolescent and adolescent levels. However, exposure can be promoted through activities such as listening to "Books on Tape;" watching movies, home videos, or Public Broadcasting System literary presentations based on books that interest older students; and listening to old-time radio dramatizations (e.g., Orson Wells's "War of the Worlds").

Hoggan and Strong (1994; 1996) summarized 22 strategies that might be used to teach narrative skills and thus achieve the goals cited by Westby (1991a). The strategies are organized into the categories of "prestory presentation," "during-story presentation," and "poststory presentation." All 22 strategies are appropriate to use at the preadolescent level, and all but "dramatic play" are appropriate for use during adolescence.

Prestory presentation strategies include establishing a preparatory set, summarizing the story before it is presented, engaging in semantic word mapping (to help students understand word relationships and concepts), and using think-alouds (e.g., asking students to make predictions about a story's topic). A few of the during-story presentation strategies are questioning (e.g., to extend thinking, to obtain information, to engage in problem solving) and episode mapping. Poststory presentation strategies include such items as clarifying internal states of characters, story retelling, and story-grammar cuing. *Scaffolding* is the term often used for this cuing. "Scaffolding is the use of leading questions that help the speaker organize (the) story" (Page and Stewart, 1985, p. 25).

A chart or map listing major elements of a story can be used as a guide for narrators and for discussion after the story (Garnett, 1986; Hutson-Nechkash, 2001). Table 13.1 suggests the content of such a chart. Preadolescents, or those less skilled in narration, should be guided to use the concrete scaffolding items first (e.g., setting, events), both when listening to stories and when telling them. As narrative skills emerge, abstract elements of a story (e.g., theme, moral) should receive focus. When these more skilled adolescents hear stories that they retell, they should be able to answer all of the questions listed in Table 13.1. When they tell stories, the beginning is marked by a description of setting and the ending is marked by a conclusion, but the elements listed in between vary in sequence and may not even need to be included.

As students become familiar with various elements of narration and practice logical sequencing of the elements, they should be encouraged to remind themselves of the questions to be answered during the narration. Long-term reliance on a visible chart or on someone to ask the questions of them should be avoided.

Table 13.1

Story Elements Guide for Narrators

Story Grammar Elements	Questions
Beginning Setting of Story	Who are the main characters? Where does the story take place? When does the story take place?

Middle
  Theme of the Story
  Events of the Story
  Goal(s) of the Characters
  Motive(s) of the Characters
  Attempts of the Characters
  Reactions of the Characters
	
	What is the main idea (theme) of the story?
	What happens to the characters?
	What are the characters trying to do?
	Why are the characters trying to reach the goal(s)?
	What happens when the characters try to reach the goal?
	What are their feelings? What are their plans?

Ending Conclusion	How does everything turn out? What lesson (moral) did you learn from the story?

Sources: Garnett (1986); Hutson-Nechkash (2001)

Page and Stewart (1985) and Westby (1991a) both emphasized the importance of direct instruction in improving cause-and-effect relationships as a general means to developing narration skills. Emphasis should be on relationships that are most essential to stories, including the effects of the environment on people, animals, and events; the effects of various types of people (e.g., the "do-gooder," the "villain") and animals on events; the effects of events on feelings and, conversely, the effects of feelings on events; and the knowledge that much behavior is intentionally planned. Through mediation and discussion, students should be presented with questions such as these:

- "How do you identify emotions?"
- "What causes feelings?"
- "What do people do when they feel a certain way?"
- "What would you predict [character name] will do in this situation? Why?"

At the highest level of narration, late adolescents should discuss themes, plots, and/or morals of stories (Westby, 1991a). They should talk about the structure of narratives and how to vary structure intentionally for different purposes (i.e., metanarrative skills). Adolescents might tell stories from the perspective of different characters, or tell a similar story with different endings. For example, *Choose Your Own Adventure* books, *Twist-A-Plot* books, and similar series allow each story to be completed in several dozen ways. A *Choose Your Own Adventure* book could

be read to the student, followed by informational and critical listening questions concerning characters and events. At the frequent decision points within the story, the student can be asked which choice to select and why. Following completion of the story once, or in a number of different ways, the student can reformulate it using the assistance of self-imposed scaffolding questions.

Adolescents might tell stories from the perspective of different characters, or tell a similar story with different endings.

Throughout narrative storytelling activities, professionals should be particularly aware of oral expression difficulties that interfere with clear formulation or reformulation (e.g., word-retrieval problems, verbal mazes, inappropriate use of sentence fragments, and nonspecific language—including lack of pronoun references). These problems must be addressed before adequate oral narrative skills can be expected. Equivalent difficulties should be addressed when working on written narrative skills (e.g., nonspecific language, sentence fragments).

Materials

The primary materials needed for narrative skill building activities are books, audiotapes, videotapes, and playback equipment. The books and tapes selected should provide models for well-structured narrations. Selection might be based on what is currently being studied in the student's classroom. Middle- and secondary-level English teachers are a good resource for selecting quality literature that is of interest to most preadolescents and adolescents. When the selected books are not available on tape, service groups in high schools are often willing to help out and record the necessary books. The literature chosen can be used for storyretelling activities or as a springboard for formulating a new variation of the story.

When written narratives are the focus, graphic organizers might be helpful (e.g., Inspiration software (1997) or *Map It Out* (Wiig and C. Wilson, 2001). A word processor may also be desirable.

Areas of Emphasis

Speaking and listening are the most often emphasized areas during oral narrative skill building activities. Listening is primary when reformulation tasks are presented; speaking is necessary during both formulation and reformulation tasks. Written language skills can be emphasized by requesting the student to formulate or reformulate a story in writing.

By analyzing and discussing various aspects of stories, meta- skills are emphasized.

Thinking and nonverbal communication can be focused on if the tasks are structured appropriately. For example, requesting the student's underlying reasoning for why a particular choice was made within a *Twist-A-Plot* story places emphasis on thinking during the activity. Asking the student to predict how the facial expression just described in the story will affect the feelings of another character places emphasis on nonverbal communication.

Bridging Questions

Consider asking these bridging questions during or after narrative storytelling activities:

- "In the story, one of the main characters felt very (emotion). When is a time you felt that way? What event led to your feeling that way?"

- "What happens when the setting of a story is never explained? Think of a time someone tried to tell you something and you did not know the setting. Think of a time you tried to tell someone else a story and forgot to tell the setting."

- "In some stories, you can predict how the characters will feel or act next. When (besides in stories) do you predict something that will happen? How can predictions help you?"

- "I prepared you for listening to the story by telling you the title and the topic of the story. How did that help you understand what the story was about? How could knowing the titles and topics of stories (or sections of your textbook) help you in social studies class? In science class?"

- "The group has been talking about cause and effect. Tell me something funny that happened in the story. Together, let's figure out what caused it to be funny."

Strategies to Mediate

A partial list of strategies to mediate for youth during narrative storytelling activities includes these:

- Asking key questions of yourself to help organize the narrative (i.e., scaffolding)

- Listening for the major organizational structure of a narrative

- Using cohesion devices to connect ideas in the narrative together (i.e., to make the narrative easier for listeners to understand)

- Predicting outcomes of events as a way to remember "what happens next"

- Describing the setting of a story first, before much action is begun

- Pretending you are a character in the story, and everything happens to you as you retell the story from the character's perspective

Expository Discourse Activities

When someone explains the rules of a game, delineates how to make something, engages in "show-and-tell" communicative behavior, or describes the characteristics of an object or idea, expository discourse skills are being used. N. Nelson (1993) defined *expository discourse* as "discourse that conveys factual or technical information" (p. 358). Referential communication, which was summarized earlier, is one aspect of expository discourse.

Success in school relies on expository discourse competence because expository text structure is used in most content textbooks and teacher lectures (N. Nelson, 1993). When students understand expository text structures, they can follow the outline of a teacher's lecture, organize their notes, apply mnemonic strategies, and prepare their own papers more efficiently. Students are at risk when they do not understand the complex language of expository discourse (e.g., directions, predictions, facts, specifications, dates, and conclusions).

> *Success in school
> relies on expository
> discourse competence
> because expository text
> structure is used in most
> content textbooks and
> teacher lectures.*

Procedure

Expository text can be viewed from both comprehension and production perspectives. Older students are simultaneously expected to listen to lectures; to derive main ideas and relevant details from their textbooks while reading; to write expository texts of their own (e.g., book reports, answers to essay questions); and to engage in activities such as oral report giving, discussing, and defining.

Intervention might begin with teaching students to recognize different discourse structures, beginning with narrative structure (N. Nelson, 1988; Wallach, 1990; Westby, 1989). Students could then be taught to contrast narrative and expository texts (N. Nelson, 1993). Expository text structures could be visually displayed for students, as in the poster shown in Figure 13.1. N. Nelson (1993) and Westby (1991b) also include two additional expository text macrostructures:

- By description
- By matrix (i.e., the intersection of several categories)

Figure 13.1 **Organize Your Information Poster**

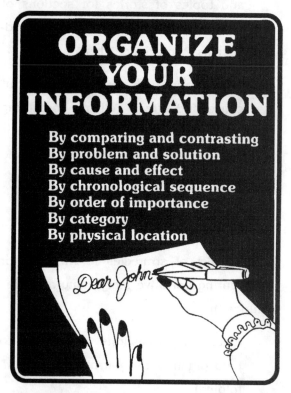

From *Language Disorders in Older Students: Preadolescents and Adolescents* (p. 193), by V. Lord Larson and N.L. McKinley, 1995, Eau Claire, WI: Thinking Publications. © 1995 by Thinking Publications. Reprinted with permission.

Initially, the adult providing intervention may set up the expository text structure, then coach the student to fit additional pieces of information into the organization. Mediation may be provided to explain the structure that is chosen and why it is an appropriate choice for the factual or technical information presented.

Students should receive practice in inferring structures, first with assistance, then without. Text excerpts from the student's curriculum and/or classroom lecture snippets could be used. While expository discourse skills are being acquired, be sure to frame the structural cues so that the student can recognize them as independently as possible. Scaffolding support should be offered (e.g. "Why did ____ happen?"; "List the features of ____;" "Give examples of ____;" or Give the steps in doing ____").

Westby (1991b) emphasized that the framing-of-cues process should help students recognize key words that may signal different kinds of expository text. Sample key words are listed in Table 13.2 for the expository text structures cited earlier. These key

Key Words and Phrases for Signaling Expository Text Structures

Table 13.2

Text Structure	Key Words and Phrases
Comparing and Contrasting	same, different, however, but, on the contrary, similar, dissimilar, yet, still, common, alike, rather than, instead of, compare, contrast
Problem and Solution	one problem, the problem is, the issues are, a solution(s) is (are)
Cause and Effect	if, then, because, reason, affected, influenced, result, resulted in, since, therefore, thus, hence, consequently, cause, caused, effect, net effect, consequence
Chronological Sequence (episodic sequence)	first, second, third, after that, antecedent, before that, preceding, next, last, in order, subsequent, proceeding, finally, eventually, gradually
Order of Importance (hierarchical)	first, second, third, most, least, all, none, some, always, never, more, less, ____ +*er*, ____ +*est*, frequent, infrequent
Category (topical cluster or list)	group, set, for instance, another, an illustration of, such as, an example of, like, category, class
Physical Location	here, there, left, right, above, below, north, south, east, west, around, on top, under, bottom, front, back, forward, backward, side
Description	defined as, called, labeled, refers to, is someone who, is something that, means, can be interpreted as, describe, procedure, how to
Matrix	interpret, intersection, come together, overlap, influenced by, simultaneously, at the same time, converge

Sources: Larson and McKinley (1995); N. Nelson (1993); Schreiber and McKinley (1995); Westby (1991b)

words are often in the form of conjunctions and logical connectors and serve as text cohesion devices. Intervention should include focusing on these key words and making certain that students comprehend their meaning. Key words might be stressed during oral exchanges, highlighted in discourse being read, and edited in when students are writing their own expository text.

Materials

The student's curricular materials should be used whenever possible when teaching expository discourse skills. Textbooks, supplemental reading, handouts, and tests can all be analyzed with the student for text structure and key words. Classroom lectures and teacher directions can also be used and are best captured on video or audiotape for ongoing benefit. Simulated lecture and direction segments can be created in lieu of capturing "the real thing." Still, simulations should be as realistic as possible so that students are exposed to expository text structures as they will naturally occur in their environment.

Areas of Emphasis

The most common areas of emphasis during expository discourse activities are speaking, listening, reading, and writing. Analysis of text structure also requires thinking and meta- skills. Intervention should incorporate both comprehension (listening, reading) and production (speaking, writing) aspects. As key words are identified while listening or

reading, they should be noted, then used by the student when speaking and writing.

Nonverbal communication is not generally emphasized while working on expository discourse skills. However, students might be taught that cues can be obtained by watching a teacher's nonverbal communication. For example, it would not be unusual for teachers to list items on their fingers as they are announcing them or to emphasize, "first, next, last" nonverbally when giving directions with a chronological sequence.

Bridging Questions

Consider asking these bridging questions during or after expository discourse activities:

- "We just analyzed a section in your textbook and decided it fit the organizational structure called ____. When else have you heard or read information organized by that structure?"

- "We've been reading information organized by category. Now you've been given some new information. How would you fit the new information into the existing categories?"

- "Your teacher has given you an assignment to write about some aspect of World War II. What are some choices of text structure, and how would what you write change with the structure? (For example, a student could write about the major chronological events of World War II or focus instead on the causes of the war and the net effects.)"

- "You need to organize a three-minute speech in which you introduce yourself to the class. You decide to organize your speech using a "comparing and contrasting" structure. What are some questions you could ask yourself to prepare for your speech?"

- "Sometimes reports are organized by describing the problem and then giving solutions. What are some topics you could organize that way? Sometimes it is easier to organize reports by the order of events (i.e., *first, next, last*). What are some topics you could organize that way?"

Strategies to Mediate

A partial list of strategies to mediate for youth during expository discourse activities includes these:

- Organizing information by several characteristics simultaneously (e.g., chronologically and by problem and solution) and seeing how text structure would alter accordingly

- Using relevant information once a text structure is chosen and ignoring irrelevant information

- Looking for relationships among separate objects, events, and experiences, then selecting the expository discourse macrostructure that can reflect these relationships

- Using logic to defend the text structure chosen for spoken or written discourse assignments

- Taking sufficient time to think through the text structure that is to be comprehended or produced

Word-Finding Activities

Word-finding difficulties are common in many children and adolescents with special needs. While the problem has been recognized for some time, word-finding intervention programs have not kept pace with diagnostic procedures (German, 1993). Word-finding problems affect all aspects of an individual's life in social, academic, and ultimately, vocational settings (German, 2001). The problems reveal themselves in discourse (e.g., when relating experiences or events), which has a negative impact on conversations.

Adequate word-finding ability is essential to these communication functions: to give information, to get information, to describe an ongoing event, to persuade the listener, to self-disclose, to solve problems, and to entertain. In short, word finding is one of the most pervasive communication skills that can be taught to students experiencing deficits. During word-finding activities, strategies are taught that eliminate or minimize the interference of word-finding problems during oral and written communication.

Procedure

German (1992, 1993) presented a word-finding intervention model focusing on three areas: (1) remediation, (2) self-advocacy instruction, and (3) compensatory modification.

Remediation

According to German (1992, 1993), during remediation, the student learns word-retrieval strategies such as these:

- Attribute-cuing strategies
- Semantic alternatives
- Associate cuing
- Reflective pausing

When teaching *attribute cuing strategies,* emphasis is placed on phonemic cuing (i.e., instructing how the initial sound(s) or syllables in a word can be used to cue the target word). Similarly, graphemic cuing takes advantage of the initial letter(s) or spelling to cue the target word. Another type of attribute cuing is imagery cuing, which uses visualization of the referent to cue the target word. Gesture cuing uses a mime of the action associated with the target word.

Semantic alternatives include synonym substituting and category name substituting. To use synonym substitution, the student must first understand the concept of a synonym. Students are taught it is appropriate to substitute a synonym for a word that is difficult to retrieve (e.g., *cook* for *chef*). In contrast, students who understand vocabulary categorization concepts could be taught to substitute a category name for a difficult-to-retrieve word (e.g., *vegetable* for *celery*).

In *associate cuing,* the adult planning word-finding activities for the student mediates how thinking of a word highly associated with the target word can provide a reminder of the difficult-to-retrieve word. For example, the student could think of the associated word *cake* to retrieve *birthday*. Other people can also provide associated words to cue the student when word-finding blocks occur. Associate cuing is good for building the retrieval strength of technical academic terms and names of important people, places, and events.

Reflective pausing is a good strategy for students who are fast but inaccurate namers. Students are taught to use pausing with the goal of reducing the retrieval of inappropriate words. When using reflective pausing, the student stops when trying to retrieve a word, remains silent rather than blurting out a competing (inaccurate) response, and applies one of the attribute-cuing or semantic-alternatives strategies described. The student might also admit to the listener that he or she "can't remember the word right now" to minimize the effects of the pause.

Students are taught to use pausing with the goal of reducing the retrieval of inappropriate words.

Techniques that help to reinforce word-finding strategies include segmenting, rhythm, rehearsal, and rapid-naming exercises. For students who understand syllabication, the use of segmenting can assist in retrieving multisyllabic words. Students divide words into syllables, then rehearse saying them. Likewise, a rhythm technique can be used with students who have syllabication skills. Again, using multisyllabic words, students tap for each syllable as they are rehearsing aloud.

When students do not have syllabication skills, a straight rehearsal technique can still help them improve word retrieval. Multisyllabic words are repeated five times, for example. For students with slow retrieval speed, rapid-naming exercises might be used (e.g., practice 10 target words written or pictured on cards and attempt to improve the overall time it takes to flip through and name the 10 cards). Words used for practicing word-retrieval strategies and techniques should come from the student's world. Words should be relevant to school, home, work, and recreational settings.

Self-Advocacy Instruction

In addition to the direct remediation activities with students just described, focus should also cross over to self-advocacy instruction (German, 1992, 1993). First, students should become knowledgeable about the retrieval strategies that are best for their particular word-finding deficits; mediation from the involved professional(s) assists this process. Students are then taught self-monitoring techniques (e.g., tallying when and how many times they engage in a particular gesture) and self-instruction sequences (e.g., what self-talk message might be used to cue a semantic alternative word choice, such as "Let me think. To what category does the word that I'm trying to find belong? Oh, yes, it's a country in South America").

Another aspect of self-advocacy is teaching students to identify the impact of language settings, contexts, times of day, and the vocabulary itself on word-retrieval skills (German, 1993). Some situations will trigger more word-finding problems than others, and students should become knowledgeable about their progress during intervention for word-retrieval deficits. They should gradually learn to self-apply retrieval strategies and techniques and establish knowledge of the compensatory modifications that can be made for them.

Compensatory Modification

The compensatory modification focus within word-finding activities should be implemented concurrently with the self-advocacy component (German, 1992, 1993); in this way, the student takes ownership of the word-retrieval problem. Instructional modifications can be made that facilitate a student's word-finding skills.

Collaboration with teachers, parents, and work supervisors identifies modifications that can be made in the classroom, at home, and on a job site. Older students, particularly those in high school and in postsecondary educations settings, should participate in conversations with teachers about modifications. Some compensatory modifications that might be used include altering tests to put less demand on retrieval skills (e.g., having an open-book exam), allowing additional time to complete a task, and providing multiple-choice formats when a retrieval block occurs. Similarly, family members and employers might allow more time for responses and reduce the number of stressful speaking situations that precipitate word-finding problems.

Materials

The primary materials needed for word-finding activities are relevant vocabulary lists derived from a student's school, home, work, and community settings. Using words that are immediately meaningful for the student motivates that individual to learn word-retrieval strategies and to engage in word-finding techniques that will generalize to new terms that constantly surface.

Maintaining a notebook of words being studied is critical. Many helpful recording forms are also available in German's (1993) *Word-Finding Intervention Program*.

Reinforcement materials may be needed to motivate younger students. For example, while engaged in the rehearsal technique, students may say a word five times and then get to move ahead on a game board, or perhaps

they toss a pair of dice and say a word the number of times specified on the dice.

Areas of Emphasis

Thinking and speaking are the most often emphasized areas during word-finding activities. Self-advocacy instruction, encompassing self-monitoring and self-instruction sequences, involves primarily thinking and meta- skills. Speaking skills are paramount to demonstrate word-finding ability orally. Writing skills may also be emphasized if word-retrieval problems are present in written communication.

Nonverbal communication is focused on when gestures are taught as an attribute-cuing strategy. Also, students may be asked to self-monitor inappropriate gestures (i.e., secondary characteristics) that sometimes occur during word-finding blocks.

Bridging Questions

Consider asking these bridging questions during or after word-finding activities:

- "How can developing word-finding skills help you in school?"

- "Tell about a time when you didn't use your word-retrieval strategies. What were the consequences?"

- "You've asked your teachers to make some compensatory modifications in their classrooms. When you get a job, could you ask your employer to modify anything? If so, what? How would you ask?"

- "When else could you use self-monitoring skills besides while retrieving words?"

- "You've identified situations when it's harder for you to retrieve words and why. Is it ever hard for you to do other communication tasks, like listening? If so, describe the situations. What are some strategies you could use to listen better?"

Strategies to Mediate

A partial list of strategies to mediate for youth during word-finding activities includes these:

- Organizing information by several characteristics simultaneously (e.g., recognizing that numerous categories could be used when applying the semantic alternative strategy, such as ice cream fitting into the categories of desserts, dairy, and frozen foods)

- Knowing when it is important to be precise and accurate (e.g., there are times when only the exact word will do, such as the password to certain computer files)

- Using relevant information and ignoring irrelevant information (e.g., picking out the key words to remember from a teacher's instructions)

- Considering different alternatives (e.g., if one strategy fails, can another one be substituted?)

- Restraining from saying something that will be regretted later

Emotional Intelligence

Emotional intelligence includes these five dimensions: self-awareness, self-regulation, motivation, empathy, and social skills (Goleman, 1998). Appendix G defines the dimensions and lists the 25 competencies they encompass. For example, the dimension of self-awareness is comprised of these competencies: emotional awareness, accurate self-assessment, and self-confidence. Goleman has stated that intelligence accounts for about 20% of one's successes in life and that the other 80% is accounted for by other factors, which he believes to be emotional intelligence. Psychologists have demonstrated that "interventions designed to target the specific deficits in emotional and social skills that undergird problems such as aggression or depression can be highly effective as buffers for children" (Goleman, 1995, p. 262). Given that emotional intelligence can be learned or taught, and that it is a predictor of being successful in the workplace, it is imperative that speech-language pathologists be aware of the dimensions of emotional intelligence and how best to teach them to, or enhance them in, older students with communication disorders. Advancing emotional intelligence will enhance students' employment success and post-secondary achievements.

[I]t is imperative

that speech-language

pathologists be aware of

the dimensions of emotional

intelligence and how best

to teach them to,

or enhance them in,

older students with

communication disorders.

Procedure

The development of emotional intelligence can be a combination of addressing the 25 competencies within the context of other intervention activities, or focusing directly on the competencies through structured activities and discussions. Adolescents who remain at the concrete period of cognitive development will likely respond better to real-life problems that result in thinking through responses and rationales or answers. An example of this type of activity is shown in the sidebar that follows.

Appropriate questions to ask while mediating each of the 25 competencies (in Appendix G) were proposed by Larson and McKinley (1999). The discussion questions and other activities for each competence are reproduced in Appendix G. Be prepared to

give students ample time to think after asking a question, then coach students through appropriate responses. Revisiting questions periodically during the intervention process is advisable rather than a once-only approach, since emotional intelligence emerges gradually as students mature and their communication skills improve.

Materials

Materials for emotional intelligence activities include any that would support oral discussion activities. For example, the range of responses to a given question might be captured on a white board, on a flip chart, on a transparency, or in an individual journal. As students become familiar with the types of discussion questions asked, they might be assigned to write their responses in a journal or a paper that gets captured for a portfolio. Alternatively, responses can also occasionally be audio- or videotaped to become part of a portfolio record and as a way to document changes in thinking and expressing thoughts over time.

Areas of Emphasis

Thinking, listening, and speaking are the most often emphasized areas during emotional intelligence activities. Most appropriate responses to the discussion questions require thoughtful consideration and formulation of ideas.

Taking a Stand

Directions: Read a situation below. Participants should move to the left side of the room to indicate agreement (yes), go to the right side of the room to indicate disagreement (no), or remain in the center of the room to indicate that they are neutral or have no opinion.

1. Your friend is in a car accident and is in a coma. She is on life-support equipment. Before the accident, she had told you she would not want to be kept alive by machines. The family opposes pulling the plug on the equipment. Do you agree with the family?

2. Your friend is pregnant. Her parents have made it clear that she if she ever got pregnant, she would be thrown out of the house. The father, a 17-year-old football player, has said he will not support her. Would you advise her to keep the baby?

3. You're concerned about the environment. When you take your car into a mechanic, he tells you your cooling system is leaking Freon (a potential hazard to the ozone layer). It will cost $250 (which you don't have) to repair the leak or about $10 every two months to replace the Freon. Do you repair the leak?

4. There are many homeless people in the city where you live. You feel sorry for them, especially for their children. You are asked by a teacher to help prepare and serve a meal to the homeless twice a month. It would cost you nothing but time. Do you help out?

5. A student in your school is always being picked on by others because she has a disability. Would you confront the students who are picking on her?

6. Your sister's boyfriend wants to move in with her. He's out of work and treats your sister rudely. Should she let him move in?

7. You go to a controversial movie with an older, more sophisticated friend. When you arrive at the theater, there are picketers outside. Their desire is to have the movie banned. You go past them into the theater. Ten minutes into the movie, you realize it is extremely offensive to you and people of your race. Do you leave and join the protesters?

8. You are walking along the street and find a wallet containing an I.D., credit cards, and $100 in cash. Would you return it to the owner without taking anything out?

9. A teacher misgrades your test. Instead of receiving a D, you receive an A. Would you tell your teacher?

10. You're at a party where alcohol is being served. Your friend Tom has had several drinks. He insists that he is not drunk and can drive himself home. Do you let him?

From Social Communication: Activities for Improving Peer Interactions and Self-Esteem (pp. 340–341), by M.A. Marquis and E. Addy-Trout, 1992, Eau Claire, WI: Thinking Publications. © 1992 by Thinking Publications. Adapted with permission.

As presented in Appendix G, the emphasis is on discussion between the professional and the student, or among all group participants. For students to stay engaged in the activity, they must carefully listen to each other's comments, to compare the perceptions of others with their own, and to contribute in a meaningful way their own thoughts on a given topic.

As mentioned in the "Materials" section on page 384, the emotional intelligence questions are easily adapted to writing tasks. Thus, emotional intelligence activities are flexible for written language assignments and simulate the types of essays that are frequently required in the general education curriculum.

Bridging Questions

Consider asking these bridging questions during or after emotional intelligence activities:

- "Why is it important for us to discuss the kinds of ideas we have been talking about? When else will you need to participate in such discussions?"

- "We have discussed these emotional intelligence competencies so far: (list them for a student; this will vary from group to group). Which competency do you think you are best at right now? Please defend your answer. When has it been helpful for you to have this competency?"

- "Who do you know that has most, if not all, of these emotional competencies? How do the competencies seem to be helping that person?"

- "What might be some of the consequences of not developing emotional intelligence competencies?"

- "Name 1 of the 25 competencies for emotional intelligence and describe a situation when it would be really helpful for you to show competency."

Strategies to Mediate

A partial list of strategies to mediate for use during emotional intelligence activities includes these:

- Considering different alternatives and what would happen if one or another were chosen

- Using logic to defend opinions

- Being clear and precise in language so that listeners (readers) understand the message

- Thinking through a response instead of immediately trying to answer

- Defining problems and determining what needs to be done

Social Skill Activities

Social skill activities emphasize the skills that allow people to interact appropriately with others. Much like referential communication was a subset of expository text, social skills are a part of emotional intelligence, but encompass a very broad, far-reaching group of behaviors. As highlighted previously under what to assess (see Appendixes J and K), social skills are broken down into dozens of individual skills that can be taught. The preferred classification system we have used organizes social skills into these categories: introductory skills, general interaction skills, peer interaction skills, and emotional expression skills (Gajewski, Hirn, and Mayo, 1998a, 1998b).

Social skill activities

emphasize the skills that

allow people to interact

appropriately with others.

Social skill breakdowns may result from a variety of reasons (Elliott and Gresham, 1991):

• A lack of knowledge

• A lack of practice or feedback

• A lack of cues or opportunities

• A lack of reinforcement

• The presence of interfering problems (e.g., word-retrieval difficulty, impulsivity, or hyperactivity)

Regardless of the reason, the consequence is impaired interaction with others that ultimately interferes academically, socially, and vocationally.

Procedure

Seven critical elements are needed for social skill instruction (Gajewski et al., 1998a, 1998b):

1. Introduction

2. Guided instruction

3. Modeling (teacher role-plays)

4. Rehearsal (student role-plays)

5. Feedback

6. Cognitive planning

7. Transfer and generalization

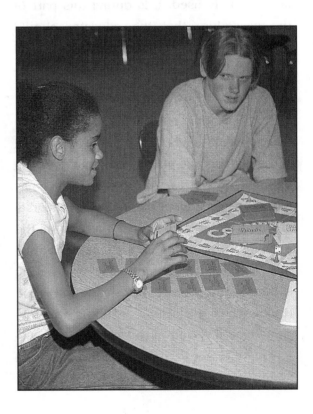

Communication Solutions
for Older Students

The *introduction* begins by giving students an opportunity to think about the skills being introduced and taught. This is the time for the professional to mediate the importance of the target skill, to share when the skill has been important, and to invite students' past experiences related to a given social skill.

The basic components of the target social skill are taught during *guided instruction.* The skill is defined and skill steps are listed and described. Activities should be planned so that students can write about, act on, or discuss the social skill being taught.

Next the professional demonstrates how to use a social skill appropriately during *modeling.* Students should observe appropriate use of this skill and specify both what the skill "looks like" and "sounds like" when appropriately used. It is during this part of the procedure that the educator should model self-talk (i.e., what the professional says in his or her mind to use the appropriate communication for the situation).

An essential element for adolescents to learn social skills is to use behavioral *rehearsal* or role-plays. Note that jumping immediately to use of role-plays typically fails. The procedures leading up to rehearsal are critical for students to succeed in the role-play situation. If students begin to role-play incorrectly, or not taking role-playing seriously, the professional should intervene (Gajewski et al., 1998a, 1998b). Students should be involved in role-playing with several people, not just one person, and should switch roles.

Feedback, the fifth component, should be provided in a positive, nonthreatening manner, and should occur not only during intervention-specific activities, but any time the opportunity presents. To the extent possible, feedback should be provided by the professional, and also by other adults who come into contact with the student. Feedback should be both encouraging (for social skills that are used correctly) and corrective (for those used inappropriately). When specific encouragement is given, the appropriate behavior the student used should be described. When corrective feedback is given, the appropriate behavior that could have been used should be described.

Cognitive planning as implemented by Gajewski et al., (1998a, 1998b) consists of the formula STOP, PLOT, GO, SO. First students STOP to think in their minds to stay calm and to use self-control strategies. Next, they PLOT what the problem is, brainstorm options, consider consequences for each option, then choose the best option. In essence, they plot which social skill is needed to carry out their plan. GO represents the student implementing his or her plan. The SO step involves the student self-evaluating the plan by asking, "How did it work?"

Finally, *transfer and generalization* rewards the real-life use of newly learned skills. Students think through roadblocks that might interfere with the use of a communication skill. Also, students have the opportunity to discuss with their families each new social skill. Students are given the opportunity to use their newfound skills outside of intervention time. These opportunities are discussed and, in some cases, might be observed first-hand through community outings.

Materials

The materials for teaching social skills involves the set of communication skills to be taught, the skill steps for teaching each skill, and any paper-and-pencil activity that might be used to support the learning of the skills. Various excellent commercial resources exist (e.g., *Social Skill Strategies: A Social-Emotional Curriculum for Adolescents (Books A* and *B;* 2nd ed.; Gajewski et al., 1998a, 1998b); *Primal Leadership* (Goleman, Boyatzis, and McKee, 2002)). Professionals may also create their own unique materials based on the student's needs.

For the rehearsal stage, it may be helpful to have scripts written for the initial phases of this step. A prepared dialog takes initial pressure off students to create the exchange themselves. An excellent resource for scripts is *Scripting: Social Communication for Adolescents* (2nd ed.) (Mayo and Waldo, 1994). The professional teaching social skills also needs a vehicle for communicating what skills are being taught with families and with colleagues in a school setting, so that others can become involved in the feedback stage. Since social skills are pervasive across all settings, widespread awareness and involvement are critical for transfer and generalization.

Areas of Emphasis

Social skill activities emphasize thinking, listening, and speaking. The cognitive planning component of social communication underlies the necessity of having students think through which skill to use, and when, why, and how to use it.

Social skills are most often demonstrated during an oral exchange with another person. However, some skills also need to be demonstrated through written language (e.g., learning to offer help, whether it be through spoken or written language). While the procedures imply spoken language, the prudent professional will include transfer and generalization activities that also emphasize the application through written language, as appropriate.

A number of social skills (e.g., making a good first impression and dealing with anger) assume intact nonverbal communication skills. Other social skills (e.g., making an apology and giving constructive criticism) rely on intact paralinguistic skills for appropriate use.

Bridging Questions

Consider asking these bridging questions during or after social skill activities:

- "What are the positive consequences of using the social skill of _____?"

- "What are the consequences of failing to use the social skill of _____?"

Communication Solutions
for Older Students

- "You're invited to stay over with a friend whose house you've never been at and whose parents you've never met. What are some of the social skills you should think about?"

- "How will you know if you used a social skill appropriately or inappropriately? Give some examples."

- "You think your friend treats you and others very rudely. What are your options for handling this situation? What social skills will you need to communicate your feelings to your friend?"

Strategies to Mediate

A partial list of strategies to mediate for use during social skill activities include these:

- Restraining from saying or doing something that will be regretted later

- Making a plan that includes steps needed to reach a goal

- Comparing objects and experiences to determine what is similar and what is different

- Finding the step to which new experiences belong

- Describing events in terms of where and when they occur

390

Points of Discussion

1. Describe additional specific intervention methods that would modify an older student's oral, written, or nonverbal language behaviors.

2. What bridging questions could you ask students when working on these language skills:

   • Detecting fact from opinion in a listening situation

   • Interrupting politely when others are talking

   • Writing a clear set of step-by-step instructions while engaged in a barrier game (i.e., referential communication task)

   • Telling a story about what happened over the weekend

Suggested Readings

Gajewski, N., Hirn, P., and Mayo, P. (1998). *Social skill strategies: A social-emotional curriculum for adolescents (Books A and B; 2nd ed.).* Eau Claire, WI: Thinking Publications.

Schreiber, L., and McKinley, N. (1995). *Daily communication: Strategies for adolescents with language disorders* (2nd ed.). Eau Claire, WI: Thinking Publications.

Points of Discussion

Suggested Readings

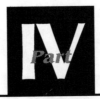

Transitions
of Adolescents

Transitions to the Future

Goals

- Discuss the three major transition points from preadolescence to adulthood

- Present the school-to-work transition

- Present the school-to-postsecondary-education transition

"Transition is a natural process of disorientation and reorientation, caused by an event or nonevent, that alters the individual's perception of self and the world, demands a change of assumptions or behavior, and may lead either to growth or to deterioration; the choice rests with the individual" (Krupp, 1987, as cited in Michaels, 1994, p. 1). This is an excellent definition to keep in mind while discussing the various transition points for preadolescents and adolescents. The definition clearly emphasizes the confusion that can result from transitions and how the individual resolves to either move forward or to retreat. The end result rests solely with each person.

Preadolescence and adolescence are developmental periods in which numerous transitions occur. Transitions can be trying, challenging, and exciting as they mark points of risk and opportunity within the students' development. As illustrated in Figure 14.1, three major transition points occur for preadolescents and adolescents.

There is some discrepancy in the literature as to whether students make these transitions with ease or difficulty. Researchers such as Simmons, Blyth, Van Cleave, and Bush (1979) have suggested that students face serious problems making multiple simultaneous transitions. Others (e.g., Offer, Ostrov, Howard, and Atkinsen, 1988) have found that most students make most changes in their lives successfully. Because students vary as to how or if they make these

Major Transition Points for Preadolescents and Adolescents

Figure 14.1

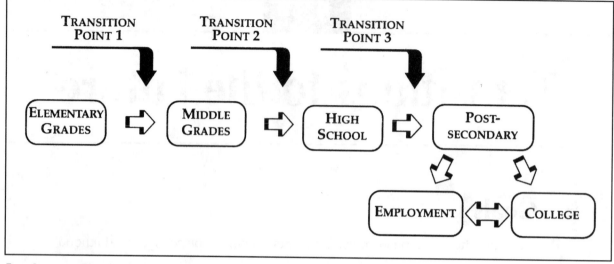

From *Language Disorders in Older Students: Preadolescents and Adolescents* (p. 222), by V. Lord Larson and N.L. McKinley, 1995, Eau Claire, WI: Thinking Publications. © 1995 by Thinking Publications. Reprinted with permission.

transitions, it is important to analyze and discuss ways to assist students in making these changes (Michaels, 1994). One primary way is the use of transition activities, which are activities scheduled to occur at the time of the transitions. The purpose for such activities is to inform and prepare students, families, and educators about current educational practices and future educational expectations (J. Epstein and MacIver, 1990).

Transition Points: A Time to Retain or Dismiss Students?

As students move from elementary schools to middle schools (or junior high schools) or from middle schools to high schools, there is often pressure from colleagues and supervisors to "clean up the caseload." By this, they mean "please dismiss all students you possibly can before the transition."

The dismissal request at transition points appears to be rooted in several underlying assumptions. First, the professionals at the building where the student is currently enrolled have learned the students' strengths and weaknesses and are deemed to be in the best position to decide if further intervention services are warranted. (Keep in mind that these same professionals are in a disadvantaged position for knowing the curriculum and language demands at the next level. Even when the demands are known, the student with a language disorder may not successfully orient to the higher level expectations without assistance.) Second, the assumption is made that the older the student, the less likely he or she will benefit from intense language intervention, and thus administrators are reluctant to schedule more professional time than currently exists in middle schools and high schools. On the contrary, older students are often ready to learn skills that previously eluded them. (See "Rationale for Services by Speech-Language Pathologists," on page 290 in Chapter 11.) Third, if students are dismissed before the transition occurs, there will be fewer disruptions in staffing needs at the next level, and the assumption is made that new personnel demands are unnecessary. Professionals who fail to dismiss students before the transition points may even be accused of shirking their duties and passing along unnecessary work to the receiving building staff.

Indeed, failing to dismiss students at transition points may affect staff distribution. We view this redistribution as necessary and positive for students who have language disorders. Professionals may need to remind supervisors and administrators of the federal laws that ensure free, appropriate public education services for all students, and how this may involve additional personnel, particularly for underserved populations like adolescents with language disorders. Until a demand exists for more services for students at the middle and high school levels, additional staff will not be added. And the need for this additional staff will not be felt as long as older students with language disorders are inappropriately dismissed at transition points.

We have found that the best strategy is to retain the student on the speech-language caseload until the transition process into middle grades (or junior high school) is successful. This ensures that the student has made the transition to the next level, understands the new rules and procedures, and is adjusting to the higher language demands that are undoubtedly present.

With each new transition in the educational sequence, the assumption is made that students can handle higher level concepts, more advanced vocabulary, and greater independence as learners. Students with language disorders have a better probability of succeeding after a transition if their speech-language pathologists remain involved throughout the process.

When students fail to adjust to the transition, and dismissal has already occurred, the process of referral, reassessment, and placement in intervention takes precious time. Clearly, this time lag is not desirable and is preventable if dismissal decisions are postponed until after major transition points in students' educational careers.

Three Major Transitions

Transition Point One: Elementary to Middle Grades

The first transition point marks the change from elementary to middle grades. (Schools that encompass grades 5–8 or 6–8 are considered middle schools, in contrast to junior high schools, which encompass grades 7–8 or 7–9 (Alexander and McEwin, 1989).

Communication Solutions for Older Students

According to Whitmire (2000), "the rising importance of peer relationships during adolescence coincides with the transition into middle or junior high school" (p. 4). This school transition results in a larger student body, varied class schedules without former friends, and numerous teachers with whom students spend only an hour a day or a couple of hours a week. Whitmire noted that "membership in a peer group can be a way of coping with the depersonalized and complex routine of secondary school" (p. 4). And yet we know that it is difficult for older students with language disorders to make and maintain friendships (Fujiki, Brinton, Hart, and Fitzgerald, 1999).

Adolescents with language disorders experience a myriad of difficulties trying to cope with the expectations of junior high (Whitmire, 2000). As youth make the transition from elementary grades to the next level, professionals should instruct students about their upcoming school program and its requirements, procedures, and opportunities. The nature of this information changes depending on whether the transition is into a middle school or a junior high school. The list of differences between the two systems is presented in the sidebar and might be helpful in planning for the students' transition. Table 14.1 further describes the middle school, junior high school, and high school settings and academic expectations.

Middle Schools vs. Junior High Schools

- An interdisciplinary plan of instruction is used more in the middle school; a departmentalized plan of instruction is used more in the junior high school.

- Flexible scheduling is used more in the middle school; uniform daily periods are used more in the junior high school.

- Reasons for establishing middle schools are program and student related; reasons for establishing junior high schools are administratively related.

- Traditional exploratory subjects are required more in middle schools than in junior high schools.

- Random assignment for grouping in basic subjects and advisory programs is more common in middle schools than in junior high schools.

- Foreign languages are offered less frequently in middle schools than in junior high schools.

- A higher percentage of teachers and principals are involved in the decision to organize middle schools than junior high schools.

Source: W. Alexander and McEwin (1989)

Descriptions of Middle School
Table 14.1 (or Junior High School) and High School

Environment	Descriptions
Instructional Setting	• Increasingly demanding curriculum, in terms of both breadth and depth of content area knowledge • Uniform standards allowing less flexibility in adapting the curriculum for students with special needs • Scheduling that encompasses a multitude of classrooms and teachers, each with differing styles and expectations • Lecture-style classroom communication • Increasingly complex instructional discourse regarding syntax, lexical meanings, and figurative language and a more rapid pace • Increasing importance of print material, resulting in higher demands for competent reading and writing
Academic Expectations	• Ability to consider more than one point of view and reconcile divergent points of view • Independent mastery of content area knowledge • The use of writing to demonstrate attainment of knowledge • Effective organization of time and materials • Efficient and effective note taking • Completion of assignments outside of class

From "Adolescence as a Developmental Phase: A Tutorial," by K. Whitmire, 2000, *Topics in Language Disorders, 20*(2), 11. © 2000 by Lippencott. Reprinted with permission.

The most common activities used in the transition from elementary to middle (or junior high) grades are these (J. Epstein and MacIver, 1990):

• Elementary school students visit their next school for an information session or assembly.

• Elementary administrators and the middle (or junior high) school administrators meet together to discuss transitioning and programs.

• Middle-grade counselors meet with elementary counselors or staff.

Less frequent transition practices include parents visiting their children's next school for orientation, teachers' meeting about courses and requirements, "big brother/big sister" programs (in which a new student is guided by an older student at the new level), and elementary students attending regular (sample) classes at the middle (or junior high) school.

Transition Point Two: Middle Grades to High School

The second transition point marks the change from middle grades (or junior high school) to senior high school. According to J. Epstein and MacIver (1990), the same primary activities occur during this transition as they did from elementary to middle grades (or junior high school): students visit the high school for an information session or assembly, administrators meet together on programs, and counselors meet together or with staff.

In many parts of the United States, particularly in urban areas, a very noticeable difference between middle schools and high schools is sheer size. "Experts repeatedly reaffirm the merits of smallness, and yet urban high schools remain Goliaths, as though there was virtue in bigness" (Maeroff, 1988, p. 638). George, Stevenson, Thomason, and Beane (1992) argue that the best high schools apply middle-school philosophy, citing exemplary programs around the country. Unfortunately, these high schools remain in the minority to date.

A realistic picture of high school has been painted by Sizer (1991), who describes it as a place where teachers need to interact with one hundred or more students each day, where teachers present material and expect students to reflect the information back to them, and where the school schedule is marked by rapid changes of subjects each period (each subject is planned by its teacher without any relation to any other subject). Add to this the growing concern in our high schools over violence and safety issues (American Association of University Women [AAUW] Foundation, 2001; Furlong and Morrison, 1994; Moore-Brown and Montgomery, 2001; Sanger, Moore-Brown, and Alt, 2000). The AAUW Foundation stated that although sexual harassment policies are in place in our high schools, the enforcement of these policies is lacking; 4 out of 5 girls say they experience harassment. This figure has not changed since 1993. The study went on to note that bullying, teasing, and harassment are common patterns experienced by students who turn to violence to solve problems or gain attention. It continues to be a challenge to find constructive means to reduce the hostility in our high school hallways.

Precisely because high school campuses are so large, and the changes to be made are so consuming, the transition of students receiving speech-language services from middle school to high school is typically not a topic of concern to administrators. If anything, pressure may again be exerted on professionals to dismiss as many students as possible from caseloads before they transition to a new school.

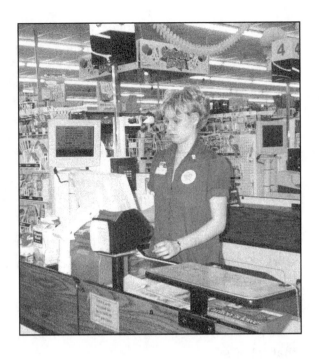

Once more, we urge clinicians to assist students through the transition and to make dismissal decisions after the transition. For students with language disorders, high school brings a new set of demands and expectations: the acquisition of credits for high school graduation, the passing of minimal competency testing (in many states), and the planning of future years beyond high school (or at least the expectation that such planning should occur). Students with language disorders may need a modified graduation plan, direct assistance to meet minimum competency requirements, and counseling to make appropriate vocational choices based on their strengths and weaknesses. A knowledgeable speech-language pathologist can greatly assist with these issues.

Students with language disorders are also at great risk for dropping out of high

school. They need the intervention, advocacy, and support that speech-language pathologists can provide. A significant reduction in the dropout rate is not only important to the students involved but should help solidify with administrators the importance of having speech-language services at the high school level.

Transition Point Three: High School to Postsecondary Life

The transition from high school to postsecondary life is the last major change made by older students. In the mid-1980s, the term *transition* became popular among educators working to prepare students for life after high school. According to the Transition Resource Guide (Heath Resource Center, 1992), "The objective of transition is to prepare students to go directly into the job market, or to enter into higher education or training, to assist them in living independently, and to enable them to become contributing members of the community" (p. 1). Furthermore, in 1990 the Individuals with Disabilities Education Act (IDEA, P.L. 101-467) began to place special emphasis on transition services. This emphasis was expanded in the 1997 amendments of IDEA. This legislation clearly defines transition services:

> "(T)ransition services" means a coordinated set of activities for a student with a disability that—

(A) is designed within an out-come-oriented process, which promotes movement from school to post-school activities, including post-secondary education, vocational training, integrated employment (including supported employment), continuing and adult education, adult services, independent living, or community participation;

(B) is based upon the individual student's needs, taking into account the student's preferences and interests; and

(C) includes instruction, related services, community experiences, the development of employment and, other post-school adult living objectives, and when appropriate, acquisition of daily living skills and functional vocational evaluation. (§ 602 [30])

Speech-language pathologists should be part of the transdisciplinary team because "language and communication skills contribute to success, whether a person's transition plan is aimed primarily toward higher education or employment" (N. Nelson, 1998, p. 59). Further, when writing the individualized education program (IEP) the team must "...include a statement that will describe how in school instruction, community-based instruction, work experiences and employment, independent living skills training, and vocational evaluation will be used to ensure positive transition outcomes for each student" (Michaels, 1994, p. 48).

Furthermore, the team should write an individualized transition plan (ITP) that actively involves them in every segment of the adolescent's life, so that the adolescent is assisted in moving from high school to work or postsecondary education (Rhea Paul, 2001). The responsibilities of secondary school personnel in individualized transition planning are presented in the sidebar that follows.

IDEA '97 mandates that students with disabilities begin preparing for transition by age 14. Transition services are to be written into each student's IEP or a separate ITP must be developed. The speech-language pathologist should be a member of the team writing these plans, since communication problems may be one of the disabilities that will need to be worked with or accommodated for in the student's postsecondary life.

Successful transition planning, according to Everson and Goodall (1991), is a visionary, individualized, and longitudinal process involving interagency and transdisciplinary processes. The remainder of this chapter will discuss two general types of postsecondary life transitions: (1) school to employment (work) and (2) school to postsecondary education.

Responsibilities of Secondary School Personnel in Individualized Transition Planning

- Form a transition team consisting of a coordinator, the student, the family, administrators, teachers, and related service personnel

- Include the student and parents in the entire planning process

- Demonstrate sensitivity to the culture and values of the student and family

- Develop an appropriate packet of materials to document the student's secondary school program and to facilitate service delivery in the postsecondary setting

- Provide administrative support, resources, and time to foster collaboration among team members

- Inform the student about laws, rules, and regulation that ensure his or her rights

- Provide appropriate course selection, counseling, and academic support services

- Ensure competence in literacy and mathematics

- Ensure that the student learns effective studying, time-management, test-preparation, and test-taking strategies

- Help the student use a range of academic accommodations and technological aids

- Help the student evaluate the need for external supports and adjust the level of assistance when appropriate

- Help the student develop appropriate skills and interpersonal communication abilities

- Help the student develop self-advocacy skills, including an understanding of his or her disability and how to use this information in communication with others

- Foster independence through increased responsibility and opportunity for self-management

- Encourage the student to develop extracurricular interests and participate in community activities

- Inform the student and family about admission procedures for diverse postsecondary settings

- Inform the student and family about services that postsecondary settings provide, such as disability services, academic counseling, and so on.

- Ensure the timely development of documentation and material to meet application deadlines

- Help the student and family select and apply to postsecondary institutions that will offer both the challenge and the support necessary

- Develop ongoing communication with postsecondary personnel

Source: National Joint Committee on Learning Disabilities (1996)

School-to-Employment (Work) Transition

The Forgotten Half

Over the past three decades, increasing percentages of high school graduates have enrolled in college in the fall following their graduation (from 49% in 1972 to 63% in 2000), but that still leaves nearly 40% transitioning to the world of work immediately following high school graduation (National Center for Educational Statistics, 2002). These students are not prepared for postsecondary education nor are they prepared by the schools to enter the workforce. O'Neil (1992) referred to these students as "the forgotten half."

A report by the Commission on the Skills of the American Workforce bluntly stated, "America may have the worst school-to-work transition of any advanced industrial country" (as cited in O'Neil, 1992, p. 7). Since no one has taken the initiative to link school-to-employment transitions for young people, young people themselves are left largely to their own devices. The economic picture for the forgotten half is often one of periods of unemployment or underemployment (i.e., dead-end jobs). The absence of an effective system to assist these students in making a smooth transition from high school to the job market costs the United States dearly, both socially and economically. To ignore this problem places the United States at a disadvantage in participating in the global economy.

The transition from school to work is especially challenging for adults with learning disabilities (Sturomski, 1996). They often lack basic academic, social, and goal-setting skills needed for successful transition and employment. Once employed, they will need to learn oral communication and technical skills as technology changes and the workplace evolves. This unlearning and relearning often proves challenging (Sturomski, 1996).

Although the gap between school and the workplace is wide, there are some positive signs (O'Neil, 1992):

- Erosion of the wall separating academic and vocational programs

- Better information flowing to the schools about the skills, knowledge, and work habits that students need to be prepared for the workforce

- Development of the interdisciplinary plans for transition from high school to life beyond resulting from IDEA '97 legislation

---

Although the gap between school and the workplace is wide, there are some positive signs.

It should be noted that several transition programs have been designed specifically to prepare high school students to enter the world of work. One such program is called Tech Prep, available in some schools throughout the United States, which prepares students for careers that require some education beyond the secondary level. The program allows students to take technically oriented courses at a community college or vocational technical college while they are still in high school. Some innovative high schools even offer these courses right on their campuses.

As a nation, we have a renewed interest in linking education to economic competitiveness and employability of individual citizens. On May 4, 1994, Congress passed P.L. 103-239 (H.R. 2884), the School-to-Work Opportunities (STWO) Act of 1994. The STWO Act was the first federal legislation to declare that preparing all students, including the college bound, to earn a living is a critical role of schooling (Halperin, 1994).

School-to-work (STW) initiatives have become more pervasive since passage of the School-to-Work Opportunities Act in 1994. Between the years 1995 and 2000 states reported substantial growth in the number of local partnerships they funded (from 294 to 1,931). Because of the proliferation in these funded partnerships, the number of participating secondary schools within the geographic areas of STW partnerships rose from 5,409 to 10,268—making up nearly 40% of the nation's public secondary

schools (Medrich et al., in press). In addition, the following increases occurred in secondary schools:

- Career-related classes went from 1 million to 3.8 million—a 280% increase.

- An integrated curriculum went from 500,000 to more than 2.9 million—a 480% increase.

- A work-based learning experience tied to an integrated curriculum went from 280,000 to over 1 million—a 257% increase (Medrich, et al., in press).

Medrich et al., also reported the following:

- Employers participating in STW rose from 178,000 to nearly 319,000 or an 79% increase.

- Employers offering work-based learning experiences for students grew from 60,000 to 214,000—a 257% increase.

- Teacher internships rose from 5,800 to nearly 30,000—a 417% increase.

- Postsecondary institutions participating in local partnerships grew from 2,600 to 3,450 or a 33% increase.

Harmon (1998) noted that local partnerships need to implement programs with three key components:

1. **Work-based learning**—a program of structured job training or workplace experiences, mentoring, and apprenticeships at job sites)

2. **School-based learning**—career exploration and counseling, based on academic and occupational skills standards)

3. **Connecting activities**—matching students to work-based learning opportunities and providing a school site mentor to act as a liaison between the school, place of employment, the community, and the student)

In turn, these local partnerships must meet each state's standards. The STWO Act of 1994 was sunsetted in October 2001, and thus the emphasis on such partnerships continues. With or without a law to encourage school-to-work initiatives, it is critical that our students understand what is needed to be employed in the 21st century. According to Michaels (1994), students need to be counseled on seven employment goals. They are summarized in the sidebar.

Types of Employment Options

Students with communication disorders, who decide to work immediately after school may need support in seeking jobs, writing resumes, interviewing techniques, and following instructions for the job itself. These students might want to be aware of the types of employment options available, such as competitive employment, supported employment, and sheltered employment (Heath Resource Center, 1992). "Regular" employment (i.e., no support from outside the hiring agency) is certainly an option too.

Seven Employment Goals

Potential employees must:

1. Have realistic identifiable job goals and salary expectations for positions they have the knowledge and skills to undertake

2. Have job goals that are supported by previous voluntary or work experiences, or skills developed in formal education or training programs

3. Define geographic locations for work and transportation alternatives

4. Demonstrate physical and emotional stamina to undertake the position

5. Demonstrate the social behaviors to engage in the job interview and ultimately the job

6. Demonstrate an appropriate rate of attendance in either school or other work that exceeds 80%

7. Demonstrate a basic understanding of employer expectations and appropriate work etiquette

---

Source: Michaels (1994)

Competitive employment provides the person with a mild or moderate communication disorder with regular supervision but not extensive follow-up, because it is expected that the person will become capable of working alone. Students can be educated for competitive employment opportunities through various means:

- **Apprenticeships**—Students learn skills for specific occupations.

- **Internships**—Students are in a time-limited, paid or unpaid position in which they can sample a wide variety of jobs.

- **On-the-job training**—Students work on the job while learning job duties.

- **Transition employment**—Students engage in a three-phase program; in phase one, participants receive total support services in a low-stress work environment; in phase two, they receive on-the-job training in local firms and agencies; and in phase three, they receive six months of follow-up services.

Each of these competitive employment options carries with it the expectation that ultimately the person is capable of functioning independently.

Supported employment provides integrated work in competitive environments and it uses a place-train approach as opposed to a train-place approach (Heath Resource Center, 1992). The individual is

placed on the job and then provided intense training. There are four popular models of supported employment:

- **Individual placement**—People receive intensive on-the-job coaching from a job coach until they are proficient at the job.

- **The enclave model**—People are trained in small groups and supervised together in an ordinary work setting.

- **The benchwork model**—8 to 15 people perform contract work procured from a business.

- **The mobile crew model**—Individuals who need more support than others perform services as a team, moving from one job site to another (e.g., janitorial work or groundskeeping).

Sheltered employment occurs in settings in which people (usually those with more severe disabilities) work in a self-contained unit, such as an adult day program, work activity center, or sheltered workshop. According to the Heath Resource Center (1992):

> In an adult day program, individuals receive training in daily living skills, social skills, recreational skills, and prevocational skills. In work activity centers, workers receive similar training, but also learn basic vocational skills. In sheltered workshops, individuals

do tasks such as sewing, packaging, collating, or machine assembly, and are paid on a piece-work basis. (p. 2)

As students with communication disorders plan for their impending graduation, a vocational transition team process can

ensure a smoother transition. Everson and Goodall (1991) suggest the five-step process enumerated in the sidebar.

Preparation for the Workplace

Given the economic trends and policy issues facing the United States in the 21st century, it

---

Vocational Transition Team Process

Given the various types of employment options, it is important that the transdisciplinary team members follow a vocational transition process. This five-step process is an example of one process that could be used.

1. Convene the individualized transition planning team members. If the adolescent has a communication disorder, the speech-language pathologist should be a member of this team. (This must begin no later than age 16 for an older student with an IEP, whether or not he or she will seek employment after school.)

2. Develop personal profiles that list the types of future employment options available that are realistic for this youth (e.g., regular employment, competitive employment, supported employment, sheltered workshop). In addition, the profile should address other adult lifestyle areas, such as postsecondary education, community living arrangements, recreation/leisure activities, medical services, and advocacy/legal needs.

3. Specify desired employment objectives and activities for this adolescent. As part of this process, the speech-language pathologist should conduct an assessment of the communication behaviors needed on the job and design a communication support system for the adolescent.

4. Implement transition objectives and activities that are critical to the adolescent's success (e.g., the speech-language pathologist might develop alternative communication systems, adapt materials, develop alternative performance strategies, facilitate functional communication, increase opportunities for communication interactions with peers and workers, and show how the adolescent might infuse communication behaviors in a variety of living, work, and leisure time activities).

5. Monitor, evaluate, and revise objectives and activities as they are needed as part of the transdisciplinary process for assisting adolescents to enter the workplace.

Source: Everson and Goodall (1991)

is imperative that adolescents with communication disorders be prepared to participate in the workplace. Professionals need to examine the impact of these trends and issues to determine how to assist preadolescents and adolescents to become better prepared to enter the workplace and to become self-advocates within the workplace under such laws as the 1990 Americans with Disabilities Act (ADA, P.L. 101-336).

Old vs. New Economy

The terms *old economy* and *new economy* have been firmly entrenched into the jargon of the early years of the 21st century, especially in the business community. One can hardly pick up a business journal or magazine without seeing reference to the new economy or digital economy and globalization. According to Pollacco (2001), there are three established trends in the new economy with far-reaching impact:

1. The shift from manufacturing to the service sector

2. The upgrading of skills and gender balance of the labor force

3. The shift from domestic toward international competition

What do these economic trends suggest for adolescents with communication disorders who are about to enter the workplace? First, adolescents will need to be educated to work in the increasingly large service sector, rather than in an industrial manufacturing society. This will require more education,

more people skills, more team-building skills, and more knowledge of technology and how to use it to increase their productivity on the job. Second, adolescents will need to be flexible thinkers with transferable skills and a willingness to change jobs/positions multiple times during their work life, rather than having one job for life. Third, workers will need to work with and be part of a diverse workforce, both in terms of increased numbers of women and multicultural populations. Fourth, workers will need to think of their places of employment in terms of a global, not domestic, economy.

The National Alliance of Business (1996) discussed the differences between the old and new economy, and they conclude that the changes require a new way of working. They also reinforce the importance of education and training. They contrast the old and new economy on a number of specific parameters that are presented in the sidebar on page 410.

As the importance of education becomes elevated, it is critical that every adolescent be encouraged to achieve his or her human potential. Failure to develop human potential is very costly, as Governor Arne Carlson of Minnesota noted in his State of the State Address on January 26, 1993:

> If a young person drops out of high school, goes on the welfare rolls for five years, then commits a violent crime and is committed to a prison for twenty years, it costs the

Understanding the New Economy

That Was Then	This Is Now
Brawn/metal-bending	Brains/mind-bending
Mass production	Small lots
Standardization	Customization
Hierarchies	Teams
Job security based on seniority	Job security based on skills
Lecture/chalk-talk	Experiential learning
Narrow, job-specific skills	Broad skills
Limited competition	Global competition
Careers built with one employer	Careers built with one occupation
Benefits tied to employer	Portable benefits
Pay for time served	Pay for performance
Big, bureaucratic organizations	Smaller, flexible organizations
Televisions, newspapers	Internet, World Wide Web
Regulation	Deregulation
Government solutions	Public-private partnerships
Competitive standards based on cost	Competitive standards based on quality, variety, timeliness
Homogeneous workforce	Diverse workforce
Finite education	Lifelong learning
Integrated companies	Core competencies
"Go It Alone"	Strategic alliances
Unlimited resources	Limited resources

From "Understanding the New Economy," by the National Alliance of Business, 1996, *Workforce Economics*, 2(2), 11. © 1996 by the National Alliance of Business. Reprinted with permission.

state of Minnesota $500,000. If the same young person graduates from high school, completes technical school training, and works for twenty years at approximately a $24,000 level average over those 20 years, that individual contributes approximately $500,000 to Minnesota. The difference monetarily is approximately one million dollars per child.

If Governor Carlson's statistics are at all generalizable to states outside of Minnesota, then billions of dollars will be spent in the years ahead and a less productive workforce will be available for competing in the global economy.

The cost of America's failure to educate its people is staggering (Boyett and Conn, 1992):

- $219 billion is spent annually for formal and informal training.

- $41 billion is spent annually for welfare programs dominated by school dropouts.

- $16 billion is spent each year in additional welfare costs because of teenage pregnancies (again dominated by school dropouts).

- $25 billion each year is lost in productivity.

- $240 billion is spent each year is lost in earnings and taxes over the lifetime of each year's dropouts because they could not get jobs at all or those they did get were marginal at best.

Given Pollacco's (2001) three economic trends (cited on page 409), the coinciding policy issues, and the cost projections, it is obvious that adolescents with communication disorders will be placed at a disadvantage in entering the workforce and will likely contribute to the costs. A concerted effort must be made to educate these adolescents in the necessary thinking and language/ literacy skills (i.e., speaking, listening, reading, and writing) needed to be successful in the workplace.

In an Associated Press release (September 21, 1992) titled "Communication Skills Said Lacking: Businesses Say Workers Need Help," it was stated that most American businesses say workers need to improve their writing and talking. The business firms listed writing as one of the most valued skills, yet said that 80% of their employees at all levels needed to improve. Of particular importance to speech-language pathologists is the observation that 75% of the companies identified cited ineffective interpersonal skills, such as speaking with and listening to customers and other workers, as a key problem.

In one poll, only one-third of employers believed that high school graduates show the ability to read and understand oral instructions (O'Neil, 1992). It is becoming increasingly more difficult for employers to find entry-level workers (high school graduates) who can think on their feet, solve problems, and apply knowledge and skills to new situations. And yet, business management models (e.g., total quality management or continuous quality improvement) require workers to think and solve problems on the job, without the aid of a manager.

Preparation for the Digital Age

Older students also need to take advantage of technology, which is increasingly being used as a way to overcome communication barriers. For example, a wide variety of communication assistive devices are available to help the student with a speech or language disorder.

It is critical that professionals connect adolescents to the Internet and its potential for learning, obtaining services, buying products, and simply interacting with the global society (McKinley and Larson, 2000). According to Sikes and Pearlman (2000), the number one reason students between the ages of 9 and 17 go online is for email (67%), and while online, 48% do their schoolwork. If professionals do not help adolescents with communication disorders connect to the digital age and go online, it will only increase the likelihood of being a "have not" in a world of "haves."

One of the caveats in connecting the disconnected is that professionals must realize that with all advances can come disadvantages, among them the wide variety of inappropriate materials, as well as the inaccurate, inconsistent, and poor quality of some of the information that exists on the World Wide Web. Teaching our youth to sift and winnow through this vast amount of information and to evaluate its quality is challenging. Professionals need to teach parents to carefully monitor their children's activities on the Internet and teach them to ask their children questions such as "What's the purpose of this information?"; "Is it the truth?"; "Is someone trying to sell something?"; and "Is someone trying to get me to do something?"

Self-Advocacy

Given the economic trends and policy issues of the 21st century, the role of speech-language pathologists in preparing older students with communication disorders to enter the workforce is threefold:

1. To assess the communication pragmatic skills needed to be successful in a given workplace (discussed in Chapter 9)

2. To teach thinking, listening, speaking, reading, and writing strategies for workplace success by developing working partnerships with the business community (strategies are discussed in Chapter 12)

3. To assist adolescents in knowing their rights and becoming self-advocates under such laws as the 1990 Americans with Disabilities Act (ADA) or Sections 503 and 504 of the Rehabilitation Act of 1973 (American Speech-Language-Hearing Association, 1992a, 1992b; Carey, 1992a; Williams, 1992)

According to G. Wilson (1994), there are a number of training models available to teach older students how to engage in self-advocacy. A representative sample of these training programs are as follows:

• The Education Planning Strategy: I PLAN (Van Reusen, Bos, Schumaker, and Deshler, 1987)

• Self-Advocacy Plan for High School Students with Learning Disabilities (Phillips, 1990)

• Students in Transition Using Planning (Parent Advocacy Coalition for Educational Rights, 1988)

• Counseling the Learning Disabled Late Adolescent and Adult: A Self-Psychology Perspective (I. Rosenthal, 1992)

Of these programs, the one most representative of our philosophy is that of The Education Planning Strategy: I PLAN (Van Reusen et al.), which is a motivational metacognitive strategy approach. The purpose of this program is to have the student gain control and influence over his or her own learning and to participate in planning conferences that detail goals and activities. The plan is a five-step approach which includes the following:

1. **Inventory**—The student identifies strengths and weaknesses, as well as goals and choices for learning.

2. **Provide**—The student presents his or her inventory information at a planning conference.

3. **Listen and Respond**—The student listens to others' comments and questions and then responds to them.

4. **Ask**—The student questions others during the planning conference.

5. **Name**—The student names the goals agreed upon during the planning conference.

Another program that assists students to develop self-advocacy skills that follows our philosophy is the Self-Advocacy Plan for High School Students with Learning Disabilities (Phillips, 1990). In this program,

the adolescent is taught responsibility for planning and decision-making about his or her own unique situation. This program specifies special roles for parents, teachers, and students each year of the secondary education program from 9th through 12th grades.

Regardless of the program or the professional implementing the program, it is critical that adolescents with communication disorders be taught self-advocacy skills. These skills will be needed during postsecondary education or employment endeavors or simply in independent living in the community.

For adolescents to be self-advocates (i.e., expressing their needs in a reasonable and informed manner) under the 1990 ADA, they must first know about the ADA and what the term *disability* means. Understanding the ADA's language is crucial to obtaining a clear grasp of the purpose, provisions, and objectives of this landmark federal civil rights legislation. In the ADA, *disability* is defined as a physical or mental impairment that substantially limits one or more of the major life activities. More specifically, a person with a disability is an individual who meets one or more of the following descriptions:

• The person has a physical or mental impairment that substantially limits one or more of the major life activities. (Major life activities include such behaviors as walking, speaking, seeing, hearing, breathing, learning, working, and caring for oneself.)

- The person has a record of such an impairment.

- The person is regarded as having such an impairment.

Key regulations for nondiscrimination on the basis of disability are provided under the four ADA titles: (1) Title I—Employment; (2) Title II—Public Services; (3) Title III—Public Accommodations; and (4) Title IV—Telecommunications. Basic requirements of each are summarized in Table 14.2.

Each of the ADA titles should be discussed as it relates to the adolescent with a communication disorder. The speech-language pathologist, as a member of a team, can provide assessment and intervention procedures to assist the individual in developing communication behaviors needed to succeed in the workplace. Informing the person of his or her rights under the law is also critical.

For example, older students need to know that they have the right to ask for workplace modifications that accommodate their communication disorders. At the same time, speech-language pathologists might also serve as resource people to businesses needing to comply with the ADA (American Speech-Language-Hearing Association, 1992a, 1992b). Accommodations that might be made for those with a communication disorder are listed in the sidebar on page 416.

Under the ADA, the employer determines reasonable accommodations. This four-step process should be used:

1. Analyze the job function to determine its purpose and essential duties.

2. Consult with the individual regarding his or her limitations and need for accommodations.

3. Identify possible accommodations and assess their effectiveness in helping the individual perform essential job functions.

4. Consider the preferences of the individual and select an appropriate accommodation based on options available.

For information on the ADA law, consider the following. First, an article in the American Speech-Language-Hearing Association's journal (Asha) by Williams (1992) titled "What Do You Know?, What Do You Need to Know?" is excellent and should be read carefully. Second, the U.S. government maintains an Americans with Disabilities website at http://www.usdoj.gov/crt/ada. As of October 15, 2002, a new website called www.DisabilityInfo.gov linked to the ADA website as well as several other federal and nonfederal websites with disability-related information. It is a one-stop interagency web portal for people with disabilities, their families, employers, service providers, and other community members. Be aware that the first site is under the auspices of the Department of Justice; the second one is not, and there is a disclaimer that the Department of Justice assumes no responsibility for the accuracy of the material at www.DisabilityInfo.gov.

Table 14.2 **Americans with Disabilities Act (ADA, 1990) Requirements**

ADA Titles	Requirements
Title I: Employment	Employers may not discriminate against an individual with a disability in hiring or promotion if the person is otherwise qualified for the job. Employers can ask about one's ability to perform a job, but cannot inquire if someone has a disability or subject a person to tests that tend to screen out people with disabilities. Employers will need to provide "reasonable accommodation" to individuals with disabilities. This includes steps such as job restructuring and modification of equipment. Employers do not need to provide accommodations that impose an "undue hardship" on business operations. Who needs to comply: All employers with 25 or more employees must comply, effective July 26, 1992. All employers with 15–24 employees must comply, effective July 26, 1994. For more information about employment issues, call the Equal Employment Opportunity Commission at 1-800-669-4000.
Title II: Public Services	State and local governments may not discriminate against qualified individuals with disabilities. All government facilities, services, and communication must be accessible consistent with the requirements of Section 504 of the Rehabilitation Act of 1973. New public transit buses ordered after August 26, 1990, must be accessible to individuals with disabilities. Transit authorities must provide comparable paratransit or other special transportation services to individuals with disabilities who cannot use fixed route bus services, unless an undue burden would result. Existing rail systems must have one accessible car per train by July 26, 1995. New rail cars ordered after August 26, 1990, must be accessible. New bus and train stations must be accessible. Key stations in rapid, light, and commuter rail systems must be made accessible by July 26, 1993, with extensions up to 20 years for commuter rail (30 years for rapid and light rail). All existing Amtrak stations must be accessible by July 26, 2010. For more information on transportation issues, contact the U.S. Department of Transportation at 1-202-366-4000 (voice) or 1-202-366-4313 (TDD), or www.dot.gov.
Title III: Public Accommodations	Private entities such as restaurants, hotels, and retail stores may not discriminate against individuals with disabilities, effective January 26, 1993. Auxiliary aids and services must be provided to individuals with vision or hearing impairments or other individuals with disabilities, unless and undue burden would result. Physical barriers in existing facilities must be removed, if removal is readily achievable. If not, alternative methods of providing the services must be offered, if they are readily achievable. All new construction and alterations of facilities must be accessible. For more information on accessibility issues, call the Access Board at 1-800-872-2253 (voice) or 1-202-272-0082 (TDD).
Title IV: Tele-communications	Companies offering telephone service to the general public must offer telephone relay services to individuals who use telecommunication devices for the deaf (TDDs) or similar devices.
For more information about the ADA or to receive this information in alternative formats (e.g., Braille, large print, audiotape), contact: U.S. Department of Justice Civil Rights · Division Coordination and Review Section P.O. Box 66118 · Washington, DC 20035-6118 · 1-800-514-0301 (voice) · 1-800-514-0383 (TDD) · 1-202-514-0383 (TDD) · www.ada.gov	

**Examples of Accommodations under Title I for Employees
with Communication Disorders**

- Providing assistive listening and signaling devices, generic-type augmentative and alternative communication devices, and interpreter services

- Altering communication styles (e.g., ensuring speechreading cues, increasing patience, or using written communication if oral communication fails)

- Modifying the work environment (e.g., reducing background noise, or redesigning work space to accommodate an augmentative communication system)

- Modifying policies (e.g., permitting hearing-assistance dogs)

Source: Larson and McKinley (1995)

Nonetheless, the site is comprehensive and provides links to many agencies beyond the Department of Justice.

School-to-Postsecondary-Education Transition

High school graduation rates for students with disabilities vary considerably by disability, as shown in Table 14.3. In 1997–98, the most recent academic year for which statistics were compiled by the U.S. Department of Education, Office of Special Education (2000) at the time of printing this text, more than 30% of students with deaf-blindness, speech or language impairments, specific learning disabilities, or visual impairments received a standard diploma. Among those least likely to graduate in 1997–98 were students with mental retardation

(14%), multiple disabilities (10%), and autism (8%).

These figures should certainly alert speech-language pathologists to the role they need to play at the secondary level, as well as on the transition planning team. To take advantage of many of the postsecondary education opportunities, the student should have a high school diploma. Speech-language pathologists, who frequently serve students in the categories least likely to graduate, should be active participants in the transitional planning for these individuals.

Transition Planning

Postsecondary education is any education beyond high school (i.e., trade or business schools, vocational technical schools, colleges, universities, and adult and continuing education programs; Heath Resource Center,

Table 14.3

Number and Percentage of Students Ages 17 and Older Graduating with a Standard Diploma, 1997–98

Disability	Number	Percentage
Specific learning disabilities	99,640	30.5
Speech or language impairments	4,099	35.0
Mental retardation	15,268	13.8
Emotional disturbance	13,861	22.3
Multiple disabilities	2,061	10.3
Hearing impairments	2,761	29.0
Orthopedic impairments	2,037	25.8
Other health impairments	5,052	29.6
Visual impairments	1,157	30.6
Autism	384	8.4
Deaf-blindness	132	39.2
Traumatic brain injury	671	27.7
All disabilities	147,123	25.5

Source: U.S. Department of Education, Office of Special Education (2000)

Note: The percentages in this table were calculated by dividing (1) the number of students age 17 and older in each disability category who graduated with a diploma by (2) the total number of students with disabilities age 17 and older in each disability category.

1994a). "Education is not just about making a living; it is also about making a life" (Byrne, Constant, and Moore, 1992, p. 26). Regardless of the type of postsecondary education experiences that adolescents or young adults are seeking, early individualized transitional planning is imperative. Career awareness built in across all grade levels (K–12) can greatly assist this planning.

Getzel (1990) noted that without a coordinated transition plan, few students with disabilities are able to take advantage of postsecondary education opportunities. A good transition plan begins when students make the transition from elementary school to middle school (or junior high school), and it continues beyond the senior year in high school. Table 14.4 provides a checklist of some variables that parents, students, and educators should consider, starting at the junior high school level (Heath Resource Center, 1992).

Guidelines for Success in Postsecondary Education

The sidebar on pages 420–421 presents suggestions for helping students with communication disorders prepare for the transition to college. Additionally, the following major ideas may help adolescents or young

Communication Solutions
for Older Students

Table 14.4   **Transition Planning**

Plan	Steps
Junior High School — **Start Transition Planning**	• Become involved in career exploration activities. • Participate in vocational assessment activities. • Use information about interests and capabilities to make preliminary decisions about possible careers: academic vs. vocational, or a combination. • Visit with a school counselor to talk about interests and capabilities. • Make use of books, career fairs, and people in the community to find out more about careers of interest.
High School — **Define Career/ Vocational Goals**	• Work with school staff, family, and people and agencies in the community to define and refine the transition plan. Make sure that the IEP includes transition plans. • Identify and take high school courses that are required for entry into college, trade schools, or careers of interest. • Identify and take vocational programs offered in high school, if a vocational career is of interest. • Become involved in early work experiences, such as job try-outs, summer jobs, volunteering, or part-time work. • Reassess interests and capabilities, based on real world or school experiences. Is the career field still of interest? If not, redefine goals. • Participate in ongoing vocational assessment and identify gaps of knowledge or skills that need to be addressed. Address these gaps. **Students who have decided to pursue postsecondary education prior to employment, may wish to consider these suggestions:** • Identify postsecondary institutions (e.g., colleges, vocational programs in the community, and trade schools) that offer training in careers of interest. Write or call for catalogs, financial aid information, or applications. Visit the institution. • Identify what accommodations would be helpful to address disability-specific needs. Find out if the educational institution makes, or can make, these accommodations. • Identify and take any standardized tests (e.g., PSAT, SAT, and ACT) necessary for entry in postsecondary institutions of interest. • In senior year, contact Vocational Rehabilitation (VR) and/or Social Security Administration (SSA) to determine eligibility for services or benefits.

Table 14.4–Continued

	Plan	Steps
Post-High School	Pursue Goals	• If eligible for VR services, work with a VR counselor to identify and pursue additional training or to secure employment (including supported employment) in your field of interest. • If not eligible for VR services, contact other agencies that can be of help: state employment offices, social services offices, mental health departments, disability-specific organizations. What services can these agencies offer? • If eligible for SSA, find out how work incentives apply. • Find out about special projects in your vicinity (e.g., Projects with Industry, Project READY, and supported employment models) Determine eligibility to participate in these training or employment programs. • Follow through on decisions to attend postsecondary institutions or obtain employment.

Source: Heath Resource Center (1992)

adults make the most of their postsecondary opportunities (Heath Resource Center, 1994b):

- **Be capable of expressing needs to others and be open to change—** Students should consider new and different ways to do things and be involved.
- **Plan ahead—**If in high school, adolescents should take time to think about their academic and career goals, main interests, and favorite subjects in school; to talk with appropriate educational personnel about their plans; and to take vocational tests that explore and identify their career interests, strengths, and weaknesses. If out of high school, adolescents should speak with a person at a local vocational rehabilitation office, community college, vocational technical college, or university.
- **Look for the best schools—**Gather information about schools that offer education in the students' areas of interest. Beware of the accommodations needed, given the students' communication disorders. Beware of the accommodations and services available at the schools that adolescents are most interested in attending. Can they accommodate students' needs? Visit, if possible, the school(s) that students are most interested in attending and get a preadmission interview with an appropriate faculty member or administrator. The sidebar on page 422 presents the types of adjustments

Helping Students Who Want to Go to College

Those students with communication disorders who are going on to college should consider the following recommendations.

1. **Get the basics in place.** Speech-language pathologists can assist older students in:

    *   Developing disability awareness (by encouraging self-advocacy)

    *   Understanding their language and learning disabilities

    *   Understanding how their disabilities affect social interactions with a wide array of individuals

    *   Comprehending Section 504 of the Rehabilitation Act of 1973 and how it compares to IDEA, (e.g., the student seeks and requests appropriate services under Section 504, whereas it is the responsibility of the schools (working with parents) to provide services under IDEA)

    *   Developing personal and skill development (by encouraging students to develop work-related skills and interests if college is delayed for some reason; making sure students' knowledge of study skills is adequate)

    *   Increasing independent living skills

    *   Seeking part-time jobs or volunteer positions

    *   Requesting assessments, records, and course options in high school (requesting the high school to provide vocational assessment starting in the seventh grade)

    *   Planning a four-year selection of college prep courses sufficient to allow the option of entering college

    *   Contacting the local vocational rehabilitation agency before graduating from high school

    *   Taking advantage of testing provided under IDEA and in obtaining all special testing records before graduation

2. **Complete the college applications process** (i.e., getting ready to apply and deciding where to apply).

    First, in getting ready to apply to a college, the student with the help of professionals, should:

    *   Consult with advisors to understand how much support was needed in high school and, therefore, how much help will be needed in college

    *   Consider how highly motivated he or she is to accomplish college work

    *   Decide whether arrangements for special testing conditions for the PSAT, SAT, and/or ACT are needed

    *   Consider a wide array of postsecondary options, including community colleges, technical colleges, and universities

Second, in deciding where to apply, the student should:

• Visit colleges while in session

• Enroll in summer orientation sessions

• Take summer study skill courses

• Search out personal contacts or follow other leads to find an appropriate advisor, friend, mentor, or teacher on campus

Source: Heath Resource Center (1994a)

and accommodations that can be made at the postsecondary level.

• **Inquire about the admissions process**—Do students need to take standardized admission tests? Are there special test-taking accommodations available that fit students' needs? Are preparatory courses required before students qualify for admission?

• **Learn the services available**—The school should provide auxiliary aids, accommodations, and services that enhance access to persons with disabilities. A number of federal laws require that access be available, such as the Rehabilitation Act of 1973 (Section 504), the Carl D. Perkins Vocational and Technical Education Act of 1998 (P.L. 105-332), and the 1990 Americans with Disabilities Act (ADA, P.L. 101-336). It should be noted that the ADA does not replace Section 504 but reaffirms the Section 504 regulations for colleges and universities.

According to DuChossois and Michaels (1994), some of the nonacademic areas that are often difficult for students with disabilities to make the transition from high school to postsecondary education are as follows: problem solving, organizing, prioritizing, studying, self-monitoring, following through on a task, managing time, and interacting socially in new situations. They go on to state that in selecting a college to attend, the student should review college catalogs, textbooks, and course outlines, and interview college students who have language and learning disabilities. In addition, the secondary school should provide direct instruction to these students about what postsecondary support services are available to them and what skills they need to have to transition into the postsecondary curriculum and environment.

Ganschow, Philips, and Schneider (2001) discuss the role of the speech-language pathologist on the transition team. They recommend that the speech-language pathologist administer the appropriate language

Types of Adjustments and Accommodations Many Postsecondary Schools Will Make for Persons with Disabilities

- Preregistration well in advance of classes so that the classes can be scheduled in such a way as to give students sufficient time to get from class to class (e.g., if transportation is an issue)

- Flexibility in class scheduling so that if a class has been scheduled in a location that is not accessible, students may request that it be moved or, if not, a way is found for them to attend the class

- Flexibility in course requirements so that students may ask that one course be substituted for another (e.g., a deaf student might take an art course rather than a music course to fulfill the fine arts requirements)

- Extended time for coursework or to complete a degree

- Test modifications such as extended time, oral versus written examinations, and use of tape recorders

- Notetakers for students having difficulty writing or listening to lectures and taking notes at the same time

- Special help for students with language and learning disabilities

- Interpreter services for students who are deaf or hard of hearing (it should be noted that interpreters are scarce, so determine ahead of time if the school can accommodate such a request)

- Special orientation programs for new students who have disabilities

In addition, physical access to places should be carefully considered (e.g., classrooms, libraries, student unions, dormitories, and recreational facilities). It is the responsibility of students with disabilities to request the auxiliary aids, accommodations, and services listed above. Likewise, these requests should come well before the semester begins.

Source: Heath Resource Center (1994b)

tests and explain the results to university administrators; help the student understand his or her communication strengths and weaknesses; help the student develop self-advocacy skills; and help the student develop realistic postsecondary and career goals.

Once the student is at the university, they recommend that the speech-language pathologist (if close to that university) remain involved by serving as a resource to the student with a language disorder and also serving on universitywide petition committees.

Points of Discussion

1. Describe how you could use computer technology to assist you in following students as they make the transition from:

   • The elementary to the middle school (or junior high school) level

   • The middle school (or junior high school) level to the high school level

   • The high school level to postsecondary experiences

2. Analyze the key communication skills needed to engage in self-advocacy. How would you teach these skills?

Suggested Readings

Heath Resource Center. (1994). *Make the most of your opportunities: A guide to postsecondary education for adults with disabilities.* Washington, DC: Author.

Ganschow, L., Philips, L., and Schneider, E. (2001). Closing the gap: Accommodating students with language learning disabilities in college. *Topics in Language Disorders, 21*(2), 17–37.

15

Merging the Futures

Goals

- List the evolving roles of speech-language pathologists

- Present contrasts among the generations, which may influence how they work together

- Summarize changes in personnel preparation related to speech-language pathologists' service to older students

- Encourage more research related to efficacy and effectiveness of service for preadolescents and adolescents

- Sound a call to action on behalf of older students

Evolving Roles of Speech-Language Pathologists

The roles of speech-language pathologists have shifted and will continue to adjust in response to trends (such as the nationwide movement calling for more standardized testing at multiple grade levels) and paradigm shifts (such as school choice vs. students being forced to stay in their own school districts; American Speech-Language-Hearing Association (ASHA) 2001b; Apel, 1999a; Goldberg, 1996; Montgomery and Herer, 1994; Moore-Brown and Montgomery, 2001). In response to paradigm shifts, the following professional roles have already emerged, or will emerge in the coming decade, for clinicians who serve older students:

- **Speech-language pathologists as consultants in addition to or instead of direct service providers—** The consultant role is receiving a great deal of attention, but little research supports its efficacy (N. Nelson, 1993).

- **Speech-language pathologists as teachers—**In this role, clinicians "assume responsibility for conveying the curriculum to children whose language problems make it largely inaccessible to them under ordinary circumstances" (N. Nelson, 1998, p. 171). The professional's attention extends beyond the student's ability to use language for social and academic purposes to include the learning of information and skills targeted in the general education curriculum. This casts the speech-language pathologist into the role of assuming responsibility for academic development and behavior management.

- **Speech-language pathologists as co-teachers—**They "...co-teach with other professionals, who assume a major responsibility for teaching the regular curriculum" (N. Nelson, 1998, pp. 171–172).

- **Speech-language pathologists as community educators—**In this role, they help administrators, parents, school boards, employers, and the students themselves understand the evolving roles that clinicians play, the importance of speech-language services, and their commitment to youth with communication disorders.

- **Speech-language pathologists as diversity experts and professionals with expertise interacting with students who speak English as a second language—**Authentic, descriptive assessment and practical results will be in demand for students from diverse backgrounds.

- **Speech-language pathologists as literacy advocates—**In addition to focusing on oral language ability, professionals will assess and intervene with written language goals (ASHA, 2001b; Casby, 1988; Catts and Kamhi, 1999; N. Nelson, 1998; Rhea Paul, 2001).

- **Speech-language pathologists as researchers—**As the demand for documentation of results grows, professionals must find creative ways to use computer technology, portfolios, and other data-gathering methods to substantiate that relevant goals are being achieved. There will be increasing demands to be accountable and to demonstrate the efficacy of services (Amiot, 1998; Apel, 1999a; Baum, 1998; Gallagher, Swigert, and Baum, 1998; Kamhi, 1999; Logemann, 1998; Logemann and Baum, 1998; O'Toole, Baum, and Logemann, 1998; O'Toole, Logemann, Baum, 1998; Slater and Baum, 1998). Apel (2001) also strongly endorsed developing evidence-based practices and research collaborations in school settings.

- **Speech-language pathologists as transition monitors—**As students move from the demands of elementary to middle school (or junior high school), then to high school, and then to employment or postsecondary education, different language expectations surface. Speech-language pathologists can be key players in helping students make the adjustments necessary to survive the transitions. They will be part of a multidisciplinary team, which fulfills the 1997 Individuals with Disabilities Education Act (P.L. 105-17, known as IDEA '97) mandates to have transition services written into individualized education programs (IEPs) in place by age 16, or to develop separate individualized transition plans (ITPs).

- **Speech-language pathologists as advisors to the corporate world—**They will work with employees on:

> presentation skills, accent modification, minor fluency/ articulation problems in management; training and supervising support personnel; supervising multi-skilled or cross-trained health care and/or educational professionals; administering across a cluster of clinical disciplines and in technology; designing computer treatment programs, consulting on augmentative, alternative communication devices. (Goldberg, 1996, p. 23)

In addition, they might work with Directors of Human Resources to develop support programs for employees who have language and/or learning disabilities.

- **Speech-language pathologists as recruiters and mentors of other speech-language pathologists—**Because of the severe shortage of speech-language pathologists (Busacco, 2001b; Holiday, 2001; Rosa-Lugo, Rivera, and McKeown, 1998), especially at the Ph.D. level (Geffner and Kuehn, 1998), and of minority students and professionals at all levels of the

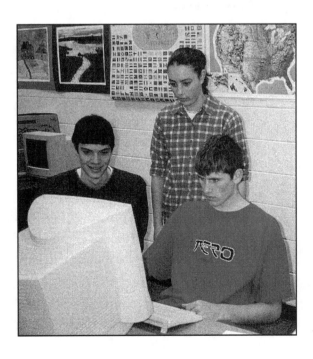

profession, a more assertive recruitment and retention campaign must be undertaken (Saenz, Wyatt, and Reinard, 1998).

- **Speech-language pathologists as supervisors of speech-language pathology assistants (SLPAs)**—As the profession moves more toward the education and employment of SLPAs, there will be an increased need to carefully educate and monitor SLPAs' activities. SLPAs must be supervised directly at least 10% of the time and even more (up to 30%) initially (Moore-Brown and Montgomery, 2001). The American Speech-Language-Hearing Association's policy and guidelines on support personnel, as well as a list of states that have SLPA degree programs, can be found at the American Speech-Language-Hearing Association's website (www.asha.org).

- **Speech-language pathologists as counselors/advocates for older students with communication disorders**—There will be an increased need under IDEA '97 for speech-language pathologists to assist students with their employment and postsecondary education opportunities.

- **Speech-language pathologists as case managers**—This will ensure that the family/students are informed and engaged, thus getting a chance to ask questions and to contribute to the IEP process (Rhea Paul, 2001). According to Moore-Brown and Montgomery (2001), speech-language pathologists who serve as case managers in the school setting will serve a number of functions, including, but not limited to, serving as a contact person for the student, family members, and professionals; scheduling, coordinating, and monitoring the service delivery model; helping to select the most appropriate service delivery model for students, given their strengths, weaknesses, age, and type of disability; and facilitating the development of transition plans.

- **Speech-language pathologists as life-long learners**—Change has come and will continue to come rapidly to the discipline. The only way to accommodate these advances will be to engage in continuing education activities. Technology will play a critical role as more and more professionals become involved in distance education/ learning opportunities to advance their learning (Busacco, 2001a; Chial, Sobolevsky, and Flahive, 2000).

- **Speech-language pathologists as technology users/integrators**—More than ever, speech-language pathologists will need to know how to use technology to enhance assessment and advance intervention goals and service delivery models. Simultaneously, they need to help students with language disorders develop information literacy, or those students will be unemployed or underemployed. *Information literacy* is "a new liberal art that extends from knowing how to use computers and access information to critical reflection on the nature of information itself, its technical infrastructure, and its social, cultural and even philosophical context and impact" (Shapiro and Hughes, 1996). Speech-language pathologists serving older students need to advocate for their clients to have a curriculum designed to address the standards shown in the sidebar. Helping to teach

The Nine Information Literacy Standards for Student Learning

Information Literacy

Standard 1: The student who is information literate accesses information efficiently and effectively.

Standard 2: The student who is information literate evaluates information critically and competently.

Standard 3: The student who is information literate uses information accurately and creatively.

Independent Learning

Standard 4: The student who is an independent learner is information literate and pursues information related to personal interests.

Standard 5: The student who is an independent learner is information literate and appreciates literature and other creative expressions of information.

Standard 6: The student who is an independent learner is information literate and strives for excellence in information seeking and knowledge generation.

Social Responsibility

Standard 7: The student who contributes positively to the learning community and to society is information literate and recognizes the importance of information to a democratic society.

Standard 8: The student who contributes positively to the learning community and to society is information literate and practices ethical behavior in regard to information and information technology.

Standard 9: The student who contributes positively to the learning community and to society is information literate and participates effectively in groups to pursue and generate information.

From *Information Power: Building Partnerships for Learning* (¶ 2–9), by American Library Association and Association for Educational Communications and Technology, 1998, Chicago, IL: Author. © 1998 by American Library Association and Association for Educational Communications and Technology. Reprinted with permission.

information literacy is part of the evolving role of the speech-language pathologist who serves older students.

From this extensive list, it is clear that the role of the speech-language pathologist is ever-evolving in response to changes in other systems (e.g., legal, corporate, and educational). At the same time our roles are shifting, the generational gap is widening. The next section addresses this gap by contrasting the values and beliefs of today's professionals (who were born between 1940 and 1980) and the older students who are the focus of this text.

Generational Contrasts

Students ages 9 to 19 in the early 2000s were born between the early 1980s and 1990s. Their generation is called the Millennials (also called Nexters, Echo Boom, Generation Y, and the Baby Busters). Between 1982 and 2000, 76 million of them were born. They are being served predominantly by professionals who are Generation Xers or Baby Boomers. Table 15.1 displays the predominant groups in our society.

Recognition of and appreciation for each generation is critical because the age groups are motivated by different forces. Professionals who fail to understand the mindset of Millennials run the risk of alienating them during the assessment or intervention processes. Table 15.1 outlines major contrasts of the groups.

As Baby Boomers and Generation Xers assist the Millennials with their communication skills, care should be taken to deliver services in a manner that is consistent with what is important to the youngest generation. For example, when providing reasons for learning language skills needed for employment, professionals might talk about the importance of communication within meaningful work experiences.

Understanding the contrasts between the generations can also be helpful in professional-to-professional communication. Baby Boomers, who tend to be in supervisory roles over Generation Xers, would do well to understand the Xers' career goals and what they find rewarding. At the same time, Generation Xers might gain some insight on why their supervisors react to situations differently than they do.

Personnel Preparation at Universities

The attitude of a speech-language pathologist toward serving older students with communication disorders, and that professional's approach to service delivery, are influenced by university professors. As university faculty members involved in personnel preparation, we have been interested in determining the extent to which preservice students are being taught to work with older students. One of our premises is that older students remain unserved or underserved, in part,

Comparison of Beliefs and Motivations of Four Generations

Table 15.1

Generation	Work/Life Balance	Career Goals	Rewards	Training
Traditionalists (born prior to 1945) 75 million	"Support me in shifting the balance."	"Build a legacy."	"The satisfaction of a job well done."	"I learned it the hard way; you can, too."
Baby Boomers (born 1946–1964) 80 million	"Help me balance everyone else and find meaning myself."	"Build a stellar career."	"Money, title, recognition, the corner office."	"Train 'em too much and they'll leave."
Generation Xers (born 1965–1981) 46 million	"Give me balance now, not when I'm 65."	"Build a portable career."	"Freedom is the ultimate reward."	"The more they learn, the more they stay."
Millennials (born 1982–2000) 76 million	"Work isn't everything; I need flexibility so I can balance all my activities."	"Build parallel careers."	"Work that has meaning for me."	"Continuous learning is a way of life."

Source: Lancaster and Stillman (2002)

because speech-language pathologists have not learned how to provide effective services to them.

To check out this premise, we developed a questionnaire that inquired about course content and faculty attitudes toward the need for teaching students about adolescents with communication disorders. In 1985, we surveyed all the programs in communication disorders in the United States by sending this questionnaire to the department chairs. The results were reported in *Communication Assessment and Intervention Strategies for Adolescents* (Larson and McKinley, 1987). The main findings were summarized as follows:

University personnel expect their students to interact clinically with adolescents, yet they do not consistently provide them with necessary

Communication Solutions
for Older Students

information on this population. Perhaps this phenomenon is partially explained by the fact that only 52% of the respondents envisioned an employment market for speech-language pathologists with adolescents with communication disorders. Another explanation is that 58% of the programs mentioned insufficient research data, and 52% mentioned insufficient assessment instruments and intervention strategies. Whatever the explanation, many students majoring in communication sciences and disorders are not receiving the curriculum to prepare them to work with adolescents in junior and senior high schools, juvenile detention centers, prisons, graduate equivalency degree (GED) programs, and academic skill resource centers for marginal students in vocational-technical institutes, colleges, and universities. Too often, graduates are ill-prepared for these jobs. Furthermore, they are inadequately prepared to create jobs in those settings. (p. 54)

In preparing for this, our latest, book, we resurveyed the programs in communication disorders that offer masters degrees. Again we mailed a questionnaire to each department chair across the United States. The results of the more recent survey are reported in Table 15.2 alongside the 1985 data, so they can be compared. Several notable gains have been made in the last 17 years. As can

be seen in question 4 in Table 15.2, most programs (i.e., 86%) do now provide specific course content on adolescent communication disorders. This is a dramatic shift from the 51% level in 1985. Likewise, a significant positive gain occurred for question 6, "Does your faculty feel that it is important to train students specifically in assessment and intervention of adolescents?" Nearly all programs (i.e., 93%) now answer in the affirmative for that question, compared to 58% in 1985.

Despite these changes, the percentages remained nearly the same for question 10, still citing the lack of a sufficient database with regard to research. Only moderate gains were reported with regard to having a database of assessment instruments and intervention strategies. These results show some progress in the last 17 years, but at a level that is disappointingly slow. Despite our most fervent efforts for the last 20 years, it remains a challenge to appropriately prepare students for serving the older student population.

The 2002 data were also examined based on the configuration of the university programs, an analysis not completed in 1985. The survey results were compiled by programs that had doctoral level degrees, non-doctoral programs that had more than 30 students pursuing masters degrees, and non-doctoral programs that had fewer than 30 students pursuing masters degrees. Results are shown in Table 15.3.

Survey of University Programs in Communication Sciences and Disorders

Table 15.2

Questions Regarding Current Emphasis on Speech-Language Services for Older Students	1985 Responses[a] (%)		2002 Responses[b] (%)	
	Yes	No	Yes	No
1. Do you provide specific courses on adolescent development?	16	80	10	86
2. Do you provide specific courses on adolescent communication disorders?	4	93	28	70
3. Do you provide specific course content on adolescent development?	39	54	75	23
4. Do you provide specific course content on adolescent communication disorders?	51	45	86	12
5. Do your students have any opportunity to assess and/or remediate adolescents with communication disorders?	95	2	99	2
6. Does your faculty feel that it is important to train students specifically in assessment and intervention of adolescents?	58	26	93	6
7. Does anyone on your faculty have an interest and/or expertise in the assessment and intervention of adolescents with communication disorders?	66	26	81	16
8. Have students in your training program expressed an interest in being trained to work with adolescents with communication disorders?	35	63	44	48
9. Is there an employment market for persons trained to work with adolescents with communication disorders?	54	25	72	15
10. Is there a sufficient database to draw upon for serving the adolescent population with regard to:				
a. Research	28	60	29	62
b. Assessment instruments	33	54	44	48
c. Intervention strategies	31	54	41	50

Source: Larson and McKinley (1987)

Note: Cells do not total to 100%, because some programs chose not to respond to certain items or gave answers that could not clearly be classified as yes or no.

[a] N = 96; 42% response rate.
[b] N = 101; 39% response rate.

2002 Survey Data
Table 15.3   ## Comparing Degree Program Responses

Questions Regarding Current Emphasis on Speech-Language Services for Older Students	Doctorate Programs[a] (%)		>30 Masters[b] (%)		<30 Masters[c] (%)	
	Yes	No	Yes	No	Yes	No
1. Do you provide specific courses on adolescent development?	4	95.2	10.4	85.4	8.7	82.6
2. Do you provide specific courses on adolescent communication disorders?	19.0	81.0	27.1	68.8	34.8	65.2
3. Do you provide specific course content on adolescent development?	85.7	14.3	75.0	22.9	65.2	26.1
4. Do you provide specific course content on adolescent communication disorders?	100	0	85.4	12.5	78.3	13.0
5. Do your students have any opportunity to assess and/or remediate adolescents with communication disorders?	100	0	100	0	100	0
6. Does your faculty feel that it is important to train students specifically in assessment and intervention of adolescents?	85.7	14.3	93.8	4.2	100	0
7. Does anyone on your faculty have an interest and/or expertise in the assessment and intervention of adolescents with communication disorders?	85.7	9.5	77.1	16.7	78.3	21.7
8. Have students in your training program expressed an interest in being trained to work with adolescents with communication disorders?	47.6	38.1	45.8	50.0	39.1	52.2
9. Is there an employment market for persons trained to work with adolescents with communication disorders?	71.4	19.0	77.1	16.7	60.9	13.0
10. Is there a sufficient database to draw upon for serving the adolescent population with regard to:						
a. Research	38.1	57.1	20.8	68.8	30.4	60.9
b. Assessment instruments	47.6	47.6	39.6	54.2	43.4	43.4
c. Intervention strategies	57.1	38.1	35.4	58.3	34.8	47.8

Table 15.3—Continued

Questions Regarding Current Emphasis on Speech-Language Services for Older Students	Doctorate Programs[a] (%)		>30 Masters[b] (%)		<30 Masters[c] (%)	
	Yes	No	Yes	No	Yes	No
11. Has your training program changed within the past decade with regard to:						
a. Curriculum emphasis on adolescent development	66.7	33.3	58.3	39.6	52.2	39.1
b. Curriculum emphasis on adolescent communication disorders	71.4	28.6	64.6	33.3	69.6	21.7
c. Students with clinical practicum experience with adolescents	61.9	38.1	58.3	35.4	56.5	30.4
d. Faculty's perspective on the importance of training students to work with this population	76.2	19.0	52.1	41.7	56.5	26.1
e. Your faculty's interest/expertise with this population	76.2	19.0	70.8	22.9	60.9	26.1
f. Student interest in being trained to work with this population	47.6	42.9	45.8	39.6	52.2	39.1
g. Employment opportunities with communicatively handicapped adolescents for your graduates	42.9	47.6	52.1	35.4	34.8	34.8
12. Currently, is anyone in your training program applying creative and innovative procedures (e.g., computer application, etc.) with the adolescent population?	28.6	57.1	18.6	70.8	30.4	65.2

Note: Cells do not total to 100%, because some programs chose not to respond to certain items or gave answers that could not clearly be classified as yes or no.

[a] $N = 21$.
[b] $N = 47$.
[c] $N = 30$.

While the personnel preparation programs offering doctoral degrees are the most likely to offer some course content on the topic of communication disorders in adolescents, it is the smallest programs that seem most likely to provide whole courses on the topic (see the responses to questions 2 and 4 in Table 15.3). Interestingly, the smallest programs have the greatest proportion of faculty who feel it is important to train students specifically in assessment and intervention of adolescents, yet it is the doctoral-level programs that have the most faculty with an interest and/or expertise in the assessment and intervention of adolescents with communication disorders (see question 6).

Question 11 was added to the 2002 survey to measure changes in personnel preparation over the preceding 17 years. Encouraging is the fact that the first five of seven items were answered affirmatively by more than half the programs responding to the survey. Unfortunately, student interest in older students and employment opportunities are not perceived to have changed as much as the first five items.

Efficacy and Effectiveness of Service

Documenting both the efficacy and effectiveness of service remains essential as professionals adjust to their evolving roles and embrace the differing generational viewpoints that surround them. If a professional has entered the discipline after being in a university program that had minimal course content on older students, figuring out how to document efficacy and effectiveness is even more challenging. Yet they must be demonstrable to administrators and decision makers for funding of programs that serve older students with language disorders if they are to be created and/or continued.

Clinical efficacy is "the ability to produce desired clinical results" (J. Damico, 1988, p. 51). It is the obligation of speech-

language pathologists to provide services for preadolescents and adolescents with language disorders that are based on valid and reliable assessment data, that are humane, and that are offered in a cost-effective manner. Ultimately, these services should contribute to the quality of the student's life and to society as a whole (Vetter, 1991).

It is the obligation of speech-language pathologists to provide services for preadolescents and adolescents with language disorders that are based on valid and reliable assessment data, that are humane, and that are offered in a cost-effective manner.

Last (as cited in Baum, 1998) noted that:

An *efficacy* study examines the extent to which a specific intervention, procedure, regimen, or service produces a beneficial result under ideal conditions. Ideally, the determination of efficacy is based on the results of randomized clinical trials. An effectiveness study examines the extent to which a specific intervention, procedure, regimen, or service, when employed in routine practice, does what it is intended to do. (p. 247)

In summary, a randomized clinical trial represents efficacy, whereas a treatment outcomes study represents effectiveness. Both types of studies contribute to the knowledge base in the discipline and help to determine best treatments for clients, which in the case of this book, are older students with language disorders.

O'Toole, Logemann, and Baum (1998) discuss the importance of public school speech-language pathologists conducting clinical trials that demonstrate the efficacy of their services. The issues raised by such trials are not only clinical, but legal and ethical as well. Carefully following guidelines is critical not only to demonstrating the efficacy of our services but also to the advancement of the discipline and new treatment procedures for our students.

Indeed, a plethora of pleas exist for professionals to examine efficacy of service (Amiot, 1998; Apel, 1999a, 2001; Baum, 1998; Gallagher, Swigert, and Baum, 1998; Kamhi, 1995, 1999; Logemann, 1998; Logemann and Baum, 1998; O'Toole, Baum, and Logemann, 1998; O'Toole, Logemann,

Baum, 1998; Slater and Baum, 1998). Students, parents, related professionals, employers, and third-party providers will question the efficacy and the effectiveness of service to students with language disorders until speech-language pathologists make the investigation and documentation of their clinical services a high research priority (Apel, 1999a, 2001; J. Damico, 1988; Kamhi, 1999; Larson and McKinley, 1987, 1995; Logemann, 1994, 1998; McKinley and Larson, 1990; Vetter, 1985, 1991).

Unfortunately, there has been a lack of research on and demonstration of efficacy of services to preadolescents and adolescents with language disorders (J. Damico, 1988; Larson and McKinley, 1987, 1995; McKinley and Larson, 1990; Vetter, 1985, 1991). Vetter (1991) proposed two reasons for the lack of investigation of the efficacy of intervention procedures. First, because the research takes so long, most people writing dissertations and those working toward tenure do not have the time for such investigation. Second, the clinicians closest to the students feel that they are not qualified to do clinical research. Vetter presents a strong argument for clinicians conducting research to determine the efficacy of their language intervention activities. She cites several research strategies to be considered (i.e., large sample size, precise definitions of what a language disorder is, single-subject designs, practical vs. statistical significance, and the use of criterion-referenced tests to replace norm-referenced standardized tests that fragment language).

The lack of data has started to be ameliorated because the American Speech-Language-Hearing Association has several efficacy and effectiveness projects in progress (Baum, 1998; Gallagher, Swigert, Baum, 1998; Logemann, 1998; O'Toole, Logemann, and Baum, 1998). The most notable effort is the NOMS (National Outcomes Measurements Systems) project in speech-language pathology and audiology.

Gallagher, Swigert, and Baum (1998) strongly advocate that public school speech-language pathologists get involved in collecting data for the NOMS project. Schooling (2000) discussed the importance of clinicians collecting treatment outcome data and sending these data to the American Speech-Language-Hearing Association to be analyzed. They, in turn, will use these data to justify treatment practices, additional positions, and third-party payments. NOMS data also provide an objective measure on which to base decision-making (Schooling).

Amiot (1998) stated that the old 1990 IDEA established a right to education, whereas the new IDEA '97 emphasizes accountability for student outcomes. This speaks volumes for the need to do outcome-based or effectiveness studies and clinical trials to determine the efficacy of our services.

As mentioned in Chapter 11, we propose a follow-up component to our comprehensive delivery model (see Appendix V) to document the effectiveness of services to older students. Once follow-up data have been collected, they must be analyzed carefully.

These data should be used to make modifications in the delivery of speech-language services to preadolescents and adolescents with language disorders. Likewise, these data should be shared with colleagues so that they, too, can make appropriate alterations in their programs.

Regardless of the investigator (J. Damico, 1988; Larson and McKinley, 1987, 1995; Vetter, 1985, 1991; Weiner, 1985), it is clear that speech-language pathologists can no longer fail to investigate and report the efficacy and effectiveness of their services to older students. To do so is unconscionable.

A Call to Action

We wrote "Students Who Can't Communicate: Speech-Language Services at the Secondary Level" (McKinley and Larson, 1989) as a call to action for secondary school principals. It was reinforced a year later among our own colleagues so that speech-language pathologists could become a united voice for older students with language disorders (Larson and McKinley, 1990). We reiterate that call to you now.

Older students with language disorders have a right to services. Our society can no longer afford to waste the human potential of youth with language disorders who, given adequate intervention and transition services, can become taxpayers rather than tax takers. Beyond dollars, society can also reap the benefit of creating adult citizens who have problem-solving strategies, communication skills, and increased self-esteem when adequate services are delivered during their school careers by speech-language pathologists, including during the critical preadolescent and adolescent periods. Once the vision for and the commitment to services for older students are set, the time and resources needed for implementation become attainable.

Our society can no longer afford to waste the human potential of youth with language disorders who, given adequate intervention and transition services, can become taxpayers rather than tax takers.

The "vision" includes seeing how speech-language pathologists are an integral part of students' school programs, sometimes all the way through to high school graduation. The "commitment" includes standing up for what is fair and just, not to mention legally mandated, for students with language disorders, even in the face of odds.

"Commitment" may include not dismissing students from intervention when that is clearly the popular choice. It may mean providing advocacy for students at risk of being dropouts or throwaways in our schools. Our level of commitment to at-risk youth needs to intensify. Judge Janice Brice Wellington (1994), speaking at The International Adolescent Conference, stated, "If we continue to operate at the same level of commitment that we currently are, we'll lose more kids than we save." She also explained, "We are engaged in a war (for at-risk youth) where there are few back-up troops.... It's a war we won't win unless we do something different (than what we're currently doing)."

By law, all students are entitled to a free, appropriate educational program that meets their individual needs. When the focus is on the needs of students under the existing laws, and when the commitment is there, time and money can be found. High school administrators are not going to invite speech-language pathologists to create jobs for themselves in their buildings. But they will defend those positions once our profession has created them in response to students' needs.

You are needed to apply the vision and the commitment in your community. Keep students' needs first, address those needs, and diminish the waste of human potential of individuals with language disorders. The preadolescents and adolescents who struggle with communication are depending on you.

Points of Discussion

1. How could you document the effectiveness or efficacy of your services to older students with language disorders?

2. As you project into the future, what new roles do you see speech-language pathologists fulfilling?

Suggested Readings

Lancaster, L., and Stillman, D. (2002). *When generations collide*. New York: HarperCollins.

Schooling, T. (2000). NOMS bears fruit: Clinicians collect treatment outcomes data. *The ASHA Leader,* 5(10), 4–5.

Appendixes

Secondary-Level Referral Form—
Communication Disorders

Educator: _____   Course or Specialty: _____

Date Completed: _____   Total of All Ratings: _____

Using the following scale, rate the statements regarding the communication behavior of _____ in your classroom.
(student's name)

   5—Almost Always   2—Infrequently

   4—Frequently   1—Almost Never

   3—Sometimes   NA/NO—Not Applicable or Not Observed

Thinking

_____   1. The student organizes and categorizes information from experiences.

_____   2. The student sequences data in a logical order.

_____   3. The student identifies and solves problems independently.

_____   4. The student finds, selects, and uses information for assignments.

_____   5. The student thinks about ideas and events that are not just in the "here and now."

_____   6. The student thinks about his or her thinking.

_____   7. The student evaluates his or her thinking.

_____   8. The student improves or revises his or her thinking strategies.

_____   9. The student benefits from scaffolding or providing a framework for thinking.

_____   10. The student demonstrates that information learned in one situation can be generalized to new situations.

_____   **TOTAL**

Comments: _____

_____

Listening

_____   1. The student understands multiple-meaning words.

_____   2. The student understands complex sentences.

_____ 3. The student comprehends main ideas during lectures and discussions.

_____ 4. The student identifies relevant supporting details as they relate to main ideas during lectures and discussions.

_____ 5. The student records main ideas and supporting details in a notebook.

_____ 6. The student follows directions of at least three steps, after listening to them one at a time.

_____ 7. The student knows how to get information by asking questions.

_____ 8. The student uses critical listening skills (e.g., detecting fact from opinion and evaluating a speaker's argument).

_____ 9. The student understands humor, jargon, and slang used by peers.

_____ 10. The student uses effective listening skills during conversations (e.g., head nodding and commenting).

_____ **TOTAL**

Comments: _____

_____

Speaking

_____ 1. The student plans what to say, sequences it in a logical way, and speaks in sentences when appropriate.

_____ 2. The student uses grammatically intact utterances.

_____ 3. The student uses accurate, precise words and avoids low-information words (e.g., *things, stuff,* and *it).*

_____ 4. The student gives directions clearly and accurately.

_____ 5. The student makes reports, tells or retells stories, and explains processes clearly and accurately.

_____ 6. The student converses by following rules of conversation (e.g., turn taking and initiating and maintaining conversations).

_____ 7. The student provides relevant and complete answers to questions.

_____ 8. The student displays normal voice characteristics with regard to pitch, volume, and quality.

_____ 9. The student displays normal fluency or flow of speech.

_____ 10. The student talks about his or her talking and can revise or repair communication breakdowns.

_____ **TOTAL**

Comments: _____

_____

Reading

_____ 1. The student is aware of phonological rules (e.g., sound-letter associations).

_____ 2. The student has knowledge of morphological rules (e.g., root words and affixes).

_____ 3. The student comprehends figurative and literal meanings in multiple-meaning words, idioms, and other ambiguous language forms.

_____ 4. The student comprehends simple and complex sentences and a variety of sentence types.

_____ 5. The student relates word knowledge and experiences to the material being read.

_____ 6. The student reads for main ideas and supporting details.

_____ 7. The student can predict the outcome of a story.

_____ 8. The student reads with various purposes in mind (e.g., skimming, outlining, analyzing, making inferences, making predictions, and critiquing).

_____ 9. The student reads differently depending on genre (e.g., narration, expository text, and persuasion).

_____ 10. The student can analyze, summarize, and critique readings.

_____ **TOTAL**

Comments: _____

_____

Writing

_____ 1. The student plans, organizes, and gathers information before writing about a selected topic.

_____ 2. The student outlines information on a selected topic before writing.

_____ 3. The student writes the first draft decisively and fluently and with a variety of grammatically correct sentences.

_____   4. The student changes writing style dependent on the purpose for writing, (e.g., formal or informal style).

_____   5. The student takes the audience/reader into account when writing.

_____   6. The student takes into account discourse genre (e.g., narration, conversation, expository text, descriptive text, and persuasive text) when writing.

_____   7. The student edits/revises content of writing for clarity, brevity, and accuracy.

_____   8. The student edits/revises the mechanics of writing (e.g., spelling, punctuation, and capitalization).

_____   9. The student writes using a variety of words with multiple meanings.

_____   10. The student enjoys the writing process.

_____   **TOTAL**

Comments: _____

_____

TOTAL OF ALL 5 RATINGS (A): _____

TOTAL NUMBER OF
POSSIBLE POINTS (B):   *250*

PERCENTAGE ([A÷B] × 100): _____

Please share your overall perception of the student by rating this item on the same scale of 1 to 5 (1 = Almost Never; 5 = Almost Always).

_____   I feel confident in this student's ability to function independently once his or her school experience is over.

If you rate this item "1" or "2," please comment on how the student's communication is contributing to the problem.

Thank you for taking time to complete this form. Please return it to the speech-language pathologist who asked you to complete it. If the student has fewer than 80% of the possible points that you could have scored, referral for additional assessment may be made. Your written comments will also be heavily considered. Even if your numerical percentage exceeds 80%, the student may still undergo further assessment based on expressed concerns that are not captured by this referral form's ratings.

Self-Evaluation of Teacher Language

Name: _____

Class: _____ Date: _____

Directions: Rate yourself on the class, lecture, or instructions you just gave by circling the item that best matches your opinion. Add each column to compute your total score and write that number in the box. (Help students total their scores on Appendix C if necessary.)

Rating

	1	2	3	2	1
Length of instructions or lecture	very long and hard to follow	somewhat long	just right	somewhat short	too short
Complexity of instructions or lecture	too hard	somewhat hard	just right	somewhat easy	too easy
Level of vocabulary	too hard	somewhat hard	just right	somewhat easy	too easy
Organization of ideas	very hard to follow	somewhat hard to follow	just right	—	—
Ease of listening	very hard to listen to	somewhat hard to listen to	just right	—	—
Rate of speech	very fast rate of speaking	somewhat fast rate of speaking	just right	somewhat slow rate of speaking	very slow rate of speaking
Tone of voice	very irritating tone of voice	somewhat irritating tone of voice	just right	—	—

TOTAL [____] = _____ + _____ + _____ + _____ + _____

_____ Mean (Total ÷ 7)

_____ Class Total

_____ Class Mean (Class Total ÷ Class Number ÷ 7)

Compare your mean total with the averages reported by your students: _____

_____

_____

_____

_____

Student Evaluation of Teacher Language

Name: _____   Date:_____

Teacher: _____   Class: _____

This is not a test. Answers will NOT affect your grade.
Answer honestly.

Directions: Rate the class lecture or instructions your teacher just gave by circling the item that best matches your opinion. Add each column to compute your total score and write that number in the box.

Rating

	1	**2**	**3**	**2**	**1**
Length of instructions or lecture	very long and hard to follow	somewhat long	Just right	somewhat short	too short
Complexity of instructions or lecture	too hard	somewhat hard	Just right	somewhat easy	too easy
Level of vocabulary	too hard	somewhat hard	Just right	somewhat easy	too easy
Organization of ideas	very hard to follow	somewhat hard to follow	Just right	—	—
Ease of listening	very hard to listen to	somewhat hard to listen to	Just right	—	—
Rate of speech	very fast rate of speaking	somewhat fast rate of speaking	Just right	somewhat slow rate of speaking	very slow rate of speaking
Tone of voice	very irritating tone of voice	somewhat irritating tone of voice	Just right	—	—

TOTAL [   ] = _____ + _____ + _____ + _____ + _____

What would help you understand the class material better?_____
_____

Do you have other comments about the teacher's language? Write your comments on the back side of this form.

Thank you.

 Communication Solutions for Older Students © 2003 by Thinking Publications
Duplication permitted for educational use only.

Curriculum Analysis Form

Student's Name:_____   Date(s) of Analysis: _____

Instructor:_____   Grade Level: _____

Examiner Completing Analysis:_____   Class: _____

TEXTBOOK ANALYSIS

Identifying Information

1. Title of Primary Text in the Class: _____

2. Author(s):_____

3. Copyright: _____

4. Year Adopted by School: _____

5. Readability Level: _____

    How was readability determined? _____

    • Is the readability level of the text appropriate for the student?

    _____ No   _____ Yes

    • Is the readability similar to that of the student's other textbooks?

    _____ No   _____ Yes

6. Is this textbook significantly different from others the student is reading?

    _____ No   _____ Yes

    If "Yes," how is it different? _____

    _____

    _____

Communication Solutions
for Older Students

Student Familiarity with the Textbook

1. Check the features included in the textbook. For any that are present, determine whether the student can locate these features upon request and state how the feature can help.

Organizational Feature	Feature Present in the Textbook?		Can the Student Locate the Feature?		Student Response to "How Can This Organizational Feature Help You?"
	Yes	No	Yes	No	
Table of Contents					
Index					
Glossary					
Appendix					
Bibliography					
Unit or Chapter Objectives					
Review Questions and/or Practice Exercises					
Varying Print Styles (use of italics, bold print, color)					
Graphic Aids (charts, tables, graphs, maps)					

CLASSROOM ANALYSIS

Course Organization

1. Which topical arrangement typifies the curriculum from this class? (Check one.)

_____ Sequential (independence among topics)

_____ Spiral (dependence among topics)

- If "sequential" arrangement is primary, have all units been problematic for the student, or only some? (Check one.)

_____ All   _____ Some

2. Does the class have significantly different requirements in comparison with the student's other classes?

    _____ No   _____ Yes

    If "Yes," explain: _____

    _____

    _____

Student's Comprehension of Lecture/Instructions

Enlist the assistance of a "good student" in the classroom. Indicate to that student that you would like him or her to take notes during the first 10 minutes of a lecture or note a set of instructions given in the class. Have the student you are evaluating take notes as well. Compare the notes taken by the two students. Use the "good student's" notes to answer the first 2 items below; for the remaining items, use the notes from the individual being assessed.

- What was the main idea presented (or sequence of instructions)? _____

  _____

- What were the relevant supporting ideas?_____

  _____

  _____

- Did the student's main idea(s) match the one(s) the "good student" identified?

  _____ No   _____ Yes   _____ Somewhat

- Did the student's relevant supporting details match the ones the "good student" identified?

  _____ No   _____ Yes   _____ Somewhat

- Did the student indicate verbally or nonverbally any words that were not understood?

  _____ No   _____ Yes

  If "Yes," list them: _____

  _____

- Does the student report having difficulty comprehending the lectures/instructions only in this class or also in others? (Check one.)

  _____ Only this class   _____ This class and others

Student's Comprehension of Tests/Evaluations

1. Obtain a recent test or other evaluation tool administered to the student. Ask the student the following questions.

- What questions were most difficult to answer? _____
_____

  Why were they more difficult? _____
_____

- What vocabulary items were unfamiliar? _____
_____

- How did you prepare for this test? (Circle one.)

  Not at all   Some   Enough   More than usual   A great amount

- Are the tests in this class significantly different from those in other classes that you are taking?

  _____ No   _____ Yes

2. Using Bloom et al.'s (1956) taxonomy (see page 45), what level(s) of thinking were required most often during this test?

_____ Knowledge	_____ Analysis
_____ Comprehension	_____ Synthesis
_____ Application	_____ Evaluation

STUDENT ATTITUDE TOWARD THE CLASS

Ask the student the following questions and record responses.

- Do you think the ideas presented in this class are important to learn?

  _____ No   _____ Yes   _____ Sometimes

- Do you think this class is interesting?

  _____ No   _____ Yes   _____ Sometimes

- Do you think this class is taught simply enough so that you can learn the information?

  _____ No   _____ Yes   _____ Sometimes

- Do you think the information you learn in this class is useful?

  _____ No   _____ Yes   _____ Sometimes

- Do you think the information in this class is presented clearly by the teacher?

  _____ No   _____ Yes   _____ Sometimes

- Do you think the information in this class is presented clearly by the textbook?

  _____ No   _____ Yes   _____ Sometimes

• Do you feel motivated to do well in this class?

_____ No   _____ Yes   _____ Sometimes

CURRICULUM ANALYSIS SUMMARY

1. Analyze results to determine the following:

   • Does the textbook for the class appear to be interfering significantly with the student's comprehension?_____
   _____

   • Does the student appear to be having difficulty understanding the teacher's lectures/ instructions in the classroom compared with other students at the same level? _____
   _____

   • Do the tests in the class seem to be interfering with class performance because the student does not understand the language in them? _____
   _____

   • Does the student show any positive attitude toward the class or attempt to perform well?
   _____

2. Compare results with the student's performance on informal assessment tasks that require the student to use informational listening for short, simulated lectures. If the classroom teacher has conducted a *Student* or *Self-Evaluation of Teacher Language* (see Appendices B and C), compare results with those findings (i.e., Is the student undergoing assessment the only student experiencing difficulty understanding the teacher?). _____
_____

INTERPRETATION

If the first three bullet points of the Curriculum Analysis Summary are answered affirmatively, and the data match those obtained during direct assessment of the adolescent, then the problem rests primarily within the student. However, if data mismatch (e.g., the student demonstrated appropriate information listening skills in an informal assessment task, but poor informational listening skills in the classroom), the problem may lie within the educational system. Note, however, that students should demonstrate a positive attitude before you conclude that the problem rests primarily within the educational system (see the fourth bullet point under #1 above).

Case History Interview
(Student Form)

Directions: Gather the "Student Form" information by interviewing the student and reading each item. Gather the "Family Form" information by interviewing one or more family members.

Information

Name: _____

Birth Date: _____ Age: _____ Gender: M   F

Education: (Highest grade completed) _____

Address: _____

Home Phone:_____ Email: _____

Work Phone of Parent/Guardian: _____

Environmental History

1. Name the members of your immediate family. Are there any speech, hearing, or language problems present among members of your household?

Name	Relationship	Communication Problem

2. Name two friends you enjoy talking to.

_____

_____

Educational and Vocational History

1. Which school subjects are your best ones? _____

2. Which school subjects do you enjoy the most? _____

3. Which school subjects are your most difficult ones? _____
   Why do you feel you are having difficulty with these subjects? _____
   _____

4. Are you involved in activities outside of school?   No   Yes
   If "Yes," describe: _____

5. Do you have any future vocational goals?   No   Yes
   If "Yes," describe: _____

6. Do you hold a full- or part-time job?   No   Yes
   If "Yes," describe: _____

Health History

1. Describe: (a) Major illnesses, diseases, or accidents
             (b) Age at the time of each
             (c) Resulting health complications or handicaps

Illnesses/Diseases/Accidents	Age	Resulting Complications

2. Were you hospitalized for any of the named conditions?   No   Yes
   If "Yes," where? _____
   For how long? _____

3. Have you received, or are you now receiving rehabilitation treatment (e.g., radiation therapy, physical therapy, or occupational therapy)?   No   Yes
   If "Yes," describe the reason for, type, duration, and result of treatments: _____
   _____

4. Are you currently under a doctor's care?   No   Yes

   If "Yes," for what? _____

5. Are you currently taking any medication?   No   Yes

   If "Yes," what kind? _____

   For what? _____

   How much? _____

   How often? _____

6. Do you have any known allergies?   No   Yes

   If "Yes," describe: _____

7. Do you have any known drug sensitivities?   No   Yes

   If "Yes," describe: _____

8. Have you had seizures?   No   Yes

   If "Yes," how often? _____

   When was the most recent seizure? _____

9. Do you have any known hearing problems?   No   Yes

   If "Yes," describe: _____

10. Have you had a past history of ear infections?   No   Yes

    If "Yes," describe: _____

11. Do you have any known visual problems?   No   Yes

    If "Yes," describe: _____

    Do you wear glasses or contact lenses?   No   Yes

Communication History

1. Describe your present communication problem: _____

   _____

2. How long has there been a problem? _____

3. What do you think caused the problem? _____

4. What types of speech and language services have you received? _____

   How long did you receive them? _____

   How do you feel about the services you received? _____

5. Were you ever dismissed from speech and language services?   No   Yes

   If "Yes," why? _____

6. How do you feel about your present speech and language problem? _____

7. Are you understood when you speak?   No   Yes

   If "No," describe:_____

8. Do you understand when others talk to you?   No   Yes

   If "No," describe:_____

9. Do you avoid speaking situations?   No   Yes

   If "Yes," describe: _____

10. Are there times or situations when your problem is better or worse?   No   Yes

    If "Yes," describe: _____

    _____

    _____

    _____

11. Tell any additional information that would be useful in evaluating your communication skills

    and in planning an intervention program. _____

    _____

    _____

    _____

    _____

    _____

    _____

Communication Solutions
for Older Students

(Family Form)

Name of Parent(s)/Guardian(s): _____ Date: _____

Name of the family member(s) who were interviewed.

Name   Relationship

_____

_____

_____

_____

Communication History

1. Describe your child's present problem: _____

   _____

2. How long has there been a problem? _____

3. What do you think caused the problem? _____

4. What types of speech and language services has he or she received? _____

   _____

   For how long? _____

   How do you feel about the services your child received? _____

5. Was your child ever dismissed from speech and language services?   No   Yes

   If "Yes," why? _____

Family Members' Perceptions of Their Child's Communication

1. Do you feel that a problem exists, or do you feel that the school or someone else is fabricating
   the problem? _____

   _____

2. If you feel a communication disorder exists, is it a primary or secondary concern? _____

    _____

    _____

3. If you feel that a problem exists, do you feel frustrated, embarrassed, guilty, and ashamed, or are you accepting of your child's communication? _____

    _____

    _____

4. How do or don't you attempt to cope with your child's communication disorder (e.g., by talking for your child, by excluding the child from the mainstream of family life and decision-making, or by ignoring the disorder)?_____

    _____

    _____

5. What are your goals and expectations for your child?

    _____

    _____

    _____

Name of Interviewer Completing This Form: _____

Listening Questionnaire

Directions: Decide if each statement is true or false. Then write your answer in the blank next to each item.

_____ 1. Teachers or friends who don't listen to me are too stupid to appreciate my ideas.

_____ 2. Teaching students to listen is as foolish as trying to teach them to breathe.

_____ 3. I already have developed good listening skills because I have to listen all the time in school.

_____ 4. It is more important to be a good speaker than a good listener because we learn by talking.

_____ 5. It is more important to be a good reader than a good listener because we can go back to check material we have read.

_____ 6. I think I have been adequately taught to listen at school and at home.

_____ 7. Students should not have to work at listening to class lectures.

_____ 8. I can't stand to listen to people who talk about ideas that sound crazy.

_____ 9. It doesn't matter if I stop listening because I don't miss much.

_____ 10. I'm a good listener when I want to be.

Each true answer reveals a misconception about listening. Count the number of true responses and compare it to the scale below.

0, 1 = Free of false information about listening.

2, 3, 4 = You have a positive attitude toward learning about listening.

5, 6, 7 = You are aware of listening as a topic, but misconceptions are warping your thinking.

8, 9, 10 = BRICK WALL. Misconceptions have kept listening information from being useful to you.

Compare and discuss results within the group.

From *Daily Communication: Strategies for the Language Disordered Adolescent* (pp. 55–56), by L. Schreiber and N. McKinley, 1995, Eau Claire, WI: Thinking Publications. © 1995 by Thinking Publications. Adapted with permission.

Emotional Intelligence Protocol

Student: _____   Date: _____

Directions: Emotional intelligence (Goleman, 1998) can be assessed by engaging individual students in discussions concerning 5 major dimensions and 25 competencies. Circle "Adequate" or "Inadequate" for each competency. Mark a competency you perceive to be penalizing, absent, or marginally present as "Inadequate." Comment on the impact of the competency on the student's academic, social, and vocational performance. Emotional intelligence capacities build on one another (i.e., they are hierarchical). For example, if the student is demonstrating inadequate competencies within the first dimension (i.e., self-awareness), then questioning should be suspended. Once the dimension in which the student is functioning has been determined, use the questions for the competencies within that dimension for intervention activities.

Check (✔)the dimensions discussed and indicate where the student reached a ceiling:

_____   I. Self-Awareness

_____   II. Self-Regulation

_____   III. Motivation

_____   IV. Empathy

_____   V. Social Skills

I. Self-Awareness

The dimension of self-awareness is a critical foundation skill for the three emotional competencies of emotional awareness, accurate self-assessment, and self-confidence.

1. *Emotional awareness* is the ability to recognize what we are feeling and why and how these feelings affect our performance in the workplace. Also, we need to be aware of how our values and goals guide our decision-making. This competence is the most fundamental of the emotional competencies. To address this competency, discuss the following:

   • What is a strong feeling? Give examples of strong feelings (e.g., rage, despair, and ecstasy).

   • Why do people feel a certain way?

   • When have you last felt anger, sadness, or happiness?

Communication Solutions
for Older Students

- Tell about situations in which you felt a particular emotion, for example, anger. When you felt that way, how did it influence your ability to complete schoolwork, talk with a friend, do jobs around the house, or do jobs outside the home?

Adequate   Inadequate

Comment on how this competency is impacting academic performance, personal-social interactions, and vocational potential: _____

_____

_____

2. *Accurate self-assessment* is the ability to be aware of one's strengths and weaknesses; to reflect on one's experiences; to be open to new perspectives, continuous learning, and self-development; and to have a sense of humor. To address this competency, discuss the following:

- What are your strengths and weaknesses?
- What experiences have been positive in your life, and how have they made you a stronger person?
- What experiences have not been positive in your life, and how have they made you a stronger person?
- What have you done to continue to learn new skills?
- Why is a sense of humor important?

Adequate   Inadequate

Comment on how this competency is impacting academic performance, personal-social interactions, and vocational potential: _____

_____

_____

3. *Self-confidence* is the ability to have a strong sense of one's self-worth and abilities. People who have this competency are self-assured to the point that they stand up for what is right even if it is unpopular. They are capable of making sound decisions despite uncertainties and pressures. To address this competency, discuss the following:

- Tell about all the abilities that make you a worthwhile person.

• When did you stand up for an unpopular idea knowing that it was the right thing to do? How did you feel about yourself when you did this? What were some positive outcomes of this experience? Were there any negative outcomes of this experience, and if so, what were they?

Adequate   Inadequate

Comment on how this competency is impacting academic performance, personal-social interactions, and vocational potential: _____

_____

_____

II. Self-Regulation

Self-regulation is the ability to manage impulsiveness and to handle upsetting situations. Five emotional competencies support this dimension: self-control, trustworthiness, conscientious-ness, adaptability, and innovation.

1. *Self-control* is the ability to manage impulsive feelings, to delay gratification, and to stay com-posed and focused—even in trying situations. To address this competency, do the following:

• Discuss options for students in this scenario: A person disagrees with you and starts yelling at you. Do you:
   a. Stay calm?
   b. Yell back?
   c. Calmly point out information that supports your position?

• Have students share how they handle stress in their lives (e.g., talk to a friend or listen to music).

• Have students answer this question: How do you manage your time?

Adequate   Inadequate

Comment on how this competency is impacting academic performance, personal-social inter-actions, and vocational potential:_____

_____

_____

2. *Trustworthiness* is the ability to act in an ethical fashion (e.g., acting openly, honestly, and consistently, regardless of the situation). To address this competency, discuss the following:

Communication Solutions
for Older Students

- What does it mean to be ethical and/or honest?

- In which situations is it difficult to be ethical and/or honest? Why is it difficult?

- Under what circumstances (if any) is it ethical to:

    a. Cheat on a test?

    b. Copy someone else's paper?

    c. Take someone else's lunch ticket?

    Adequate   **Inadequate**

Comment on how this competency is impacting academic performance, personal-social interactions, and vocational potential: _____

_____

_____

3. *Conscientiousness* is the ability to meet commitments, to keep promises, and to be well organized and careful in work outcomes. To address this competency, discuss the following:

- What is a commitment?

- When have you made a commitment?

- Have you ever broken a commitment? What was the consequence?

- Is it easier to keep a commitment if you are well organized? Why or why not?

    Adequate   **Inadequate**

Comment on how this competency is impacting academic performance, personal-social interactions, and vocational potential: _____

_____

_____

4. *Adaptability* is the ability to change responses, procedures, or approaches in a given situation (i.e., to be flexible and to handle multiple demands). To address this competency, discuss the following:

- What does it mean to be flexible?

- What are several situations in which you were flexible, and what were the consequences?

- How well do you handle multiple demands within a single situation?

- What strategies do you use to handle multiple demands across several situations?

Adequate   **Inadequate**

Comment on how this competency is impacting academic performance, personal-social inter-actions, and vocational potential: _____

_____

_____

5. *Innovation* is the ability to seek out new ideas, to generate new approaches, and to be will-ing to take risks to implement original solutions to problems. To address this competency, discuss the following:

- How do you search out new ideas?

- Are you willing to try new ideas? If so, when?

- Are there times when you are unwilling to try new ideas? If so, when and why?

- Do you enjoy coming up with new solutions?

Adequate   **Inadequate**

Comment on how this competency is impacting academic performance, personal-social inter-actions, and vocational potential: _____

_____

_____

III. Motivation

The third dimension is that of motivation, which is using our deepest preferences to move and guide us toward our goals. Four emotional competencies exemplify outstanding performers: achievement drive, commitment, initiative, and optimism.

1. *Achievement drive* is the ability to strive to improve or meet a standard of excellence. To do this, one must be result-oriented, set challenging goals and take risks, and pursue ways to improve. To address this competency, do the following:

- Have the student talk about what it means to be an achiever.

- Ask the student to describe someone who has a drive to be excellent.

• Have the student talk about what a goal is and how to set goals.

Adequate   **Inadequate**

Comment on how this competency is impacting academic performance, personal-social interactions, and vocational potential: _____

_____

_____

2. *Commitment* is the ability to align our goals with the goals of a group or an organization. More specifically, people with this competence are capable of sacrificing to meet organizational goals, sensing a purpose in and seeking out opportunities to fulfill the larger group mission, and making decisions and clarifying choices using the group's core values. To address this competency, discuss the following:

• What does it mean to be committed to the larger group or organization?

• How does being committed to a larger group or organization:

   a. Help you?

   b. Help the group?

• Have you gone the "extra mile" for a group or an organization? If so, how?

• Have you ever sacrificed your own goals for those of the group? If so, how did you feel?

Adequate   **Inadequate**

Comment on how this competency is impacting academic performance, personal-social interactions, and vocational potential: _____

_____

_____

3. *Initiative* is the ability to be proactive by seizing opportunities, pursuing goals beyond what is required, cutting through the bureaucracy to get the job done, and mobilizing others. To address this competency, discuss the following:

• When have you taken advantage of an opportunity?

• Have you ever gone beyond what was required? If so, when, and how did you feel?

- Have you ever gotten other people excited about an idea and helped them achieve their goal? If so, how?

Adequate   Inadequate

Comment on how this competency is impacting academic performance, personal-social interactions, and vocational potential: _____

_____

_____

4. *Optimism* is the ability to be persistent despite setbacks or barriers, and to be hopeful of successful outcomes. To address this competency, discuss the following:

- What does it mean to be optimistic? Describe someone you know who is optimistic.
- What does it mean to be pessimistic? Describe someone you know who is pessimistic.
- When you are optimistic and feel positive about accomplishing a task, are you more successful at the task? If so, why?
- Have you ever overcome a barrier? If so, how did you do it?

Adequate   Inadequate

Comment on how this competency is impacting academic performance, personal-social interactions, and vocational potential: _____

_____

_____

IV. Empathy

The fourth dimension is empathy, which is an essential "people skill" for workplace success. Empathy is our social radar; it permits us to sense what others feel without them saying so. The five emotional competencies of empathy include understanding others, developing others' abilities, advancing a service orientation, leveraging diversity, and being politically aware.

1. *Understanding others* is the ability to sense others' feelings and perspectives by listening well and being attentive to emotional cues, as well as to take an active interest in their concerns. To address this competency, do the following:

- Present a set of photos of people with various emotional expressions. Have the student describe each emotion and how the person may be feeling.

Communication Solutions
for Older Students

- Discuss what it means to be a good listener. Have the student describe someone he or she knows who is a good listener.

- Have the student discuss what it means to take the point of view of the person speaking.

- Ask the student to demonstrate how people show they understand someone's perspective.

Adequate   Inadequate

Comment on how this competency is impacting academic performance, personal-social interactions, and vocational potential: _____

_____

_____

2. *Developing others' abilities* means sensing others' needs and bolstering their abilities. This is accomplished by rewarding people's strengths, offering feedback and identifying people's needs for growth, and mentoring people. To address this competency, discuss the following:

- What have you done to recognize and reward something that someone has done that is good?

- How does coaching or mentoring help someone develop his or her abilities?

- What have you done to help someone do better at an activity?

Adequate   Inadequate

Comment on how this competency is impacting academic performance, personal-social interactions, and vocational potential: _____

_____

_____

3. *Advancing a service orientation* means anticipating, recognizing, and meeting customers' needs. To address this competency, discuss the following:

- When you were in a store and you received good customer service, how did you react and feel? Tell about the situation.

- When you were in a store and you received poor customer service, how did you react and feel? Tell about the situation.

- What is good customer service?

- Assume you are working in a fast-food restaurant. How would you give good customer service?

Adequate   Inadequate

Comment on how this competency is impacting academic performance, personal-social interactions, and vocational potential: _____

_____

_____

4. *Leveraging diversity* means cultivating opportunities by working with different kinds of people. More specifically, it is respecting, relating to, and understanding people with different backgrounds and diverse worldviews. It also means challenging bias and intolerance. To address this competency, discuss the following:

   • What is a stereotype and how does it hurt people?

   • What does it mean to have a zero tolerance level for racial and gender biases?

   • What is hate speech and why is it wrong?

   • Why is diversity among people a wonderful opportunity to learn more about our world?

   Adequate   Inadequate

   Comment on how this competency is impacting academic performance, personal-social interactions, and vocational potential: _____

_____

_____

5. *Being politically aware* means reading social and political situations. This means recognizing power relationships, detecting important social networks, understanding forces that shape viewpoints and actions of people, and being able to read organizational and external realities. To address this competency, discuss the following:

   • What does it mean to have political savvy?

   • What is a social network?

   • Do you have a social network? If so, describe it.

   • What is the informal structure or network that makes good things happen in your school? If you don't know, how could you find out?

   Adequate   Inadequate

Comment on how this competency is impacting academic performance, personal-social inter-actions, and vocational potential: _____

_____

_____

V. Social Skills

This is the final dimension of emotional intelligence and is critical to success in the workplace and in life. Eight emotional competencies undergird this dimension: influence, communication, conflict management, leadership, change catalyst, building bonds, collaboration and coopera-tion, and team capabilities.

1. *Influence* is the ability to use persuasion to affect others to perform. People with this com-petence are skilled at getting people's support and in building consensus. To address this competency, discuss the following:

   • What does it mean to persuade someone to do something?

   • What does it mean to build consensus and why is this important?

   • Have you gotten people to support one of your ideas? If so, how?

   Adequate   Inadequate

   Comment on how this competency is impacting academic performance, personal-social inter-actions, and vocational potential: _____

   _____

   _____

2. *Communication* as an emotional intelligence competence is the ability to listen openly and to send convincing messages. More specifically, it is the ability to effectively give-and-take in a conversation, note the emotional cues the speaker is sending and receiving, deal with dif-ficult issues in a straightforward manner, and foster open communication regardless of whether it is good or bad news. To address this competency, discuss the following:

   • What does it mean to be a good communicator?

   • Why is being a good communicator important to success in life?

   • Do you know any good communicators? If so, what characteristics do they have?

   • How can you be a better communicator?

   Adequate   Inadequate

Comment on how this competency is impacting academic performance, personal-social interactions, and vocational potential: _____

_____

_____

3. *Conflict management* is the ability to negotiate and resolve disagreements. More specifically, it is the ability to handle difficult people and situations tactfully, to encourage debate and open discussions, and to create win-win solutions. To address this competency, discuss the following:

   • What does it mean to negotiate with someone?

   • How do you handle:

      a. Difficult people?

      b. Difficult situations?

   • What does it mean to create a win-win situation?

   Adequate   Inadequate

   Comment on how this competency is impacting academic performance, personal-social interactions, and vocational potential: _____

   _____

   _____

4. *Leadership* is the ability to inspire and guide individuals and groups. To address this competency, discuss the following:

   • What does it mean to be a leader?

   • Name some people who are leaders. What characteristics do they have:

      a. That are similar?

      b. That are different?

   • Name a U.S. leader. What makes (made) him or her a leader?

   • What leadership characteristics do you have?

   Adequate   Inadequate

Communication Solutions
for Older Students

Comment on how this competency is impacting academic performance, personal-social interactions, and vocational potential: _____

_____

_____

5. *Change catalyst* is having the ability to initiate or manage change. More specifically, people with this competence have the ability to recognize the need for change, challenge the status quo, mobilize others to change, and model change expectations. To address this competency, discuss the following:

- What does it mean to be a change agent?

- Describe someone you know or admire who brings about positive change.

- Why and when is it important to change?

- Describe a time when it was important for you to change. Was it easy to change? Why or why not?

Adequate   Inadequate

Comment on how this competency is impacting academic performance, personal-social interactions, and vocational potential: _____

_____

_____

6. *Building bonds* is the ability to cultivate interpersonal relationships through networking, building rapport, and keeping people informed. To address this competency, discuss the following:

- What does it mean to build relationships?

- List two people with whom you have a positive relationship and describe it.

- What is the difference between a working relationship and a friendship?

Adequate   Inadequate

Comment on how this competency is impacting academic performance, personal-social interactions, and vocational potential: _____

_____

_____

7. *Collaboration and cooperation* is the ability to work with others toward shared goals. To address this competency, discuss the following:

   - What does it mean to collaborate on a project?

   - Explain how you have collaborated on a project. Was it a better project because you worked with someone, rather than working alone?

   - When you collaborate and cooperate on a project, what do you:

     a. Gain?

     b. Lose?

     c. Need to change?

   Adequate   Inadequate

   Comment on how this competency is impacting academic performance, personal-social interactions, and vocational potential: _____

   _____

   _____

8. *Team capabilities* is the ability to create group synergy in pursuing collective goals. People with this competency are capable of modeling team qualities like respect, helpfulness, cooperation, and commitment. To address this competency, discuss the following:

   - Describe characteristics you need to have to be a team member.

   - What does it mean to be a member of a team?

   - When is it an advantage to be a member of a team?

   - When is it a disadvantage to be a member of a team?

   Adequate   Inadequate

   Comment on how this competency is impacting academic performance, personal-social interactions, and vocational potential: _____

   _____

   _____

If older students with language disorders learn the 25 competencies that undergird emotional intelligence, their success in personal-social interactions and in the workplace will be greatly enhanced.

Supplemental Case History Interview

Student: _____   Age: _____

Interviewer: _____   Date: _____

Feelings and Attitudes

Thinking

1. What is thinking? _____

   _____

   _____

2. On a scale from 1 to 5, how important is thinking in your life? _____

1	**2**	**3**	**4**	**5**
Not at All Important		Sometimes Important		Extremely Important

3. Whom do you know that you consider to be a good thinker? _____

   What makes you think that he or she is a good thinker? _____

   _____

4. Have you ever felt that you would like to think better? _____ No _____ Yes

   If "Yes," in what situations? _____

   _____

5. What interferes with your ability to think clearly? _____

   _____

Listening

1. What is listening? _____

   _____

2. On a scale from 1 to 5, how important is listening in your life? _____

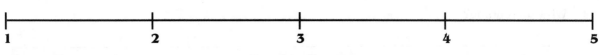

1   2   3   4   5

Not at All Important   Sometimes Important   Extremely Important

3. Whom do you know that you consider to be a good listener? _____

What makes you think that he or she is a good listener? _____

_____

4. Have you ever felt that you would like to listen better? _____ No _____ Yes

If "Yes," in what situations? _____

_____

5. What interferes with your ability to listen? _____

_____

Speaking

1. What is speaking? _____

_____

2. On a scale from 1 to 5, how important is speaking in your life? _____

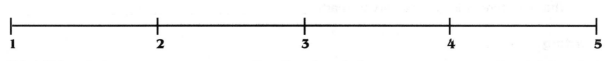

1   2   3   4   5

Not at All Important   Sometimes Important   Extremely Important

3. Whom do you know that you consider to be a good speaker? _____

What makes you think that he or she is a good speaker? _____

_____

4. Have you ever felt that you would like to speak better? _____ No _____ Yes

If "Yes," in what situations? _____

_____

5. What interferes with your ability to speak? _____

_____

Communication Solutions
for Older Students

Reading

1. What is reading?_____

_____

2. On a scale from 1 to 5, how important is reading in your life? _____

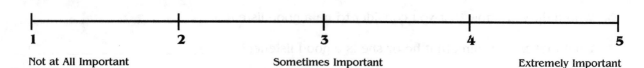

1   2   3   4   5

Not at All Important   Sometimes Important   Extremely Important

3. Whom do you know that you consider to be a good reader?_____

_____

   What makes you think that he or she is a good reader? _____

_____

4. Have you ever felt you would like to read better? _____ No   _____Yes

   If "Yes," in what situations? _____

_____

5. What interferes with your ability to read? _____

Writing

1. What is writing? _____

_____

2. On a scale from 1 to 5, how important is writing in your life? _____

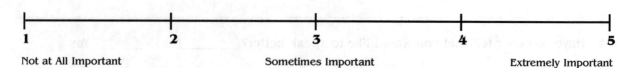

1   2   3   4   5

Not at All Important   Sometimes Important   Extremely Important

3. Whom do you know that you consider to be a good writer? _____

_____

What makes you think that he or she is a good writer? _____

_____

4. Have you ever felt that you would like to write better? _____ No _____Yes

   If "Yes," in what situations? _____

   _____

5. What interferes with your ability to write? _____

   _____

Current Needs for Thinking, Listening, Speaking, Reading, and Writing

Academic Environment

How often are you required to think, listen, speak, read, and write in classroom situations? Use this scale:

   1 = Frequently   2 = Occasionally   3 = Seldom   4 = Never

Classes/Subjects	Think	Listen	Speak	Read	Write

Comments: _____

_____

_____

Communication Solutions
for Older Students

Social Environment

How often are you required to think, listen, speak, read, and write in daily living situations (e.g., with friends or with family members)? Use this scale:

	1 = Frequently	2 = Occasionally	3 = Seldom	4 = Never	

Daily Living Situations	Think	Listen	Speak	Read	Write

Comments: _____

_____

_____

Vocational Environment

How often are you required to think, listen, speak, read, and write in a job situation (e.g., with co-workers or with customers)? Use this scale:

	1 = Frequently	2 = Occasionally	3 = Seldom	4 = Never	

Job Situations	Think	Listen	Speak	Read	Write

Comments: _____

_____

_____

Intervention: Past and Future

1. What intervention have you received in the past:

For thinking? _____
_____

For listening? _____
_____

For speaking? _____
_____

For reading? _____
_____

For writing? _____
_____

2. Do you feel you need to improve:

Your thinking? _____ No _____Yes

Comments: _____
_____

Your listening? _____ No _____Yes

Comments: _____
_____

Your speaking? _____ No _____Yes

Comments: _____
_____

Your reading? _____ No _____Yes

Comments: _____
_____

Your writing? _____ No _____Yes

Comments: _____
_____

Learning Style Questionnaire

Name: _____

Date: _____ Gender: M   F   Grade: _____

Birth Date: _____ School: _____

Directions: This is NOT a test. There are no right or wrong answers. The following items are simply a way to find out how you learn best. If an item is unclear, feel free to ask questions.

The purpose of this questionnaire is to determine how you learn best, not how much you like to learn a subject. For example, you might like to have the TV on while you are studying, but you study best when it is quiet. Also, you might like to study at night, but you are more productive if you study in the morning. *Learn best* means how you remember information the longest, pay attention to a task the most, and recall details and main ideas easiest. Knowing how you learn best will help your teachers to help you be more successful in school.

Before you begin to answer the questions, write your name, the date, and other iden-tification information requested in the space provided above. Then answer the fol-lowing statements honestly about when, how, where, why, and with whom you learn best.

My most difficult subject is: _____

I learn my most difficult subject best: When?

1. Time (Check only 1 box.)   ☐ Morning   ☐ Afternoon   ☐ Night

   Other (explain): _____

2. Timing (Check only 1 box.)   ☐ Before meals   ☐ After meals

I learn my most difficult subject best: How?

1. Sound (Check only 1 box.)   ☐ When quiet   ☐ Radio on   ☐ When talking
   ☐ TV on   ☐ Music on   ☐ When noisy

   Other (explain): _____

2. Light (Check only 1 box.)   ☐ Dim   ☐ Moderate   ☐ Bright

   Other (explain): _____

3. Temperature (Check only 1 box.) ☐ Cold   ☐ Cool
                                   ☐ Warm   ☐ Very Warm

   Other (explain): _____

4. Intake (Check only 1 box.)   ☐ Eat foods   ☐ Drink liquids   ☐ Chew on
                                                                     something

   ☐ Not eat, drink, or chew on anything

   Other (explain): _____

I learn my most difficult subject best: Where?

1. Place (Indicate your first and second choices.)

   Home: Which two rooms/places within your home (e.g., bedroom, kitchen, or living room)?

   _____

   _____

   School: Which two rooms within the school (e.g., library, study hall, or classroom)?

   _____

   _____

2. Conditions (Rank these locations from 1 to 6. 1 = The location where you learn best.)

   Home

   _____ Desk/Table   _____ Bed   _____ Floor
   _____ Straight chair   _____ Soft chair _____ Couch

   Other (explain): _____

   _____

   School

   _____ Student desk   _____ Floor   _____ Study carrel
   _____ Straight chair   _____ Soft chair _____ Table

   Other (explain): _____

   _____

Communication Solutions
for Older Students

I learn my most difficult subject best: Why?

(Rank these reasons from 1 to 4. 1 = Your strongest reason for learning your most difficult subject.)

_____ I want to.

_____ My teacher expects me to/demands it.

_____ My parents/guardians expects me to/demand it.

_____ I'll get a reward such as:

☐ Money   ☐ Better grades   ☐ Privileges

Other (explain): _____

_____

I learn my most difficult subject best: With Whom?

(Rank these items from 1 to 7 as to with whom you learn best. 1 = The best way to learn your most difficult subject.)

_____ Alone   _____ Partner

_____ Small group (3–7)   _____ Large group (8 and above)

_____ Teacher(s)   _____ Parent(s)/Guardian(s)

_____ Sibling(s)

Other (explain): _____

_____

Inside the Classroom

1. Participating in the class (Rank the ways you learn best in the classroom from 1 to 6.
   1 = The best way to learn your most difficult subject.)

   _____ Listening   _____ Reading

   _____ Writing   _____ Speaking

   _____ Doing   _____ Combination of the above

   Other (explain): _____

   _____

2. Participating in assignments within the classroom (Rank the assignments that help you learn
   information best from 1 to 7. 1 = The best way to learn via an assignment.)

   _____ Worksheet questions   _____ Experiments

   _____ Demonstrations   _____ Group projects

   _____ Individual projects   _____ Written reports

   _____ Oral reports

Other (explain): _____

_____

3. Remembering main points from what the teacher says (Rank from 1 to 4 your top four strategies. 1 = The best way to remember main points from what the teacher says.)

_____ Repeat the material to yourself

_____ Think of a picture in your mind

_____ Make up words to remember main points in order

_____ Break ideas into smaller chunks

_____ Outline what the teacher says in writing

_____ Follow an outline that the teacher has provided

_____ Use rhyming words to recall main points

_____ Put main points into categories

_____ Audiotape what the teacher is saying and replay it later

Other (explain): _____

_____

4. Remembering main points from a textbook (Rank from 1 to 4 your top four strategies. 1 = The best way to remember main points from a textbook.)

_____ Look at headings and subheadings

_____ Outline important ideas from the textbook

_____ Underline/Highlight main points

_____ Write down questions to anticipate what a teacher will ask on a test

_____ Answer the questions at the end of each chapter (if available)

_____ Follow along in the textbook while listening to an audiotape of the textbook

Other (explain): _____

_____

5. Taking notes (Check only 1 box.)

While listening to a lecture, I take notes when learning my most difficult subject as follows:

❑ Notes are key words   ❑ Notes are attempts at complete sentences

❑ Notes are "doodles"/drawings

Other (explain): _____

_____

Communication Solutions
for Older Students

6. Asking questions of the teacher (Check only 1 box.)

   I learn my most difficult subject best if I ask questions:

   ☐ During class   ☐ After class   ☐ Before class

   Other (explain): _____

   _____

Outside the Classroom

1. Participating in outside classroom assignments (Rank from 1 to 4 the assignments that help you to learn a difficult subject best. 1 = The best way to learn via an assignment.)

   _____ Preparing a written report

   _____ Preparing an oral report

   _____ Answering questions from the textbook or worksheet

   _____ Reading assigned information

   Other (explain): _____

   _____

2. Studying for a test (Rank the top four strategies from 1 to 4. 1 = The way you study best for a test in your most difficult subject.)

   _____ Read or reread the textbook the day before

   _____ Read or reread the textbook 2–3 days before

   _____ Listen or re-listen to audiotapes of what the teacher said

   _____ Review the outline of my notes

   _____ Review the outline provided by the teacher

   _____ Predict questions to be on the test and answer them

   _____ Rework problems assigned by the teacher

   Other (explain): _____

3. I learn my most difficult subject best when I study for _____ minutes each hour before taking a break.

Now look back over all your answers. You have just described how you learn best. Whenever you need to learn something new or study really hard, try to modify your surroundings to match how you describe them in this questionnaire.

484 Communication Solutions for Older Students © 2003 by Thinking Publications
Duplication permitted for educational use only.

Social Skills Rating Scale—Adult Form

Name of Student: _____

Grade: _____   Age: _____   Date: _____

Name of Person Completing Rating Scale: _____

Relationship to Student (e.g., parent, teacher, coach): _____

Directions: Rate this student on his or her use of the following social-emotional skills.

Circle:

    1—if the skill is SELDOM used appropriately.

    2—if the skill is SOMETIMES used appropriately.

    3—if the skill is ALMOST ALWAYS used appropriately.

For example, if a student usually complains and begs when he or she is told "No" by an authority figure, rate the student as follows:

ACCEPTING "NO"—Responds appropriately when   ①   2   3
               told "No" by an authority figure.

Write examples and comments in the margin areas when appropriate (e.g., if you give a SELDOM rating for ACCEPTING "NO," you might explain that the student argues with you when he or she is told "No").

Social-Emotional Skill	SELDOM	SOMETIMES	ALMOST ALWAYS
1. USING BODY LANGUAGE—Uses body language (components of the body that communicate messages) that is appropriate to the situation.	1	2	3
2. USING MANNERS—Speaks and acts politely in social situations.	1	2	3
3. CHOOSING THE RIGHT TIME AND PLACE—Chooses an appropriate time and place before beginning a conversation with another person.	1	2	3

	SELDOM	SOMETIMES	ALMOST ALWAYS
4. STAYING ON AND SWITCHING TOPICS—Sticks to the topic of conversation or prepares the listener for a topic shift.	1	2	3
5. LISTENING—Gives his or her full attention to a speaker in order to hear and think about the message.	1	2	3
6. CONVERSING—Takes the initiative to start a conversation. Begins with a greeting, participates in talking and listening, and ends conversations smoothly with a closing.	1	2	3
7. MAKING A POSITIVE FIRST IMPRESSION—His or her words, actions, appearance, and personal qualities make other people think favorably about him or her.	1	2	3
8. USING FORMAL AND INFORMAL LANGUAGE—Talks in a more traditional way by using the longer forms of words, when speaking to people in authority positions. Talks in a more casual way, by using shorter forms of words and slang, when speaking to peers and adults whom he or she feels close to.	1	2	3
9. GIVING REASONS—Gives explanations that are specific and relevant when answering questions.	1	2	3
10. PLANNING WHAT TO SAY—Thinks about and chooses what he or she will say before speaking.	1	2	3
11. INTERRUPTING—Interrupts in an appropriate way and only when necessary.	1	2	3
12. GIVING A COMPLIMENT—Remembers to compliment others and is honest and sincere when doing so.	1	2	3

	SELDOM	SOMETIMES	ALMOST ALWAYS
13. ACCEPTING A COMPLIMENT—Accepts compliments in a sincere way.	1	2	3
14. SAYING "THANK YOU"—Expresses genuine appreciation when someone has done something nice.	1	2	3
15. INTRODUCING YOURSELF—Remembers to give his or her name when introducing himself or herself to a new person.	1	2	3
16. INTRODUCING PEOPLE—Helps two or more people who do not know one another to learn one another's names. Makes the introduction reciprocal. For example, "Steve, meet Beth. Beth, this is Steve."	1	2	3
17. MAKING A REQUEST—Remembers to ask instead of demand when he or she wants something.	1	2	3
`18. OFFERING HELP—Offers help to people in need. Remembers to ask first instead of just taking over for the other person.	1	2	3
19. ASKING FOR HELP—Asks for help when needed, but attempts something on his or her own first. Asks for help in an appropriate way.	1	2	3
20. ASKING FOR PERMISSION—Asks for permission to do things whenever necessary.	1	2	3
21. ACCEPTING "NO"—Responds appropriately when told "No" by an authority figure.	1	2	3

Communication Solutions
for Older Students

	SELDOM	SOMETIMES	ALMOST ALWAYS
22. MAKING AN APOLOGY—Says he or she is sorry when necessary.	1	2	3
23. EXPRESSING AN OPINION—Does not try to suggest that his or her opinions are facts.	1	2	3
24. AGREEING OR DISAGREEING—Disagrees without putting down the other person's idea or opinion. Doesn't get angry when someone disagrees with him or her.	1	2	3
25. CONVINCING OTHERS—Provides relevant and enticing reasons when trying to get others to share in his or her opinion.	1	2	3
26. GIVING INFORMATION—Provides precise and easy-to-understand details when giving information (e.g., explaining a problem, giving directions).	1	2	3
27. DEALING WITH CONTRADICTIONS—Knows when he or she is receiving messages that are opposite in meaning and asks for clarification.	1	2	3
28. BEING HONEST—Tells the truth and understands the consequences of losing someone's trust.	1	2	3
29. BEING OPTIMISTIC—Looks on the bright side. Expects good things to happen. Has a positive attitude.	1	2	3
30. HAVING A POSITIVE REPUTATION—Has a positive reputation in the home, at school, and in the community.	1	2	3
31. STARTING A FRIENDSHIP—Starts new friendships with people based on common interests.	1	2	3

	SELDOM	SOMETIMES	ALMOST ALWAYS
32. MAINTAINING A FRIENDSHIP—Treats friends appropriately in order to maintain relationships.	1	2	3
33. GIVING EMOTIONAL SUPPORT—Listens and provides encouragement to a friend who is making a difficult decision or who is feeling depressed.	1	2	3
34. GIVING ADVICE—Gives advice only when asked and only in areas he or she is qualified to give advice.	1	2	3
35. IGNORING—Ignores disruptions and negative behaviors of other people.	1	2	3
36. DEALING WITH TEASING—Responds appropriately to friendly teasing and ignores unfriendly teasing.	1	2	3
37. DEALING WITH PEER PRESSURE—Says "No" to negative peer pressure.	1	2	3
38. JOINING IN—Joins in an activity or a conversation without disrupting those involved.	1	2	3
39. DEALING WITH BEING LEFT OUT—Copes with being left out of an activity in an appropriate way.	1	2	3
40. TELLING ON OTHERS—Does not tell on others for unimportant reasons. When telling on others for important reasons, he or she does so discretely.	1	2	3
41. BEING ASSERTIVE—Makes comments in a confident and firm way, without making threats.	1	2	3

Communication Solutions
for Older Students

	SELDOM	SOMETIMES	ALMOST ALWAYS
42. MAKING A COMPLAINT—Makes a complaint to the appropriate person in a nonaggressive manner.	1	2	3
43. RECEIVING A COMPLAINT—Listens appropriately when receiving a complaint. Suggests a solution when he or she is responsible for a complaint received.	1	2	3
44. GIVING CONSTRUCTIVE CRITICISM—Is specific about behaviors he or she would like to see improved without making personal insults.	1	2	3
45. ACCEPTING CONSTRUCTIVE CRITICISM—Accepts constructive criticism without getting defensive.	1	2	3
46. MAKING AN ACCUSATION—Seeks proof before accusing someone.	1	2	3
47. DEALING WITH A FALSE ACCUSATION—When falsely accused, he or she offers proof and/or offers another explanation without getting angry.	1	2	3
48. NEGOTIATING AND COMPROMISING—Makes sincere attempts to solve disputes with others. Meets others "halfway" when working to solve a problem.	1	2	3
49. ACCEPTING CONSEQUENCES—Accepts negative consequences of his or her actions without argument.	1	2	3
50. EXPRESSING FEELINGS—Expresses his or her feelings appropriately instead of keeping them inside.	1	2	3

	SELDOM	SOMETIMES	ALMOST ALWAYS
51. DEALING WITH ANGER—Expresses his or her anger without acting impulsively or losing control.	1	2	3
52. DEALING WITH EMBARRASSMENT—Reacts appropriately when something makes him or her feel uncomfortable or self-conscious.	1	2	3
53. COPING WITH FEAR—Takes steps to reduce unrealistic fears.	1	2	3
54. DEALING WITH HUMOR—Enjoys "safe" humor and avoids "unsafe" humor (i.e., humor that hurts or upsets others).	1	2	3
55. DEALING WITH FAILURE—Deals with failure appropriately and does not let it get him or her down.	1	2	3
56. DEALING WITH DISAPPOINTMENT—Handles disappointment without getting impulsive.	1	2	3
57. UNDERSTANDING THE FEELINGS OF OTHERS—Is perceptive to the way other people are feeling.	1	2	3

List the social-emotional skills you believe this student most needs to improve.

1. _____
_____

2. _____
_____

3. _____
_____

4. _____
_____

5. _____
_____

From *Social Skill Strategies (Book A;* pp. 325–329), by N. Gajewski, P. Hirn, and P. Mayo, 1998, Eau Claire, WI: Thinking Publications. © 1998 by Thinking Publications. Adapted with permission.

Social Skills Rating Scale—Student Form

Name: _____

Grade: _____ Age: _____ Date: _____

Directions: Rate yourself on how well you use the following skills. Please be honest.

Circle:

    1—if you ALMOST NEVER use the skill appropriately.

    2—if you SOMETIMES use the skill appropriately.

    3—if you ALMOST ALWAYS use the skill appropriately.

For example, if you usually argue and beg when your parent tells you that you can't do something you really want to do, you would rate yourself as follows:

ACCEPTING "NO"—I act mature when I am told "No" by an authority figure.	(1)	2	3

Please give examples and comments when necessary (for example, if you give an Almost Never rating for ACCEPTING "NO," you might write on this form that you usually argue when told "No" by your mother or father).

Social-Emotional Skill	ALMOST NEVER	SOMETIMES	ALMOST ALWAYS
1. USING BODY LANGUAGE—I know which body actions and facial expressions to use to show my feelings.	1	2	3
2. USING MANNERS—I use appropriate manners (for example, saying "Please" and "Thank you" and using polite table manners).	1	2	3
3. CHOOSING THE RIGHT TIME AND PLACE—I choose an appropriate time and place to talk to others.	1	2	3
4. STAYING ON AND SWITCHING TOPICS—My comments deal with the main topic when I have a conversation. I warn others before I switch topics.	1	2	3

 Communication Solutions for Older Students © 2003 by Thinking Publications
Duplication permitted for educational use only.

	ALMOST NEVER	SOMETIMES	ALMOST ALWAYS
5. LISTENING—When someone is talking to me, I give that person my full attention.	1	2	3
6. CONVERSING—I feel comfortable starting conversations. I begin with a greeting. I end conversations smoothly.	1	2	3
7. MAKING A POSITIVE FIRST IMPRESSION—I try to make a positive impression by how I look, what I say, and what I do when I meet new people.	1	2	3
8. USING FORMAL AND INFORMAL LANGUAGE—When I speak to people in respected positions, I talk in a more "traditional" way. I use longer forms of words (for example, "Thank you very much"). When I speak to people my own age or adults I feel close to, I talk in a more "relaxed" way. I use shorter forms of words (for example, "Thanks a lot").	1	2	3
9. GIVING REASONS—When someone asks me to explain something, I give reasons that are specific and relevant.	1	2	3
10. PLANNING WHAT TO SAY—I think about what I am going to say before I speak.	1	2	3
11. INTERRUPTING—I only interrupt people when it is necessary. I interrupt others appropriately.	1	2	3
12. GIVING A COMPLIMENT—I give people compliments about the way they look, the items they own, and what they say and do. I don't give compliments just to get people to like me.	1	2	3

Communication Solutions
for Older Students

	ALMOST NEVER	SOMETIMES	ALMOST ALWAYS
13. ACCEPTING A COMPLIMENT—When someone gives me a compliment, I say "Thank you" in a sincere way.	1	2	3
14. SAYING "THANK YOU"—I thank people when they do something nice for me.	1	2	3
15. INTRODUCING YOURSELF—I introduce myself to people I don't know. I remember to tell my full name.	1	2	3
16. INTRODUCING PEOPLE—I introduce people when they do not know each other. (For example, "Steve, meet Beth. Beth, this is Steve").	1	2	3
17. MAKING A REQUEST—When I want something, I ask for it in a polite way. I do not demand things from others.	1	2	3
18. OFFERING HELP—I offer help to people in need. I ask first, instead of just taking over right away.	1	2	3
19. ASKING FOR HELP—I try things on my own first. If I can't figure something out, I ask for help in an appropriate way.	1	2	3
20. ASKING FOR PERMISSION—I ask for permission from authority figures whenever I should.	1	2	3
21. ACCEPTING "NO"—I act mature when I am told "No" by an authority figure.	1	2	3
22. MAKING AN APOLOGY—I say "I'm sorry" when I have done something wrong.	1	2	3

	ALMOST NEVER	SOMETIMES	ALMOST ALWAYS
23. EXPRESSING AN OPINION—When I say something that is just my opinion, I remember to begin with statements like "I think..." or "In my opinion...."	1	2	3
24. AGREEING OR DISAGREEING—When I disagree with others, I do not put down their ideas or opinions. I do not get angry when someone disagrees with me.	1	2	3
25. CONVINCING OTHERS—I give good reasons when I try to convince someone to agree with me.	1	2	3
26. GIVING INFORMATION—I express myself clearly when I give information to others (for example, giving directions or answering questions).	1	2	3
27. DEALING WITH CONTRADICTIONS—When I hear a contradiction (statements that are opposite in meaning), I ask what is meant.	1	2	3
28. BEING HONEST—I am truthful, even when I have done something wrong. I don't want to lose people's trust in me.	1	2	3
29. BEING OPTIMISTIC—I try to have a positive attitude. I expect good things to happen. I look on the bright side when something goes wrong.	1	2	3
30. HAVING A POSITIVE REPUTATION—I have a positive reputation at home, at school, and in the community.	1	2	3
31. STARTING A FRIENDSHIP—I am good at starting new friendships with others.	1	2	3

Communication Solutions
for Older Students

	ALMOST NEVER	SOMETIMES	ALMOST ALWAYS
32. MAINTAINING A FRIENDSHIP—I keep my friends because I treat them well.	1	2	3
33. GIVING EMOTIONAL SUPPORT—When one of my friends is feeling depressed or is having a problem, I listen and give encouragement.	1	2	3
34. GIVING ADVICE—I only give advice when someone asks me to do so. I avoid giving advice about things I don't know much about.	1	2	3
35. IGNORING—I ignore disruptions. I ignore others who try to get my attention in a negative way.	1	2	3
36. DEALING WITH TEASING—I laugh when people tease me in a friendly way. I ignore people when they tease me in a mean way.	1	2	3
37. DEALING WITH PEER PRESSURE—I say "No" when others try to pressure me into doing things I don't feel comfortable doing.	1	2	3
38. JOINING IN—I feel comfortable joining conversations and activities after they have already begun. I join others in a way that is not disruptive.	1	2	3
39. DEALING WITH BEING LEFT OUT—When I am left out of an activity or a conversation, I try to decide if it happened by mistake or on purpose. If it seems like a mistake, I try to join the activity without being disruptive. If it seems like others purposely excluded me, I find something else to do.	1	2	3
40. TELLING ON OTHERS—I only tell on others for important reasons. When I do tell on others, I only tell the person who needs to know about the behavior.	1	2	3

	ALMOST NEVER	SOMETIMES	ALMOST ALWAYS
41. BEING ASSERTIVE—When someone goes against my rights, I tell the other person how I feel and what I want. I do not make threats or get aggressive.	1	2	3
42. MAKING A COMPLAINT—I only make complaints when it is fair to do so. I do not become aggressive when I make a complaint.	1	2	3
43. RECEIVING A COMPLAINT—When someone complains to me, and I know I am responsible, I apologize and offer a solution.	1	2	3
44. GIVING CONSTRUCTIVE CRITICISM—When I criticize others, I tell exactly what I think should be improved. I do not personally insult the other person. I try to say something positive about the person first.	1	2	3
45. ACCEPTING CONSTRUCTIVE CRITICISM—I can handle it when someone tells me I need to improve on something. I don't get defensive.	1	2	3
46. MAKING AN ACCUSATION—I make sure I have proof before I accuse someone of doing something wrong.	1	2	3
47. DEALING WITH A FALSE ACCUSATION—When someone accuses me of doing something wrong, and I didn't do it, I stay calm. I offer proof that I'm innocent or try to offer another explanation.	1	2	3
48. NEGOTIATING AND COMPROMISING—I am willing to give in a little to help solve a disagreement. I don't always need things to go my way.	1	2	3
49. ACCEPTING CONSEQUENCES—When I know I have done something wrong, I am willing to face the consequence.	1	2	3

Communication Solutions
for Older Students

	ALMOST NEVER	SOMETIMES	ALMOST ALWAYS
50. EXPRESSING FEELINGS—I talk about my feelings when it's appropriate. I do not hold them all inside.	1	2	3
51. DEALING WITH ANGER—When I feel angry, I can control myself. I don't lose control.	1	2	3
52. DEALING WITH EMBARRASSMENT—I handle myself well when I get embarrassed. I don't fall apart.	1	2	3
53. COPING WITH FEAR—When I am afraid of something, I don't let it control me. I face my fears and try to reduce them.	1	2	3
54. DEALING WITH HUMOR—I only use humor that is "friendly" and will not upset or hurt anyone. I avoid "unfriendly" humor.	1	2	3
55. DEALING WITH FAILURE—I don't let myself get "down" when I fail at something. I just try to do better the next time.	1	2	3
56. DEALING WITH DISAPPOINTMENT—I stay in control when I am disappointed because someone or something lets me down.	1	2	3
57. UNDERSTANDING THE FEELINGS OF OTHERS—I am sensitive to the way other people are feeling.	1	2	3

Write the social skills you think you most need to improve.

1. _____

   _____

2. _____

   _____

3. _____

   _____

From *Social Skill Strategies* (Book A; pp. 330–334), by N. Gajewski, P. Hirn, and P. Mayo, 1998, Eau Claire, WI: Thinking Publications. © 1998 by Thinking Publications. Adapted with permission.

Adolescent Conversational Analysis

Student: _____   Date: _____

Conversational Partner: _____   Age of Student: _____   Grade: ____

Setting of Conversation: _____

Materials Present to Elicit Sample: _____

Directions: Obtain a minimum of 10 minutes of conversational speech with each partner in each setting. (Use a separate analysis form for each partner.) Transcribe exactly the conversational units of each participant. Analyze for the behaviors listed below. Circle "A" for Appropriate and "I" for Inappropriate behaviors. Determine appropriateness and inappropriateness of a behavior by judging whether or not it is penalizing to the adolescent; a behavior perceived by the clinician as penalizing is marked as inappropriate (Prutting and Kirchner, 1983). Circle "N/O" if a behavior is Not Observed during the sample. Probe any behaviors marked "N/O" during directed tasks. Compile information on the Conversational Analysis Profile on the last page.

Role of the Listener in the Conversation

A   I   N/O   1. Appears to understand the vocabulary and syntactical structures of the conversational partner

Comments: _____

_____

A   I   N/O   2. Appears to follow the main idea of conversational topics

Comments_____

_____

A   I   N/O   3. Appears to listen in a nonjudgmental manner

Comments: _____

_____

A   I   N/O   4. Indicates understanding or lack of understanding of the conversational partner by use of verbal and/or nonverbal feedback

Comments: _____

_____

Communication Solutions
for Older Students

Role of the Speaker in the Conversation

Language Features

A   I   N/O   1. Produces a variety of syntactic forms

Comments: _____

_____

A   I   N/O   2. Produces a variety of questions (question forms)

Comments: _____

_____

A   I   N/O   3. Produces figurative language

Comments: _____

_____

A   I   N/O   4. Produces nonspecific language

Comments: _____

_____

5. Produces precise vocabulary

A   I   N/O   a. Demonstrates word-retrieval skills

Comments: _____

_____

A   I   N/O   b. Avoids verbal mazes

Comments: _____

_____

A   I   N/O   c. Avoids false starts

Comments: _____

_____

Paralanguage Features

A   I   N/O   1. Uses suprasegmental features appropriately (use of vocal inflection, juncture, and rate)

Comments: _____

_____

A   I   N/O   2. Has normal fluency

Comments: _____

_____

A   I   N/O   3. Is intelligible

Comments: _____

_____

Communication Functions

A   I   N/O   1. Uses language to give information

Comments: _____

_____

A   I   N/O   2. Uses language to get information

Comments: _____

_____

A   I   N/O   3. Uses language to describe an ongoing event

Comments: _____

_____

A   I   N/O   4. Uses language to persuade one's listener to do, believe, or feel something

Comments: _____

_____

A   I   N/O   5. Uses language to express one's own intentions, beliefs, and feelings

Comments: _____

_____

A   I   N/O   6. Uses language to indicate a readiness for further communication

Comments: _____

_____

A   I   N/O   7. Uses language to solve problems

Comments: _____

_____

Communication Solutions
for Older Students

A   I   N/O   8. Uses language to entertain

Comments: _____

_____

Conversational Rules

1. Uses verbal rules to govern topics and turns

A   I   N/O   a. Initiates conversation

Comments:_____

_____

A   I   N/O   b. Chooses topics of conversation

Comments:_____

_____

A   I   N/O   c. Maintains conversational topics

Comments:_____

_____

A   I   N/O   d. Switches topics using direct or indirect cues

Comments:_____

_____

A   I   N/O   e. Uses turn-taking skills

Comments:_____

_____

A   I   N/O   f. Repairs/Revises when necessary

Comments: _____

_____

A   I   N/O   g. Makes interruptions appropriately

Comments:_____

_____

2. Uses verbal rules of politeness

A   I   N/O   a. Appears not to talk too much or too little in the situation (quantity)

Comments:_____

_____

A   I   N/O   b. Appears to be honest and sincere

Comments:_____

_____

A   I   N/O   c. Appears to make relevant contributions

Comments:_____

_____

A   I   N/O   d. Appears to express ideas clearly and concisely

Comments:_____

_____

A   I   N/O   e. Appears to be tactful

Comments:_____

_____

                    3. Uses nonverbal rules

A   I   N/O   a. Uses gestures that support spoken message

Comments:_____

_____

A   I   N/O   b. Uses facial expressions

Comments:_____

_____

A   I   N/O   c. Uses eye contact/gazing

Comments:_____

_____

A   I   N/O   d. Maintains correct physical distance from partner (proxemics)

Comments:_____

_____

Communication Solutions
for Older Students

Conversational Analysis Profile	APPROPRIATE	INAPPROPRIATE	NOT OBSERVED
ROLE OF LISTENER			
Vocabulary/Syntax			
Main Ideas*			
Nonjudgmental manner			
Feedback			
ROLE OF SPEAKER Language Features			
Syntax			
Questions			
Figurative language			
Nonspecific language			
Precise vocabulary			
Word-retrieval skills*			
Verbal mazes			
False starts			
Paralanguage Features			
Suprasegmental features			
Fluency*			
Intelligibility*			
Communication Functions			
To give information			
To get information			
To describe an event			
To persuade a listener			

	APPROPRIATE	INAPPROPRIATE	NOT OBSERVED
To express one's beliefs			
To indicate readiness			
To problem-solve			
To entertain			
Conversational Rules			
Verbal (Topics/Turns)			
Initiation			
Topic choice			
Topic maintenance			
Topic switch			
Turn-taking*			
Repair/Revision			
Interruptions			
Verbal (Politeness)			
Quantity			
Sincerity			
Relevance			
Clarity			
Tactfulness			
Nonverbal			
Gestures			
Facial expressions			
Eye contact			
Proxemics			

_____38_____ Total Number of Items

_____ Total Number of Items Marked "Not Observed"

_____ Total Number of Items Rated

_____ Number Rated as Inappropriate ÷ _____ Number of Items Rated × 100 = _____%

*If consistent problems are evident in this area, conduct additional assessment.

Narration Analysis Form

Student:_____   Examiner:_____

Age:_____   Grade: _____   Date: _____

Directions: Check to reflect the highest level of narrative development for formulated and reformulated tasks.

Cognitive Period	Approximate Age of Emergence	Narrative Stage	Tasks	
			Formulated	**Reformulated**
Preoperational	2 years	Heap Stories		
	2 to 3 years	Sequence Stories		
	3 to 4 years	Primitive Narratives		
	4 to 5 years	Chain Narratives		
	5 to 7 years	True Narratives		
Concrete	7 to 11 years	Narrative Summaries		
	11 to 12 years	Complex Narratives		
Formal	13 to 15 years	Analysis		
	16 to Adulthood	Generalization		

Description of Formulated Task: _____

Description of Reformulated Task: _____

Comments: _____

_____

_____

Communication Solutions
for Older Students

Use these questions to determine the student's ability to respond to the highest levels of the developmental hierarchy.

	Questions	Formulated	Reformulated
Concrete	Tell me in one sentence what your story was about.		
	What would be a good title for this story?		
Formal	In what category would you put this story (e.g., drama, mystery, or comedy)?		
	How else could you categorize this story (e.g., short, long, exciting, or boring)?		
	How did this story make you feel?		
	Why do you think (main character) acted like he or she did?		
	What was the moral of this story?		

Comments:

Reading Skills Profile

Student: _____   Grade Level: _____

Examiner: _____   Date: _____

Directions: Obtain a content-area text that is appropriate for the student's grade level. Select a passage for the student to read. Then have the student answer the following questions or engage in the following tasks. Repeat using a passage of similar length and density that you deliver as a simulated lecture while the student listens. Note-taking is allowed. (NOTE: Do not read the passage to the student; rather, deliver the information as a teacher might in the classroom. The number of main ideas in the reading passage should match the number of main ideas in the simulated lecture.) Allow either spoken or written responses—whichever is the easiest modality for the student to demonstrate comprehension. Then complete the "Text Knowledge during Reading" section of the profile based on the passage that the student read and/or other recent observations.

Text Comprehension

1. What was the main idea(s)?

   Reading Performance   Listening Performance

   _____   _____

   _____   _____

   _____   _____

   Comparison: ____ Reading was stronger.   ____ Listening was stronger.
                  ____ Both were about the same.

2. What were the supporting details for each main idea?

   Reading Performance   Listening Performance

   _____   _____

   _____   _____

   _____   _____

   Comparison: ____ Reading was stronger.   ____ Listening was stronger.
                  ____ Both were about the same.

3. Summarize (i.e., paraphrase) what you just read (heard).

Reading Performance   Listening Performance

_____   _____

_____   _____

_____   _____

Comparison: ____ Reading was stronger.   ____ Listening was stronger.
               ____ Both were about the same.

4. What questions do you think you'd be asked on a test about what you just read (heard)?

Reading Performance   Listening Performance

_____   _____

_____   _____

_____   _____

Comparison: ____ Reading was stronger.   ____ Listening was stronger.
               ____ Both were about the same.

5. What else do you think you will learn about this topic?

Reading Performance   Listening Performance

_____   _____

_____   _____

_____   _____

Comparison: ____ Reading was stronger.   ____ Listening was stronger.
               ____ Both were about the same.

Summary of Reading Performance _____

_____

_____

Summary of Listening Performance _____

_____

_____

Tally: Reading was stronger. _____

Listening was stronger. _____

Both were about the same. _____

Text Knowledge during Reading

1. The student has knowledge of derivational morphology and orthographic patterns of irregularly spelled words.

    Most of the Time   *Sometimes*   *Not at All*   *Not Observed*

    Comments: _____

    _____

    _____

2. The student has knowledge of different text structures and genres (e.g., narratives and expository passages).

    Most of the Time   *Sometimes*   *Not at All*   *Not Observed*

    Comments: _____

    _____

    _____

3. The student has knowledge of the different purposes of text (e.g., to persuade, negotiate, inform, and entertain).

    Most of the Time   *Sometimes*   *Not at All*   *Not Observed*

    Comments: _____

    _____

    _____

4. The student has strategies for different styles of reading (e.g., skimming, overviewing, and using analytic and critical reading skills).

    Most of the Time   *Sometimes*   *Not at All*   *Not Observed*

    Comments: _____

    _____

    _____

5. The student has strategies for facilitating comprehension, storage, and retrieval of information (e.g., using headings and subheadings, table of contents, summaries, and end-of-chapter questions).

    Most of the Time   *Sometimes*   *Not at All*   *Not Observed*

    Comments: _____

    _____

    _____

Writing Analysis Profile

Student: _____ Date: _____

Examiner: _____ Age: _____

Type of Writing Sample: Narrative _____ Expository _____

Topic: _____ Selected By: _____

❑ Word Processed   ❑ Handwritten

Time Limit: ❑ None   ❑ Yes _____minutes

Directions: Obtain a written sample. Analyze the writing for each behavior listed below. Circle "A" for Appropriate and "I" for Inappropriate skills. Determine appropriateness and inappropriateness of a behavior by judging whether or not it is penalizing to the adolescent; a behavior perceived by the clinician as penalizing is marked as inappropriate (Prutting and Kirchner, 1983). Circle "N/O" if a skill is Not Observed during the sample. Probe any behaviors marked "N/O" during directed tasks.

Writing Process

A. Prewriting Strategies

A   I   N/O   Plans writing process

Comments: _____

_____

A   I   N/O   Develops a topic

Comments: _____

_____

A   I   N/O   Reviews literature

Comments: _____

_____

A   I   N/O   Takes notes

Comments: _____

_____

A   I   N/O   Organizes/Outlines information

Comments: _____

_____

A   I   N/O   Reviews notes/outline

Comments: _____

_____

B. Composing Strategies

A   I   N/O   Refers to outline or graphic organizer

Comments: _____

_____

A   I   N/O   Proceeds to efficiently write first draft

Comments: _____

_____

A   I   N/O   Uses drafting style depending on genre

Comments: _____

_____

A   I   N/O   Follows plan depending on genre

Comments: _____

_____

A   I   N/O   Revises/Edits while writing

Comments: _____

_____

C. Editing Strategies

A   I   N/O   Compares draft to outline

Comments: _____

_____

A   I   N/O   Adds necessary information

Comments: _____

_____

Communication Solutions
for Older Students

A   I   N/O   Revises ideas for content and clarity

Comments: _____

_____

A   I   N/O   Revises for mechanics (e.g., grammar, punctuation, spelling)

Comments: _____

_____

Writing Product

A. Discourse

A   I   N/O   Shows fluency in writing

Comments: _____

_____

A   I   N/O   Adapts writing to various genre

Comments: _____

_____

A   I   N/O   Takes audience into account for purpose, relevance, adequacy

Comments: _____

_____

B. Syntax

Calculate the number of communication units_____

Calculate the number of words_____

Comments: _____

_____

A   I   N/O   Writes simple sentences

Comments: _____

_____

A   I   N/O   Writes complex sentences

Comments: _____

_____

A   I   N/O   Uses varied sentence types

Comments: _____

_____

Incorporates cohesion devices:

A   I   N/O   Within sentences

Comments: _____

_____

A   I   N/O   Across sentences

Comments: _____

_____

C. Semantics

A   I   N/O   Uses literal words

Comments: _____

_____

A   I   N/O   Uses abstract words

Comments: _____

_____

A   I   N/O   Uses varied word choices

Comments: _____

_____

A   I   N/O   Uses multiple-meaning words

Comments: _____

_____

D. Conventions/Mechanics

A   I   N/O   Demonstrates spelling skills

Comments: _____

_____

Communication Solutions
for Older Students

A   I   N/O   Uses capitalization

Comments: _____

_____

Uses punctuation:

A   I   N/O   Periods

Comments: _____

_____

A   I   N/O   Commas

Comments: _____

_____

A   I   N/O   Question marks

Comments: _____

_____

A   I   N/O   Apostrophes

Comments: _____

_____

A   I   N/O   Quotation marks

Comments: _____

_____

A   I   N/O   Applies paragraph formatting

Comments: _____

_____

Writing Analysis Profile	APPROPRIATE	INAPPROPRIATE	NOT OBSERVED
WRITING PROCESS Prewriting Strategies			
Plans writing process			
Develops a topic			
Reviews literature			
Takes notes			
Organizes/Outlines information			
Reviews notes/outline			
Composing Strategies			
Refers to outline or graphic organizer			
Proceeds to efficiently write fist draft			
Uses drafting style depending on genre			
Follows plan depending on genre			
Revises/Edits while writing			
Editing Strategies			
Compares draft to outline			
Adds necessary information			
Revises ideas for content and clarity			
Revises for mechanics (e.g., grammar, punctuation, spelling)			
WRITING PRODUCT Discourse			
Shows fluency			
Adapts to genre			
Takes audience into account			

	APPROPRIATE	INAPPROPRIATE	NOT OBSERVED
Syntax			
Writes simple sentences			
Writes complex sentences			
Uses varied sentence types			
Incorporates cohesion devices			
Within sentences			
Across sentences			
Semantics			
Uses viteral words			
Uses abstract words			
Uses varied word choices			
Uses multiple-meaning words			
Conventions/Mechanics			
Demonstrates spelling skills			
Uses capitalization			
Uses punctuation			
Periods			
Commas			
Question marks			
Apostrophes			
Quotation marks			
Applies paragraph formatting			

_____ Number of Communication Units

_____ Number of Words

Number of Words ÷ Number of Communication Units = _____ Words per Unit

___*35*___ Total Number of Items

_____ Total Number of Items Marked "Not Observed"

_____ Total Number of Items Rated

_____ Number Rated as Inappropriate ÷ _____ Number of Items Rated × 100 = _____%

Example Rubric for Meta-abilities

	Meta-Linguistic	Meta-Cognitive	Meta-Pragmatic	Meta-Narrative
Consistently and appropriately…				
4 = Expert	• Recognizes phonological, syntactical, and semantic breakdowns • Analyzes phonological, syntactical, and semantic breakdowns • Revises phonological, syntactical, and semantic breakdowns	• Recognizes breakdowns in own thinking process • Analyzes the thinking process • Demonstrates ability to think about thinking • Revises own thinking strategies	• Recognizes social/cultural rules • Analyzes social/cultural rules • Uses language across and within a variety of social contexts • Switches code according to social/cultural rules	• Recognizes and evaluates story elements and structure • Recognizes various story genres • Summarizes stories • Generalizes information or concepts from one story to another
Usually appropriately…				
3 = Competent	• Recognizes phonological, syntactical, and semantic breakdowns • Analyzes phonological, syntactical, and semantic breakdowns • Revises phonological, syntactical, and semantic breakdowns	• Recognizes breakdowns in own thinking process • Analyzes the thinking process • Demonstrates ability to think about thinking • Revises own thinking strategies	• Recognizes social/cultural rules • Analyzes social/cultural rules • Uses language across and within a variety of social contexts • Switches code according to social/cultural rules	• Recognizes and evaluates story elements and structure • Recognizes various story genres • Summarizes stories • Generalizes information or concepts from one story to another
Sometimes appropriately…				
2 = Advanced Beginner	• Recognizes phonological, syntactical, and semantic breakdowns • Analyzes phonological, syntactical, and semantic breakdowns • Revises phonological, syntactical, and semantic breakdowns	• Recognizes breakdowns in own thinking process • Analyzes the thinking process • Demonstrates ability to think about thinking • Revises own thinking strategies	• Recognizes social/cultural rules • Analyzes social/cultural rules • Uses language across and within a variety of social contexts • Switches code according to social/cultural rules	• Recognizes and evaluates story elements and structure • Recognizes various story genres • Summarizes stories • Generalizes information or concepts from one story to another
Sometimes to never…				
1 = Beginner	• Recognizes phonological, syntactical, and semantic breakdowns • Analyzes phonological, syntactical, and semantic breakdowns • Revises phonological, syntactical, and semantic breakdowns	• Recognizes breakdowns in own thinking process • Analyzes the thinking process • Demonstrates ability to think about thinking • Revises own thinking strategies	• Recognizes social/cultural rules • Analyzes social/cultural rules • Uses language across and within a variety of social contexts • Switches code according to social/cultural rules	• Recognizes and evaluates story elements and structure • Recognizes various story genres • Summarizes stories • Generalizes information or concepts from one story to another

From *Structured-Multidimensional Assessment Profiles (S-MAPs) for Curriculum-Based Assessment and Intervention*, by E. Wiig and V. Lord Larson, in press, Eau Claire, WI: Thinking Publications. Reprinted with permission.

Problem-Solving Recording Form

Student: _____   Age:_____   Grade:_____

Examiner: _____   Date: _____

Directions: On a scale of 1 to 5, rate how well the student performed during each of the problem-solving steps for situations presented. Record your rating in the chart below.

1 = Independent of prompts

2 = Somewhat independent of prompts

3 = Adequate use of prompts

4 = Somewhat dependent on prompts

5 = Dependent on prompts

Problem-Solving Steps	Problem Situation #1	Problem Situation #2	Problem Situation #3	Problem Situation #4
1. Identifies the problem (by posing a question)				
2. Proposes alternative solutions				
3. Chooses the best solution				
4. Makes a plan to implement the best solution				
5. Evaluates the decision				

School Floor Plan

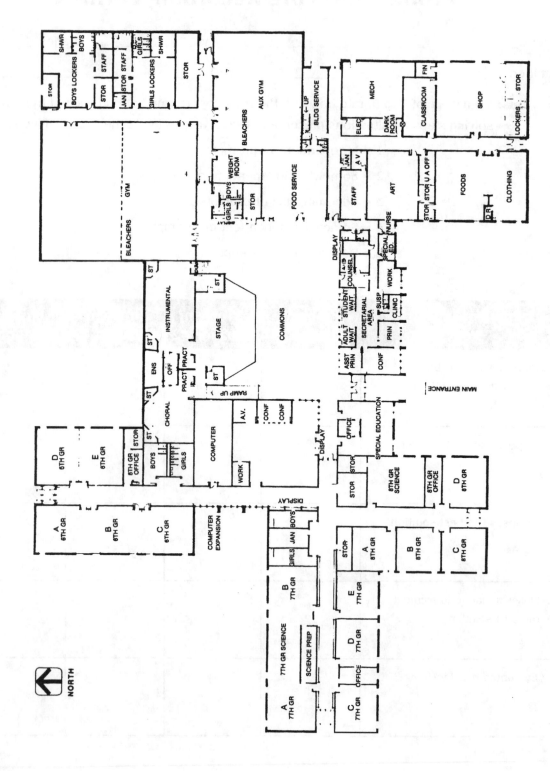

Topic Tally

Student: _____ Age: _____ Grade: _____

Examiner: _____ Date: _____

Conversational Partner (circle one): Peer   Adult

Directions: Tally the number of topics and subtopics introduced as well as the direction and manner of topics and subtopics. Tally for a 10-minute sample.

Topic Shift—Direction	Sample 1	Sample 2
Return		
New		
Topic Shift—Manner	**Sample 1**	**Sample 2**
Abrupt		
Gradual		

NOTE: Typical older students begin 2–4 new topics in 10 minutes and rarely return to a topic; they make 1–3 abrupt topic shifts and 1 gradual shift in 10 minutes (Larson and McKinley, 1998).

Other Observations

Cognitive: _____

_____

Linguistic: _____

_____

Social: _____

_____

Comments:

Listening Skill Recording Form

Student:_____ Age:_____ Grade: _____

Examiner:_____ Date: _____

Directions: Obtain 3, 5- to 10-minute taped lectures from a classroom or simulate the same. Use one for each of the following listening tasks. Ask questions about the content and record percentages of correct responses in the grid. Compare the percentages to determine how listening alters under different conditions.

Lecture

Main Idea: _____

_____

Relevant Details: _____

_____

Lecture with Listening Guide

Main Idea: _____

_____

Relevant Details: _____

_____

Lecture on a Topic of Interest to Student

Main Idea: _____

_____

Relevant Details: _____

_____

Percentage of Correct Answers

Lecture Condition	Main Idea Answers	Relevant Details Answers
Lecture	%	%
Lecture with listening guide	%	%
Lecture on a topic of interest	%	%

Progress Report

Name:_____   School Year:_____

School:_____   Grade: _____

Dear Parent,

This is a progress report for your child, who is involved in individualized programming. This progress report includes performance in academics as well as work habits. It addresses individualized classes as well as general classes. This report is intended to reflect the student's progress throughout his or her total day so that areas of strength can be recognized and assistance provided for areas of weakness. There are two scales used in this reporting system. One is for academics and one for work habits. Please see the following detailed explanation of these progress scales.

Sincerely,

_____

REPORTING SYSTEMS

Academic

Academic work is evaluated by the following criteria:

1. Attempts but does not perform with assistance

2. Performs with assistance or supervision

3. Performs without assistance

4. Performs without assistance with more than acceptable quality, speed, and accuracy

5. Performs with more than acceptable quality, speed, and accuracy with high initiative and adaptability to a variety of situations

6. Can lead or teach others

Work Habits

Work habits are evaluated by the following criteria:

Never – Unacceptable   Seldom – Needs Improvement

Usually – Good   Always – Excellent

Communication Solutions
for Older Students

Student:_____   School Year: _____

Teacher:_____   Prog. Period: _____   Gr.: _____

School:_____   Credit Area: _____

ACADEMIC WORK

Subject Area(s)_____   Credit Area _____

We are working on:	Performance					
	1	2	3	4	5	6

Quarter Grade:_____   Semester Grade:_____   Credit Earned:_____

(Grades are based on daily work)

Work Habits	Never/ Unacceptable	Seldom/ Needs Improvement	Usually/ Good	Always/ Excellent	Not Evaluated
1. Seeks help when appropriate					
2. Works independently					
3. Accepts criticism					
4. Assumes responsibility					
5. Acknowledges and accepts rights of others					
6. Observes rules and regulations					
7. Exhibits self-control					
8. Completes assignments on time					
9. Follows oral directions					
10. Follows written directions					

Student:_____   School Year: _____

Teacher:_____   Prog. Period: _____   Gr.: _____

School:_____   Credit Area: _____

ACADEMIC WORK

Subject Area(s)_____   Credit Area_____

We are working on:	Performance					
	1	2	3	4	5	6

Quarter Grade:_____   Semester Grade:_____   Credit Earned:_____

(Grades are based on daily work)

Subject Area(s)_____   Credit Area_____

We are working on:	Performance					
	1	2	3	4	5	6

Quarter Grade:_____   Semester Grade:_____   Credit Earned:_____

(Grades are based on daily work)

Comments: _____

_____

EXPLANATION OF WORK HABITS EVALUATED

1. Seeks Help When Appropriate

a. Seeks help when clarification of an academic assignment is needed

b. Seeks help in solving personal and interpersonal problems when needed

2. Works Independently

a. Completes assignments on his or her own

b. Does not seek unneeded assistance

3. Accepts Criticism (Directed toward Behavior on Academic Work) in a Positive Manner

a. Listens without overreaction

b. Initiates corrections willingly

4. Assumes Responsibility

a. Brings required materials to class

b. Maintains locker, notebooks, and work area in orderly manner

c. Accepts rightful blame and consequences for actions

d. Attends class regularly

e. Comes to class on time

5. Acknowledges and Accepts Rights of Others

a. Works without distracting others

b. Gains permission before using property of others

c. Uses materials of others and returns without damage

d. Refrains from touching others inappropriately

6. Observes Rules and Regulations

a. Observes rules of classroom, playground, and lunchroom

b. Observes rules of IMC and all other school property

c. Complies with directives given by any school staff

7. Exhibits Self-Control

a. Avoids inappropriate behaviors, even when upset

b. Refrains from engaging in excessive physical or verbal activity

c. Remains on task, even when others are misbehaving

d. Doesn't complain

8. Completes Assignments On Time

9. Follows Oral Directions

a. Attends to verbal instructions both visually and auditorily

b. Applies group directions to self

c. Follows directions the first time they are given

10. Follows Written Directions

a. Reads written directions before proceeding

b. Completes tasks according to directions

Success in life or on a job will not be achieved
without the proper work habits.

Attendance:

Quarter	1	2	3	4	Total
Days Present					
Days Absent					
Times Tardy					

Signature   **Date**

_____   _____
Parent's Signature

_____   _____
Student's Signature

_____   _____
Teacher's Signature

Dear Parent:

Please sign above so we know you have had a chance to review your child's progress report. Return only this cover sheet; keep the enclosed progress report sheets.

Return the cover sheet to:_____

Thank You!

From *Special Education Handbook for the Trempealeau Valley Cooperative.* © 1986 by Cooperative Educational Services Agency #4 (Northern Cluster), La Crosse, WI. Reprinted with permission.

Communication Follow-Up Questionnaire

COVER LETTER

Dear _____:

We are collecting information from people who were in the communication program in either middle school or high school. We would like you to help with a project that will study the benefits of the speech-language program while you were in high school. It will take you about _____ minutes to complete the questionnaire I have sent.

This questionnaire has been approved by the Review Board for the Protection of Human Subjects. If you have any complaints about your participation in this study, please contact _____ at _____.

Your participation in the project is completely voluntary. You may refuse to participate. It will not be held against you. If you decide not to participate, throw the questionnaire away.

It is all right to ask for help to read the questionnaire. You may also ask someone to explain unfamiliar words. However, you should decide the answers to the questions by yourself. Send your questionnaire back to me in the self-addressed envelope.

The questionnaire is anonymous. Please do not write your name or address anywhere on the questionnaire or the return envelope. Your information will be combined with that of others. Your cooperation is very important for the success of this study. I hope you will participate in the study. If you have any questions about this study, contact me at _____.
Thank you for your cooperation.

Sincerely,

PERSONAL DATA

Date of Follow-Up:_____

Middle School Attended:_____

High School Attended:_____

Number of Years in Secondary-Level Communication Programs:

_____ years, from calendar year _____ to _____

Are you the sole head of the household for tax purposes?

_____No _____Yes

Are you living independently from your parents? _____No _____Yes

Number of Dependents: _____

Age at Time of This Follow-Up:

_____ Less than 20 years of age

_____ 20 to 25 years of age

_____ 26 to 30 years of age

_____ More than 30 years of age

EDUCATIONAL/EMPLOYMENT DATA

Educational Status (Check one)

_____ Credits toward high school diploma, but diploma is not yet earned

_____ High school diploma

_____ 1 to 2 years of vocational/technical education after high school

_____ 1 to 3 years of college education

_____ Earned B.S. or B.A. degree from college

_____ Other (specify):_____

Communication Solutions
for Older Students

Work Experience (Check one)

_____ 3 years or fewer of part-time employment

_____ More than 3 years of part-time employment

_____ 3 years or fewer of full-time employment

_____ More than 3 years of full-time employment

_____ Other (specify):_____

Employment Skill Level (Check one)

_____ Primarily unskilled (little or no training required for the job)

_____ Semi-skilled (trained on the job)

_____ Vocationally/Technically skilled (trained in school 1 to 3 years after high school)

_____ Professional (trained at the bachelor's degree level or more)

_____ Other (specify):_____

Income Level

Per Year—Individual (Check one)

_____ $10,000 and under

_____ $10,001 to $20,000

_____ $20,001 to $30,000

_____ $30,001 to $40,000

_____ $40,001 to $50,000

_____ $50,001 and over

Per Year—Joint Income (Check one, if applicable)

_____ $10,000 and under

_____ $10,001 to $20,000

_____ $20,001 to $30,000

_____ $30,001 to $40,000

_____ $40,001 to $50,000

_____ $50,001 and over

Workplace accommodations you've asked for (Check all that apply)

_____ To receive all instructions orally

_____ To receive all instructions visually

_____ To provide a Dictaphone or tape recorder

_____ To provide an electronic reader

_____ To have voice recognition software

_____ Other: _____

My employer knows I have a speech-language disability: _____ Yes _____ No

Comments: _____

_____

SATISFACTION QUESTIONS

Use this scale for the questions below.

1	2	3	4	5
Not at All	A Little Bit	Some	Quite a Bit	A Great Amount

1. On a scale from 1 to 5, how much do you think your participation in the communication program helped you in school? _____

2. On a scale from 1 to 5, how much do you think your participation in the communication program helped you to relate better to people? _____

3. On a scale from 1 to 5, how much do you think your participation in the communication program helped you to perform better at work? _____

4. On a scale from 1 to 5, how satisfied are you with your communication skills with co-workers? _____

5. On a scale from 1 to 5, how satisfied are you with your communication skills with family members? _____

6. On a scale from 1 to 5, how satisfied are you with your communication skills with friends? _____

7. On a scale from 1 to 5, how satisfied are you with your communication skills during leisure time activities? _____

ADDITIONAL COMMENTS (Please note on the back of this sheet.)

Tutor Application Form

Identification Information

Name: _____

Address: _____

City: _____ State: _____ ZIP Code: _____

Telephone: _____ Age: _____

Email: _____

Homeroom: _____ Grade: _____

Schedule

Please attach your class schedule to this form.

How often can you tutor per week? _____

What days and time periods are you available?

Days	Time Periods
Monday	_____
Tuesday	_____
Wednesday	_____
Thursday	_____
Friday	_____

When might your available time periods change? _____

Experience

Have you ever worked with other teenagers who have disabilities? _____ Yes _____ No

If yes, describe those experiences: _____

_____

Why do you want to participate in the tutoring program? _____

_____

_____

What interests, skills, talents, or strengths do you have that you could share with the classmate you tutor? _____

_____

_____

References

Please list the names of two teachers who could provide a recommendation on your ability to tutor a peer successfully.

_____

_____

Parental Permission

Please obtain a parent's signature to indicate approval of your participation in the peer tutoring program.

My child, _____, has my permission to participate in the peer tutoring program coordinated by the speech-language pathologist _____ for _____ hours per week.

_____ _____

Parent Signature   Date

Sample Communication Contract

UNIT: Following and Generating Instructions   **GRADE**

a. (<u>Name</u>) will collect (<u>number</u>) instructions that are difficult
to follow and discuss why they are difficult.   **A   B   C   D   F**

b. (<u>Name</u>) will concisely and clearly state (<u>number</u>) specific
instructions for activities (e.g., how to open a combination
locker or how to get from school to home).   **A   B   C   D   F**

c. (<u>Name</u>) will describe (<u>number</u>) situations where precision in
giving instructions if of utmost importance.   **A   B   C   D   F**

d. (<u>Name</u>) will describe (<u>number</u>) situations where a lack of
giving instructions will cause a problem.   **A   B   C   D   F**

I, (<u>name</u>), agree to complete this contract starting on (<u>beginning date</u>) and ending on (<u>ending date</u>). I understand that my overall contract grade will be determined by averaging the letter grades for each of the four parts of the contract. Evaluation of each objective will be made by the adult who signs this contract.

If I fail to complete this contract by the date listed above, I will undergo the following consequences:

Student's Signature:_____ Date:_____

Professional's Signature: _____ Date:_____

NOTE TO PROFESSIONALS: Assist students to select an appropriate number of instructions or situations to earn specific letter grades (e.g., 10 instructions earn an "A", 8 earn a "B", 6 earn a "C", 4 earn a "D", and 2 earn an "F"). Insert these numbers where indicated. Have students project the grade they will attempt to earn for each objective and insert the number corresponding to this grade in the stated objective.

References

Aaron, P., Joshi, M., and Williams, K. (1999). Not all reading disabilities are alike. *Journal of Learning Disabilities, 32,* 120–137.

Abel, E. (1990). *Fetal alcohol syndrome.* Oradell, NJ: Medical Economics Books.

Abkarian, G., Jones, A., and West, G. (1992). Young children's idiom comprehension: Trying to get the picture. *Journal of Speech and Hearing Research, 35,* 580–587.

Ackerman, B. (1982). On comprehending idioms: Do children get the picture? *Journal of Experimental Child Psychology, 33,* 439–454.

Adams, G., Montemayor, R., and Gullotta, T. (1989). *Biology of adolescent behavior and development.* London: Sage.

Alexander, W., and McEwin, C. (1989). *Schools in the middle: Status and progress.* Columbus, OH: National Middle School Association.

Alley, G., and Deshler, D. (1979). *Teaching the learning disabled adolescent: Strategies and methods.* Denver, CO: Love Publishing.

Allington, R., and Fleming, J. (1978). The misreading of high-frequency words. *Journal of Special Education. 12,* 417–421.

American Library Association and Association for Educational Communications and Technology. (1998). *Information power: Building partnerships for learning.* Retrieved May 9, 2003, from http://www.ala.org/Content/NavigationMenu/AASL/Professional_Tools10/Information_Power/Information_Literacy_Standards_for_Student_Learning.htm

American Association of University Women Foundation. (2001). *Hostile hallways: Bullying, teasing, and sexual harassment in school.* Washington, DC: American Association of University Women.

American Educational Research Association, American Psychological Association, and National Council on Measurement in Education. (1985). *Standards for educational and psychological testing.* Washington, DC: American Psychological Association.

American Psychiatric Association. (2000). Diagnostic and statistical manual of mental disorders (4th ed., text revision). Washington. DC: Author.

American Speech-Language-Hearing Association. (1992a). Communication and the ADA. *Asha, 34*(6/7), 62–67.

American Speech-Language-Hearing Association. (1992b). Special section: Americans with Disabilities Act. *Asha, 34*(6/7), 35–61.

American Speech-Language-Hearing Association. (1993). Definitions of communication disorders and variations. *Asha, 35,* (Suppl. 10), 40–41.

American Speech-Language-Hearing Association. (1996). Inclusive practices for children and youths with communication disorders [Position statement and technical report]. *Asha, 38*(Suppl.16), 35–44.

American Speech-Language-Hearing Association. (1999). *Guidelines for the roles and responsibilities of school-based speech-language pathologists.* Rockville, MD: Author.

American Speech-Language-Hearing Association. (2000a). ASHA Special Interest Division 1: *Language Learning and Education 7*(1), 1–29.

American Speech-Language-Hearing Association. (2000b). *IDEA and your caseload: A template for eligibility and dismissal criteria for students ages 3 to 21.* Rockville, MD: Author.

American Speech-Language-Hearing Association. (2001a). *Communication facts: Incidence and prevalence of communication disorders and hearing loss.* Retrieved from http://professional.asha.org/research/children.htm

American Speech-Language-Hearing Association. (2001b). *Roles and responsibilities of speech-language pathologists with respect to reading and writing in children and adolescents.* Rockville, MD: Author.

American Speech-Language-Hearing Association Ad Hoc Committee on Instrument Evaluation. (1986, August). *Report of the committee submitted to the Executive Board.* Rockville, MD: Author.

Americans With Disabilities Act of 1990, 42 U.S.C.A. § 12101 *et seq.*

Amiot, A. (1998). Policy, politics, and the power of information: The critical need for outcomes and clinical trials data in policy making in the schools. *Language, Speech, and Hearing Services in Schools, 29,* 245.

Apel, K. (1999a). Checks and balances: Keeping the science in our profession. *Language, Speech, and Hearing Services in Schools, 30,* 98–107.

Apel, K. (1999b). An introduction to assessment and intervention with older students with language-learning impairments: Bridges from research to clinical practices. *Language, Speech, and Hearing Services in Schools, 30,* 228–230.

Communication Solutions
for Older Students

Apel, K. (2001). Epilogue: Developing evidence-based practices and research collaborations in school settings. *Language, Speech, and Hearing Services in Schools, 32*, 196–197.

Apel, K., and Masterson, J. (2000). What is the role of the speech-language pathologist in assessing and facilitating spelling skills? *Topics in Language Disorders, 20*(3), 83–93.

Apel, K., and Swank, L. (1999). Second chances: Improving decoding skills in the older student. *Language, Speech, and Hearing Services in Schools, 30*, 231–242.

Applebee, A. (1978). *The child's concept of story.* Chicago: University of Chicago Press.

Applebee, A. (1981). *Writing in the secondary school.* Urbana, IL: National Council of Teachers of English.

Applebee, A., Auten, A., and Lehr, F. (1981). *Writing in the secondary school: English and the content areas.* Urbana, IL: National Council of Teachers of English.

Aram, D., Ekelman, B., and Nation, J. (1984). Preschoolers with language disorders: 10 years later. *Journal of Speech and Hearing Research, 27*, 232–244.

Aram, D., and Hall, N. (1989). Longitudinal follow-up of children with preschool communication disorders: Treatment implications. *School Psychology Review, 18*, 487–501.

Arlin, P. (1975). Cognitive development in adulthood: "A fifth stage?" *Developmental Psychology, 11*, 602–606.

Armour-Thomas, E., and Allen, B.A. (1990). Componential analysis of analogical-reasoning performance of high and low achievers. *Psychology in the Schools, 27*, 269–275.

Arwood, E. (1983). *Pragmaticism: Theory and application.* Rockville, MD: Aspen.

Asch, S., and Nerlove, H. (1960). The development of double function terms in children: An exploratory investigation. In B. Kaplan and S. Wapner (Eds.), *Perspectives in psychological theory: Essays in honor of Heinz Werner* (pp. 47–60). New York: International Universities Press.

Ashear, V., and Snortum, J. (1971). Eye contact in children as a function of age, sex, social and intellectual variables. *Developmental Psychology, 4*, 479.

Asher, S., and Gazelle, B. (1999). Loneliness, peer relations, and language disorders in childhood. *Topics in Language Disorders, 19*(2), 16–33.

Associated Press. (1992, September 21). Communication skills said lacking: Businesses say workers need help. *Oshkosh Northwestern*, p. 12.

Atkins, C., and Cartwright, L. (1982). Preferred language elicitation procedures used in five age categories. *Asha, 24*, 321–323.

Aune, B., and Friehe, M. (1996). Transition to postsecondary education: Institutional and individual issues. *Topics in Language Disorders, 16*(3), 1–22.

Austin, J. (1962). *How to do things with words.* London: Oxford University Press.

Baggett, L. (March 30-April 3, 1969). *Behavior that communicates understanding as evaluated by teen-agers.* Paper presented at the American Personnel and Guidance Association Convention. Las Vegas, NV.

Bakan, D. (1971). Adolescence in America: From ideal to social fact. *Daedalus, 100*, 981.

Bandura, A., and Walters, R. (1963). *Social learning and personality development.* New York: Holt, Rinehart, and Winston.

Barker, L. (1971). *Listening behavior.* Englewood Cliffs, NJ: Prentice-Hall.

Barringer, H., Gardner, R.W., and Levin, M.J. (1993). *Asians and Pacific Islanders in the United States.* New York: Sage.

Bart, W. (1971). The factor structure of formal operations. *British Journal of Educational Psychology, 41*, 40–77.

Baum, H. (1998). Overview, definitions, and goals for ASHA's treatment outcomes and clinical trials activities (What difference do outcome data make to you?) *Language, Speech, and Hearing Services in Schools, 29*, 246–249.

Beatty, P., Holman, B., and Schiraldi, V. (2000). *Poor prescription: The costs of imprisoning drug offenders in the United States.* San Francisco, CA: Center on Juvenile and Criminal Justice.

Bellugi, U., Marks, S., Bihrle, A., and Sabo, H. (1998). Dissociation between language and cognitive functions in Williams syndrome. In D. Bishop and K. Mogford (Eds.), *Language development in exceptional circumstances* (pp. 177–189). Hillsdale, NJ: Erlbaum.

Benedict, R. (1954). Continuities and discontinuities in cultural conditioning. In W. Martin and C. Stendler (Eds.), *Readings in child development* (pp. 142–148). New York: Harcourt, Brace.

Benjamin, A. (2000). *An English teacher's guide to performance tasks and rubrics: High school.* Larchmont, NY: Eye on Education.

Bergman, M. (1987). Social grace or disgrace: Adolescent social skills and learning disability subtypes. *Reading, Writing, and Learning Disabilities, 3*, 161–166.

Berninger, V.W., Vaughan, K., Abbott, R.D., Brooks, A., Begay, K., Curtin, G., et al. (2000). Language-based spelling instruction: Teaching children to make multiple connections between spoken and written words. *Learning Disability Quarterly, 23*(2), 117–135.

Bernstein, D. (1989). Assessing children with limited English proficiency: Current perspectives. *Topics in Language Disorders, 9*(3), 15–20.

Berzonsky, M. (1978). Formal reasoning in adolescence: An alternate view. *Adolescence, 13,* 279–290.

Billow, R.M. (1975). A cognitive developmental study of metaphor comprehension. *Developmental Psychology, 11,* 415–423.

Birdwhistell, R. (1970). *Kinesics and context.* Philadelphia: University of Pennsylvania Press.

Blackwell, P., Engen, E., Fischgrund, J., and Zarcadoolas, C. (1978). *Sentences and other systems: A language and learning curriculum for hearing-impaired children.* Washington, DC: The Alexander Graham Bell Association for the Deaf.

Blalock, J. (1981). Persistent problems and concerns of young adults with learning disabilities. In W. Cruickshank and A. Silver (Eds.), *Bridges to tomorrow* (Vol. 2; pp. 35–56). Syracuse, NY: Syracuse University Press.

Blalock, J. (1982). Persistent auditory language deficits in adults with learning disabilities. *Journal of Learning Disabilities, 15,* 604–609.

Blanck, P., and Rosenthal, R. (1982). Developing strategies for decoding "leaky" messages: On learning how and when to decode discrepant and consistent social communications. In R. Feldman (Ed.), *Development of nonverbal behavior in children* (pp. 203–229). New York: Springer-Verlag.

Bliss, L. (1993). Pragmatic language intervention. Eau Claire, WI: Thinking Publications.

Bloom, B.J. (Ed.), Engelhart, M.D., Furst, E.J., Hill, W.H., and Krathwohl, D.R. (1956). *Taxonomy of educational objectives: The classification of education goals: Handbook I: Cognitive domain.* New York: Longman.

Bloom, L., and Lahey, M. (1978). *Language development and language disorders.* New York: Wiley.

Blosser, J., and DePompei, R. (1989). The head-injured student returns to school: Recognizing and treating deficits. *Topics in Language Disorders, 9*(2), 67–77.

Blosser, J., and Kratcoski, A. (1997). PACs: A framework for determining appropriate service delivery options. *Language, Speech, and Hearing Services in Schools, 28,* 99–107.

Blue, C. (1975). The marginal communicator. *Language, Speech, and Hearing Services in Schools, 6,* 32–37.

Botvin, G., and Sutton-Smith, B. (1977). The development of structural complexity in children's fantasy narratives. *Developmental Psychology, 13,* 377–388.

Boyce, N., and Larson, V. Lord. (1983). *Adolescents' communication: Development and disorders.* Eau Claire, WI: Thinking Publications.

Boyett, J., and Conn, H. (1992). *Workplace 2000: The revolution reshaping American business.* New York: Plume.

Bracewell, R., Scardamalia, M., and Bereiter, C. (1978). Cognitive processes in composing and comprehending discourse. *Educational Psychologist, 17*(3), 146–164.

Brinton, B., and Fujiki, M. (1999). Social interactional behaviors of children with specific language impairment. *Topics in Language Disorders, 19*(2), 49–69.

Brown, A., and Smiley, S. (1977). Rating the importance of structural units of prose passages: A problem of metacognitive development. *Child Development, 48,* 1–8.

Brown, B. Byers, and Beveridge, M. (1979). *Language disorders in children* (Monograph No. 1). London: College of Speech Therapists.

Brown, B. Byers, and Edwards, M. (1998). *Developmental disorders of language.* San Diego, CA: Singular.

Brown, R. (1973). *A first language: The early stages.* Cambridge, MA: Harvard University Press.

Bryan, T. (1977). Children's comprehension of nonverbal communication. *Journal of Learning Disabilities, 10,* 501–506.

Bryan, T., Donahue, M., and Pearl, R. (1981). Studies of learning disabled children's pragmatic competence. *Topics in Learning and Learning Disabilities, 1*(2), 29–39.

Bunce, B. (1989). Using a barrier game format to improve children's referential communication skills. *Journal of Speech and Hearing Disorders, 54,* 33–43.

Busacco, D. (2001a). Learning at a distance—Technology and the new professional. *The ASHA Leader, 6*(2), 4–5, 9.

Busacco, D. (2001b). Student/Mentor pairs announced: Program helps students make career choices. *The ASHA Leader, 6*(11), 8, 14.

Byrne, S., Constant, A., and Moore, G. (1992). Making transitions from school to work. *Educational Leadership, 49*(6), 23–26.

Cain, K., and Oakhill, J. (1998). Comprehension skill and inference-making ability: Issues of causality. In C. Hulme and R.M. Joshi (Eds.), *Reading and spelling* (pp. 343–367). Hillsdale, NJ: Erlbaum.

Carey, A. (1992). Americans With Disabilities Act and you. *Asha, 34*(6/7), 5–6.

Carl Perkins Vocational and Technical Education Act of 1998, 20 U.S.C. § 2301 *et seq.*

Carlson, A. (Governor). (1993, January 26). *State of the State Address* (Radio broadcast). St. Paul, MN: Minnesota Public Radio.

Communication Solutions
for Older Students

Carpenter, L. (1990). *Including multicultural content in the undergraduate communication disorders curriculum: A resource guide and reference document.* Unpublished manuscript, University of Wisconsin—Eau Claire.

Casby, M. (1988). Speech-language pathologists' attitudes and involvement regarding language and reading. *Language, Speech, and Hearing Services in Schools, 19,* 352–358.

Casby, M. (1992). The cognitive hypothesis and its influence on speech-language services in schools. *Language, Speech, and Hearing Services in Schools, 23,* 198–202.

Case, R. (1984). The process of stage transition: A neo-Piagetian view. In R. Sternberg (Ed.), *Mechanisms of cognitive development* (pp. 19–44). New York: Freeman.

Case, R. (1985). *Intellectual development: Birth to adulthood.* Orlando, FL: Academic Press.

Cashen, A.S. (1989). *Analogical processing skills in three modalities in fifth, eighth, and eleventh graders.* Unpublished master's thesis, Western Michigan University, Kalamazoo, MI.

Catts, H., and Kamhi, A. (1999). *Language and reading disabilities.* Needham Heights, MA: Allyn and Bacon.

Chall, J. (1983). *Stages of reading development.* New York: McGraw-Hill.

Chamberlain, P., and Medinos-Landurand, P. (1991). Practical considerations for the assessment of LEP students with special needs. In E. Hamayan and J. Damico (Eds.), *Limiting bias in the assessment of bilingual students* (pp. 111–156). Austin, TX: Pro-Ed.

Chapman, R. (1972). Some simple ways of talking about normal language and communication. In J. McLean, D. Yoder, and R. Schiefelbusch (Eds.), *Language intervention with the retarded: Developing strategies* (pp. 17–32). Baltimore: University Park Press.

Chapman, R. (1981). Exploring children's communicative intents. In J. Miller (Ed.), *Assessing language production in children* (pp. 111–136). Baltimore: University Park Press.

Chappell, G. (1980). Oral language performance of upper elementary school students obtained via story reformulation. *Language, Speech, and Hearing Services in Schools, 11,* 236–250.

Chial, M., Sobolevsky, R., and Flahive, M. (2000, March 28). Utopians, Luddites, or just plain realists? Distance education in communication sciences and disorders. *The ASHA Leader, 5*(6), 4–5, 23.

Children's Defense Fund Action Council. (2002, February). Key facts on Black youth, violence, and crime. In *Testimony and issue basics: Juvenile justice and youth development.* Retrieved February 19, 2003, from http://www.cdfactioncouncil.org/blackyvc.htm

Children's literacy: Hearings before the Committee on Education and the Workforce, U.S. House of Representatives, 105th Cong., (1997) (testimony of G. Reid Lyon)

Chomsky, C. (1969). *The acquisition of syntax in children from 5 to 10.* Cambridge, MA: MIT Press.

Cimorelli, J.M., McCready, V., Brucke, J., and Bushur, T. (November, 2000). The relationship between literacy impairments and delinquency behaviors in adolescents. Paper presented at the annual convention of the American Speech-Language-Hearing Association. Washington, DC.

Civil Rights Act of 1964, 20 U.S.C. § 1401 *et seq.*

Coats, D. (1991). America's youth: A crisis of character. *Imprimis: Journal of Hillsdale College, 20*(9), 1–6.

Cole, K., Mills, P., and Kelley, D. (1994). Agreement of assessment profiles used in cognitive referencing, *Language, Speech, and Hearing in Schools, 25,* 25–31.

Cole, L. (1983). Implications of the position on social dialects. *Asha, 25*(9), 25–31.

Committee on the Status of Racial Minorities. (1983). Social dialects: Position paper. *Asha, 25*(9), 23–24.

Conte, B., Menyuk, P., and Bashir, A. (November, 1992). Text comprehension in normal and language impaired adolescents. Paper presented at the annual convention of the American Speech-Language-Hearing Association, New Orleans, LA.

Coufal, K. (1993). Collaborative consultation for speech-language pathologists. *Topics in Language Disorders, 14*(1), 1–14.

Council for Exceptional Children. (2003, February 10). *Law and regulations: IDEA '97 law and regs.* Retrieved February 19, 2003, from IDEAPractices website: http://www.ideapractices.org/law/regulations/index.php

Cocozza, J.J. (1997). Identifying the needs of juveniles with co-occurring disorders. *Corrections Today, 59*(7), 146–149.

Cozad, R., and Rousey, C. (1966). Hearing and speech disorders among delinquent children. *Corrective Psychiatry and Journal of Social Therapy, 12,* 250–255.

Crager, R., and Spriggs, A. (1969). Development of concept utilization. *Development Psychology, 1,* 415–424.

Crago, M., and Cole, E. (1991). Using ethnography to bring children's communicative and cultural worlds in focus. In T. Gallagher (Ed.), *Pragmatics of language: Clinical practice issues* (pp. 99–131). San Diego, CA: Singular.

Craig, H. (1983). Applications of pragmatic language models for intervention. In T. Gallagher and C. Prutting (Eds.), *Pragmatic assessment and intervention issues in language* (pp. 101–128). San Diego, CA: College-Hill.

Crais, E. (1990). World knowledge to word knowledge. *Topics in Language Disorders, 10*(3), 45–62.

Creaghead, N.A., and Tattershall, S.A. (1991). Observation and assessment of classroom pragmatic skills. In C. Simon (Ed.), *Communication skills and classroom success: Assessment and therapy methodologies for language and learning disabled students* (pp. 106–122). Eau Claire, WI: Thinking Publications.

Cromer, R. (1994). A case study of dissociations between language and cognition. In H. Tager-Flusberg (Ed.), *Constraints in language acquisition: Studies of atypical children* (pp. 141–153). Hillsdale, NJ: Erlbaum.

Cruttenden, A. (1985). Intonation comprehension in ten-year-olds. *Journal of Child Language, 12,* 643–661.

Crystal, D. (1992). *Profiling linguistic disability* (2nd ed.). San Diego, CA: Singular.

Crystal, D., Fletcher, P., and Garman, M. (1991). *The grammatical analysis of language disability: A procedure for assessment and remediation.* San Diego, CA: Singular.

Culatta, B., Page, J., and Ellis, J. (1983). Story retelling as a communicative performance screening tool. *Language, Speech, and Hearing Services in Schools, 14,* 66–78.

Cummins, J. (1989). A theoretical framework for bilingual special education. *Exceptional Children, 56,* 111–119.

Curtis, M.E. (2002, May). *Adolescent reading: A synthesis of research.* Paper presented at NICHD Workshop 2: Practice models for adolescent literacy success, Baltimore, MD.

Damico, J. (1988). The lack of efficacy in language therapy: A case study. *Language, Speech, and Hearing Services in Schools, 19,* 51–66.

Damico, J. (1991). Clinical discourse analysis: A functional approach to language assessment. In C. Simon (Ed.), *Communication skills and classroom success: Assessment and therapy methodologies for language and learning disabled students* (pp. 125–150). Eau Claire, WI: Thinking Publications.

Damico, J. (1992). Using a whole language framework for language intervention. *The Clinical Connection, 6*(1), 10–13.

Damico, J. (1993). Language assessment in adolescents: Addressing critical issues. *Language, Speech, and Hearing Services in Schools, 24(1),* 29–35.

Damico, J., and Armstrong, M. (1991). Empowerment in the clinical context: The speech-language pathologist as advocate. *The NSSLHA Journal, 18,* 34–43.

Damico, J., and Damico, S. (1993). Language and social skills from a diversity perspective: Considerations for the speech-language pathologist. *Language, Speech, and Hearing Services in Schools, 24,* 236–243.

D'Arcangelo, M. (2002). The challenge of content-area reading: A conversation with Donna Ogle. *Educational Leadership, 60*(3), 12–15.

Davelaar, E. (1977). Formal operational reasoning and its relationship to complex speech patterns and tentative statement use. *Language and Speech, 20*(1), 73–79.

Davis, A. (1944). Socialization and adolescent personality. In N. Henry (Ed.), *Adolescence, yearbook of the national society for the study of education: Volume 43. Part 1* (pp. 198–216). Chicago: University of Chicago, Department of Education.

De Ajuriaguerra, J., Jaeggi, A., Guignard, F., Kocher, F., Maguard, M., Roch, S., and Schmid, E. (1976). The development and prognosis of dysphasia in children. In D. Morehead and A. Morehead (Eds.), *Normal and deficient child language* (pp. 345–386). Baltimore: University Park Press.

DePaulo, B., and Jordan, A. (1982). Age changes in deceiving and detecting deceit. In R. Feldman (Ed.), *Development of nonverbal behavior in children* (pp. 151–180). New York: Springer-Verlag.

Deshler, D., and Schumaker, J. (1983). Social skills of learning disabled adolescents: Characteristics and intervention. *Topics in Learning and Learning Disabilities, 3*(2), 15–23.

Dimitrovsky, L. (1964). The ability to identify the emotional meaning of vocal expressions at successive age levels. In J. Davitz (Ed.), *The communication of emotional meaning* (pp. 69–86). New York: McGraw-Hill.

DiSimoni, F. (1978). *Token Test for Children.* Chicago: Riverside.

Dittman, A. (1972). Development factors in conversational behavior. *Journal of Communication, 22,* 404–423.

Dollaghan, C. (1987). Comprehension monitoring in normal and language-impaired children. *Topics in Language Disorders, 7*(2), 45–60.

Dolphin, C. (1991). Variables in the use of personal space. In *Intercultural communication: A reader* (pp. 320–329). Belmont, CA: Wadsworth.

Donahue, M. (1984). Learning disabled children's conversational competence: An attempt to activate the inactive listener. *Applied Psycholinguistics, 5,* 21–35.

Donahue, M., and Bryan, T. (1984). Communicative skills and peer relations of learning disabled adolescents. *Topics in Language Disorders, 4*(2), 10–21.

Donahue, M., Pearl, R., and Bryan, T. (1980). Learning disabled children's conversational competence: Responses to inadequate messages. *Applied Psycholinguistics, 1,* 387–403.

537

Donahue, M., Pearl, R., and Bryan, T. (1982). Learning disabled children's syntactic proficiency on a communicative task. *Journal of Speech and Hearing Disorders, 47,* 297–403.

Dore, J. (1974). A pragmatic description of early language development. *Journal of Psycholinguistics, 3,* 343–350.

Dore, J. (1975). Holophrases, speech acts, and language universals. *Journal of Child Language, 2,* 21–40.

Dorval, B. (1980, April). *The development of conversation.* Paper presented at the Biennial Southeastern Conference on Human Development, Alexandria, VA.

Douglas, J., and Peel, B. (1979). The development of metaphor and proverb translation in children grades one through seven. *Journal of Education Research, 73,* 116–119.

DuChossois, G., and Michaels, C. (1994). Postsecondary education. In C. Michaels (Ed.)., *Transition strategies for persons with learning disabilities* (pp. 79–118). San Diego, CA: Singular.

Duncan, D.M. (1989). *Working with bilingual language disability.* London: Chapman and Hall.

Duncan, S., Jr., and Fiske, D. (1977). *Face to face interaction: Research, methods, and therapy.* New York: Wiley.

Dunn, R., Dunn, K., and Price, G. (1989). *Learning style inventory. LSI manual.* Lawrence, KS: Price Systems.

Duranti, A. (1988). Ethnography of speaking: Toward a linguistics of praxis. In F. Newmeyer (Ed.), *Linguistics: The Cambridge survey: Vol. 4. Language: The socio-cultural context* (pp. 210–228). Cambridge, UK: Cambridge University Press.

Eckert, P. (1990). Cooperative competition in adolescent "girl talk." *Discourse Processes, 13,* 91–122.

Edmondson, W. (1981). *Spoken discourse: A model for analysis.* New York: Longman.

Ehren, B. (2002a). Getting into the adolescent literacy game. *The ASHA Leader, 7*(7), 4–5, 10.

Ehren, B. (2002b). Speech-language pathologists contributing significantly to the academic success of high school students: A vision for professional growth. *Topics in Language Disorders, 22*(2), 60–80.

Ehri, L. (1994). Development of the ability to read words: Update. In R. Ruddell, M. Ruddell, and H. Singer (Eds.), *Theoretical models and processes of reading* (pp. 323–358). Newark, DE: International Reading Association.

Ehri, L. (2000). Learning to read and learning to spell: Two sides of a coin. *Topics in Language Disorders, 20*(3), 19–36.

Eisenberg, L. (1965). A developmental approach to adolescence. *Children, 12,* 131–135.

Eisner, E. (1965). Critical thinking: Some cognitive components. *Teachers College Record, 66,* 624–634.

Elder, G. (1975). Adolescence in the life cycle: An introduction. In S. Dragastin and G. Elder, Jr. (Eds.), *Adolescence in the life cycle: Psychological change and social context* (pp. 1–22). Washington, DC: Hemisphere.

Elkind, D. (1974). *Children and adolescents: Interpretive essays on Jean Piaget.* New York: Oxford University Press.

Elkind, D. (1975). Recent research on cognitive development in adolescents. In E. Sigmund, S. Dragastin, and G. Elder, Jr., (Eds.), *Adolescence in the life cycle: Psychological change and social context* (pp. 49–62). New York: Wiley.

Elkind, D. (1978). Understanding the young adolescent. *Adolescence, 13*(14), 127–134.

Elkind, D. (2000). *All grown up and no place to go.* Boulder, CO: Perseus Books.

Elkind, D., Barocas, R., and Johnsen, R. (1969). Concept production in children and adolescents. *Human Development, 12,* 10–21.

Elliott, S., and Gresham, F. (1991). *Social skills intervention guide: Practical strategies for social skill training.* Circle Pines, MN: American Guidance Service.

Ellis, E. (1989). A metacognitive intervention for increasing class participation. *Learning Disabilities Focus, 5*(1), 36–46.

Ellis, E., and Friend, P. (1991). Adolescents with learning disabilities. In B. Wong (Ed.), *Learning and learning disabilities* (pp. 506–563). San Diego, CA: Academic Press.

Ellsworth, P., and Sindt, V. (1991). *What every teacher should know about how students think: A survival guide for adults.* Eau Claire, WI: Thinking Publications.

Engler, L., Hannah, E., and Longhurst, T. (1973). Linguistic analysis of speech samples: A practical guide for clinicians. *Journal of Speech and Hearing Disorders, 38,* 192–204.

Epstein, H. (1974). Phrenoblysis: Special brain and mind growth periods. I. Human brain and skill development. *Developmental Psychobiology, 7,* 207–216.

Epstein, H. (1978). Growth spurts during brain development: Implications for educational policy and practice. In J. Chall and A. Mirsky (Eds.), *Education and the brain: The seventy-seventh yearbook of education* (pp. 343–370). Chicago: University of Chicago Press.

Epstein, H.J. (1979). Cognitive growth and development. Brain growth and cognitive functions. *Colorado Journal of Educational Research, 19*(1), 4–5.

Epstein, H., and Toepfer, C. (1978). A neuroscience basis for reorganizing middle grades education. *Educational Leadership, 35*(8), 656–660.

Epstein, J., and MacIver, D. (1990). *Education in the middle grades: Overview of national practices and trends.* Columbus, OH: National Middle School Association.

Erikson, E. (1968). *Identity: Youth and crisis.* New York: Norton.

Everson, J., and Goodall, D. (1991). School-to-work transition for youth who are both deaf and blind. *Asha, 33*(11), 45–47.

Fahey, K., and Reid, K. (2000). *Language development, differences, and disorders: A perspective for general and special education teachers and classroom-based speech-language pathologists.* Austin, TX: Pro-Ed.

Falconer, K., and Cochran, J. (1989). Communication skills in male institutionalized juvenile offenders. *Rocky Mountain Journal of Communication Disorders, 5,* 45–54.

Fawcett, G. (1994). Debatable issues underlying whole language philosophy: A literacy instructor's perspective. *Language, Speech, and Hearing Services in Schools, 25,* 37–39.

Farmer, S. (2000). Literacy brokering: An expanded scope of practice for SLPs. *Topics in Language Disorders, 21*(1), 68–81.

Fein, D. (1983). The prevalence of speech and language impairments. *Asha, 25*(2), 37.

Feldman, R., White, J., and Lobato, D. (1982). Social skills and nonverbal behavior. In R. Feldman (Ed.), *Developmental of nonverbal behavior in children* (pp. 257–274). New York: Springer-Verlag.

Ferguson, L. (1970). *Personality development.* Belmont, CA: Brooks/Cole.

Feuerstein, R. (1979). *The dynamic assessment of retarded performers: The learning potential assessment device: Theory, instruments, and techniques.* Chicago: Foresman.

Feuerstein, R. (1980). *Instrumental enrichment.* Chicago: Foresman.

Feuerstein, R. (1983, November). *Instrumental enrichment training workshop.* Hadassah-WIZO Canada Research Institute, Toronto, Ontario.

Feuerstein, R., Feuerstein, R., and Schur, Y. (1997). Process as content in education of exceptional children. In A.L. Costa and R.M. Liebman (Eds.). *Supporting the spirit of learning: When process is content* (pp. 1–22). Thousand Oaks, CA: Corwin Press.

Fischer, K. (1980). Learning as the development of organized behavior. *Journal of Structural Learning, 3,* 253–267.

Fischer, K., and Corrigan, R. (1981). A skill approach to language development. In R. Stark (Ed.), *Language behavior in infancy and early childhood* (pp. 245–275). New York: Elsevier/North Holland.

Fischer, K., Hand, H., and Russell, S. (1984). The development of abstractions in adolescence and adulthood. In M. Commons, F. Richards, and C. Armon (Eds.), *Beyond formal operations* (pp. 43–73). New York: Praeger Scientific.

Fischer, K., and Pipp, S. (1984). Processes of cognitive development. Optimal level and skill acquisition. In R. Sternberg (Ed.), *Mechanisms of cognitive development* (pp. 45–81). New York: Freeman.

Flavell, J. (1976). Metacognitive aspects of problem solving. In L. Resnick (Ed.), *The nature of intelligence* (pp. 231–236). Hillsdale, NJ: Erlbaum.

Flavell, J. (1977). *Cognitive development.* Englewood Cliffs, NJ: Prentice-Hall.

Foorman, B., Francis, D., Fletcher, J., Schatschneider, C., and Mehta, P. (1998). The role of instruction in learning to read: Preventing reading failure in at-risk children. *Journal of Educational Psychology, 90,* 37–55.

Foorman, B.R., Francis, D.J., Shaywitz, S.E., Shaywitz, B.A., and Fletcher, J.M. (1997). The case for early reading intervention. In B. Blachman (Ed.), *Foundations of reading acquisition and dyslexia: Implications for early intervention* (pp. 243–264). Mahwah, NJ: Erlbaum.

Forum on Child and Family Statistics. (1999). Trends in the well-being of America's children and youth. Washington, DC: U.S. Department of Health and Human Services.

Freeman, D. (1983). *Margaret Mead and Samoa: The making and unmaking of an anthropological myth.* Cambridge, MA: Harvard University Press.

French, R. (1978). Nonverbal patters in youth culture. *Educational Leadership, 35*(7), 541–546.

Freud, A. (1948). *The ego and the mechanism of defense.* New York: International Universities Press.

Freud, S. (1953). *A general introduction to psychoanalysis.* New York: Permabooks.

Fujiki, M., Brinton, B., Hart, C., and Fitzgerald, A. (1999). Peer acceptance and friendship in children with specific language impairment. *Topics in Language Disorders, 19*(2), 34–48.

Fuligni, A.J. (1997). The academic achievement of adolescents from immigrant families: The roles of family background, attitudes, and behavior. *Child Development, 68,* 351–363.

Furlong, M., and Morrison, G. (1994). Introduction to miniseries: School violence and safety in perspective. *School Psychology Review, 23*(2) 139–150.

Gajewski, N., Hirn, P., and Mayo, P. (1998a). *Social skill strategies: A social-emotional curriculum for adolescents: Book A.* (2nd Ed.) Eau Claire, WI: Thinking Publications.

Communication Solutions
for Older Students

Gajewski, N., Hirn, P., and Mayo, P. (1998b). *Social skill strategies: A social-emotional curriculum for adolescents: Book B.* (2nd Ed.) Eau Claire, WI: Thinking Publications.

Galda, S. (1981, April). *The development of comprehension of metaphor.* Paper presented at the annual meeting of the American Educational Research Association, Los Angeles, CA.

Gallagher, T. (1983). Pre-assessment: A procedure for accommodating language use variability. In T. Gallagher and C. Prutting (Eds.), *Pragmatic assessment and intervention issues in language* (pp. 1–28). San Diego, CA: College-Hill.

Gallagher, T. (1991). Language and social skills: Implications for assessment and intervention with school-age children. In T. Gallagher (Ed.), *Pragmatics of language: Clinical practice issues* (pp. 11–41). San Diego, CA: Singular.

Gallagher, T. (1999). Interrelationships among children's language, behavior, and emotional problems. *Topics in Language Disorders, 19*(2), 1–15.

Gallagher, T., Swigert, N., Baum, H. (1998). Collecting outcomes data in schools: *Language, Speech, and Hearing Services in Schools, 29,* 250–256.

Ganschow, L., Philips, L., and Schneider, E. (2001). Closing the gap: Accommodating students with language learning disabilities in college. *Topics in Language Disorders, 21*(2), 17–37.

Garnett, K. (1986). Telling tales: Narratives and learning-disabled children. *Topics in Language Disorders, 6*(2), 44–56.

Garvey, J., and Gordon, N. (1973). A follow-up study of children with disorders of speech and development. *British Journal of Disorders of Communication, 8,* 17–28.

Gates, G. (1923). An experimental study of growth of social perception. *Journal of Educational Psychology, 14,* 449–461.

Geers, A., and Moog, J. (1978). Syntactic maturity of spontaneous speech and elicited imitations of hearing-impaired children. *Journal of Speech and Hearing Disabilities, 43,* 380–391.

Geffner, D., and Kuehn, D. (1998). National Association addresses shortages of researchers and practitioners (Letter to the editor). *Topics in Language Disorders, 19*(1), 76–78.

George, P., Stevenson, C., Thomason, J., and Beane, J. (1992). *The middle school—and beyond.* Alexandria, VA: Association for Supervision and Curriculum Development.

German, D. (1992). Word-finding intervention for children and adolescents. *Topics in Language Disorders, 13*(1), 33–50.

German, D.J. (1993). *Word-finding intervention program.* Austin, TX: Pro-Ed.

German, D.J. (2001). *It's on the tip of my tongue.* Chicago: Word Finding Materials.

Gesell, A., Ilg, F., and Ames, L. (1956). *Youth: The years from ten to sixteen.* New York: Harper.

Getzel, E. Evans. (1990). Entering postsecondary programs: Early individualized planning. *Teaching Exceptional Children, 23,* 51–53.

Gillam, R., and Johnston, J. (1992). Spoken and written language relationships in language/learning-impaired and normally achieving school-age children. *Journal of Speech and Hearing Research, 35,* 1303–1315.

Gillam, R., Pena, E., and Miller, L. (1999). Dynamic assessment of narrative and expository discourse. *Topics in Language Disorders, 20*(1), 33–47.

Gillespie, P., and Lerner, N. (1999). *The Allyn and Bacon guide to peer tutoring.* Boston: Allyn and Bacon.

Gilligan, C. (1982). New map of development: New vision of maturity. *American Journal of Orthopsychology, 52*(2), 199–212.

Gilliland, H. (1988). *Teaching the Native American.* Dubuque, IA: Kendall-Hunt.

Glover, R.J. (1999). Coming of age: Developmental norms of the adolescent years. *NASSP Bulletin, 83*(603), 62–69.

Goldberg, B. (1996). Imagining tomorrow: What's ahead for our professions. *Asha, 38*(3), 22–28.

Goleman, D. (1995). *Emotional intelligence: Why it can matter more than IQ.* New York: Bantam Books.

Goleman, D. (1998). *Working with emotional intelligence.* New York: Bantam Books.

Goleman, D., Boyatzis, R., and McKee, A. (2002). *Primal leadership: Realizing the power of emotional intelligence.* Boston: Harvard Business School.

Golumbia, L., and Hillman, S. (1990, August). *A comparison of learning disabled and nondisabled adolescent motivational processes.* Paper presented at the annual meeting of the American Psychological Association, Boston, MA.

Gray, L., and House, R. (1989). No guarantee of immunity: Aids and adolescents. In D. Capuzzi and D. Gross (Eds.), *Youth at-risk: A resource for counselors, teachers, and parents* (pp. 231–270). Alexandria, VA: American Association for Counseling and Development.

Greenfield, P., and Smith, J. (1976). *The structure of communication in early language development.* New York: Academic Press.

Greene, J.F. (1996). Psycholinguistic assessment: The clinical base for identification of dyslexia. *Topics in Language Disorders, 16*(2), 45–72.

Greer, J., and Wethered, C. (1984). Learned helplessness: A piece of the burnout puzzle. *Exceptional Children, 50,* 524–531.

Gregg, N. (1983). College learning disabled writer: Error patterns and instructional alternatives. *Journal of Learning Disabilities, 16,* 334–338.

Gregg, N., Coleman, C., Stennett, R., and Davis, M. (2002). Discourse complexity of college writers with and without disabilities: A multidimensional analysis. *Journal of Learning Disabilities, 35*(1), 23–38, 56.

Grice, H. (1975). Logic and conversation. In P. Cole and J. Morgan (Eds.), *Syntax and semantics: Vol. 3: Speech acts* (pp. 41–58). New York: Academic Press.

Griffiths, C. (1969). A follow-up study of children and disorders in speech. *British Journal of Disorders of Communication, 4,* 46–56.

Gross, T. (1985). *Cognitive development.* Monterey, CA: Brooks/Cole.

Gruen, A., and Gruen, L. (1994). *Traumatic brain injury activities.* Eau Claire, WI: Thinking Publications.

Gruenwald, L., and Pollak, S. (1984). *Language interaction in teaching and learning.* Baltimore: University Park Press.

Grunwell, P. (1986). Aspects of phonological development in later childhood. In K. Durkin (Ed.), *Language development in the school years* (pp. 34–56). Cambridge, MA: Brookline.

Gullotta, T., Adams, G., Markstrom, C. (2000). *The adolescent experience* (4th ed.). New York: Academic Press.

Hains, A., and Miller, D. (1980). Moral and cognitive development in delinquent and nondelinquent children and adolescents. *Journal of General Psychology, 137,* 21–35.

Hakes, D. (1980) *The development of metalinguistic abilities in children.* New York: Springer-Verlag.

Hall, G. (1904). *Adolescence: Its psychology and its relations to physiology, anthropology, sociology, sex, crime, religion, and education.* New York: Appleton.

Halliday, M. (1975). *Learning how to mean: Explorations in the development of language.* New York: Elsevier-North Holland.

Halperin, S. (1994). *School-to-work: A larger vision.* Washington, DC: American Youth Policy Forum, The Institute for Educational Leadership.

Hamburg, D. (1992). *Today's children: Creating a future for a generation in crisis.* New York: Times Books.

Hammill, D. (1990). On defining learning disabilities: An emerging consensus. *Journal of Learning Disabilities, 23,* 74–84.

Harmon, H. (1998). *Building school-to-work systems in rural America.* Retrieved via Eric Digest: http://www.ael.org/eric/digests/edorc977.htm

Harris, K.R. and Graham, S. (1996). *Making the writing process work: Strategies for composition and self-regulation.* Cambridge, MA: Brookline Books.

Harter, S., and Connell, J. (1984). A comparison of alternative models between academic achievement and children's perceptions of competence, control, and motivated orientation. In J. Nicholls (Ed.), *The development of achievement-related cognitions and behaviors* (pp. 214–250). Greenwich, CT: JAI Press.

Hartzell, H.E. (1984). The challenge of adolescence. *Topics in Language Disorders, 4*(2), 1–9.

Havertape, J., and Kass, C. (1978). Examination of problem solving in learning disabled adolescents through verbalized self-instructions. *Learning Disability Quarterly, 1*(4), 94–100.

Havighurst, R. (1953). *Human development and education.* New York: Longmans, Green.

Hayes, J., and Flower, L. (1987). On the structure of the writing process. *Topics in Language Disorders, 7*(4), 19–30.

Hayes, J., Flower, L., Schriver, K., Stratman, J., and Carey, L. (1985). *Cognitive processes in revision* (Tech. Rep. No. 12). Pittsburgh, PA: Carnegie Mellon University, Communication Design Center.

Health Strategies. (2002). Characteristics of puberty. In *Health Teacher: Personal and Consumer Health.* Retrieved February 6, 2003, from http:// www.healthteacher.com/teachersupports/content/consumer/teacher1.asp

Heath Resource Center. (1985). *Measuring student progress in the classroom.* Washington, DC: Author.

Heath Resource Center. (1992). *Transition resource guide.* Washington, DC: Author.

Heath Resource Center. (1994a). *Getting ready for college: Advising high school students with learning disabilities.* Washington, DC: Author.

Heath Resource Center. (1994b). *Make the most of your opportunities: A guide to postsecondary education for adults with disabilities.* Washington, DC: Author.

Hechinger, R. (1992). *Fateful choices: Healthy youth for the 21st century.* New York: Hill and Wang.

Hedberg, N., and Westby, C. (1993). *Analyzing storytelling skills: Theory to practice.* Tucson, AZ: Communication Skill Builders.

Hill, J. (1970, April). *Models for screening.* Paper presented at the annual meeting of the American Educational Research Association, Minneapolis, MN.

Hoggan, K., and Strong, C. (1994). The magic of "once upon a time": Narrative teaching strategies. *Language, Speech, and Hearing Services in Schools, 25,* 76–89.

Holiday, P. (2001). Demand may exceed supply in future job market. *The ASHA Leader, 6*(8), 18.

Hoskins, B. (1996). *Conversations: A framework for language intervention.* Eau Claire, WI: Thinking Publications.

Huffman, N. (2000). The changing face of practice in communication sciences and disorders in educational settings. *The Communication Connection 14*(4), 1, 4–6.

Hughes, D., McGillivray, L., and Schmidek, M. (1997). *Guide to narrative language: Procedures for assessment.* Eau Claire, WI: Thinking Publications.

Hull, G. (1987). Current views of error and editing. *Topics in Language Disorders, 7*(4)55–64.

Hutson-Nechkash. P. (2001). *Narrative toolbox: Blueprints for storybuilding.* Eau Claire, WI: Thinking Publications.

Hymes, D. (1971). Competence and performance in linguistic theory. In R. Huxley and E. Ingram (Eds.), *Language acquisition: Models and methods* (pp. 3–28). New York: Academic Press.

Hymes, D. (1972). Introduction. In C. Cazden, V. John, and D. Hymes (Eds.), *Functions of language in the classroom* (pp. xi–lvii). New York: Teachers College Press.

Hymes, D. (1974). The ethnography of speaking. In B. Blount (Ed.), *Language, culture, and society: A book of readings* (pp. 189–223). Cambridge, MA: Winthrop.

Individuals with Disabilities Education Act (IDEA), 20 U.S.C.§ 1400 *et seq.* (1990).

Individuals with Disabilities Education Act (IDEA) Amendments, 20 U.S.C. §1400 *et seq.* (1997).

Inhelder, B., and Piaget, J. (1958). *The growth of logical thinking from childhood to adolescence: An essay on the construction of formal operational structures.* New York: Basic Books.

Inspiration Software. (1997). Inspiration (Computer software). Portland, OR: Author. (Available from Thinking Publications, 424 Galloway Street, Eau Claire, WI 54701)

IntelliTools. (1996). IntelliTalk (Computer software). Portland, OR: Author. (Available from IntelliTools, Inc., 55 Leveroni Court, Suite 9, Novato, CA 94949)

Isaacson, S. (1991). Assessing written language skills. In C. Simon (Ed.), *Communication skills and classroom success: Assessment and therapy methodologies for language and learning disabled students* (pp. 224–237). Eau Claire, WI: Thinking Publications.

Jackson, S. (1965). The growth of logical thinking in normal and subnormal children. *British Journal of Educational Psychology, 35,* 255–258.

James, S. (1990). *Normal language acquisition.* Austin, TX: Pro-Ed.

Johnson, C. (1995). Expanding norms for narration. *Language, Speech, and Hearing Services in Schools, 26,* 326–341.

Johnson, C.J., Beitchman, J.H., Young, A., Escobar, M., Atkinson, L., and Wilson, B., et al. (1999). Fourteen-year follow-up of children with and without speech/language impairments: Speech/language stability and outcomes. *Journal of Speech, Language, and Hearing Research, 42,* 744–760.

Johnson, R., Greenspan, S., and Brown, G. (1980, September). *Children's ability to recognize and improve upon socially inept communications.* Paper presented at the 88th annual convention of the American Psychologists Association, Montreal, Canada.

Johnston, J. (1982). Narratives: A new look at communication problems in older language-disordered *children. Language, Speech, and Hearing Services in Schools, 13,* 144–155.

Johnston, J. (1985). *Doing things with words.* Madison, WI: Educational Teleconferencing Network.

Jones, J., and Stone C. (1989). Metaphor comprehension by language learning disabled and normally achieving adolescent boys. *Learning Disability Quarterly, 12,* 251–260.

Jones, P. (1972). Formal operational reasoning and the use of tentative statements. *Cognitive Psychology, 3,* 467–471.

Kagan, J., Rosman, B., Day, D., Albert, J., and Phillips, W. (1964). Information processing in the child: Significance of analytic and reflective attitudes. *Psychology Monographs, 78*(1), 1–37.

Kamhi, A. (1987). Metalinguistic abilities in language-impaired children. *Topics in Language Disorders, 7*(2), 1–12.

Kamhi, A. (1991). Specific language impairment as a clinical category: An introduction. *Language, Speech, and Hearing Services in Schools, 22,* 65.

Kamhi, A. (1995). Research to practice: defining, developing, and maintaining clinical expertise. *Language, Speech, and Hearing Services in Schools, 26,* 353–356.

Kamhi, A. (1997). Three perspectives on comprehension: Implications for assessing and treating comprehension problems. *Topics in Language Disorders, 17*(3), 62–74.

Kamhi, A. (1999). Dual perspectives on choosing treatment approaches to use or not to use: Factors that influence the selection of new treatment approaches. *Language, Speech, and Hearing Services in Schools, 30*(1), 92–98.

Kamhi, A., and Catts, H. (1986). Toward an understanding of developmental language and reading disorders. *Journal of Speech and Hearing Disorders, 51,* 337–347.

Kamhi, A., and Catts, H. (Eds.). (1989). *Reading disabilities: A developmental language perspective.* Austin, TX: Pro-Ed.

Kamhi, A., and Lee, R. (1988). Cognition. In M. Nippold (Ed.), *Later language development: Ages nine through nineteen* (pp. 127–158). Boston: Little, Brown.

Kao, G. (1995). Asian Americans as model minorities? A look at their academic achievement. *American Journal of Education, 103,* 121–159.

Kaufer, D., Hayes, J., and Flower, L. (1986). Composing written sentences. *Research in the Teaching of English, 20*(2), 121–140.

Kaufman, P., Kwan, J., Klein, S., and Chapman, C. (2000). Dropout rates in the United States: 1998. *Education Statistics Quarterly, 2*(1), 43–47.

Kerr, M., and Nelson, C. (1989). *Strategies for managing behavior problems in the classroom.* Columbus, OH: Merrill.

Kett, J. (1977). *Rites of passage: Adolescence in America, 1790 to the present.* New York: Basic Books.

Killian, C. (1979). Cognitive development of college freshmen. *Journal of Research in Science Teaching, 16,* 347–350.

Kindsvatter, R., Wilen, W., and Ishler, M. (1988). *Dynamics of effective teaching.* New York: Longman.

King, R., Jones, C., and Lasky, E. (1982). In retrospect: A fifteen-year follow-up report of speech-language disordered children. *Language, Speech, and Hearing Services in Schools, 13,* 24–32.

Kishta, M. (1979). Proportional and combinatorial reasoning in two cultures. *Journal of Research in Science Teaching, 16,* 439–443.

Knapp, M. (1978). *Nonverbal communication in human interaction.* New York: Holt, Rinehart and Winston.

Knight-Arest, I. (1984). Communicative effectiveness of learning disabled and normally achieving 10- to 13-year-old boys. *Learning Disability Quarterly, 7,* 237–245.

Knowles, M. (1973). *The adult learner: A neglected species.* Houston, TX: Gulf.

Knowles, M., Holton, E., III, and Swanson, R. (1998). *The definitive classic in adult education and human resource development* (5th ed.). Houston, TX: Gulf.

Kogan, N., Connor, K., Gross, A., and Fava, D. (1980). Understanding visual metaphor: Developmental and individual differences. *Monographs of the Society for Research in Child Development, 45*(Serial No. 183).

Kohlberg, L. (1975). The cognitive-developmental approach to moral education. *Phi Delta Kappan, 56,* 670–677.

Konopka, G. (1971). Adolescence in the 1970s. *Child Welfare, 50*(10), 553–559.

Konopka, G. (1973). Requirements for healthy development of adolescent youth. *Adolescence, 8*(3), 291–316.

Koskinen, P., and Wilson, R. (1982). *Developing a successful tutoring program.* New York: Teachers College Press, Columbia University.

Kramer, P., Koff, E., and Luria, Z. (1972). The development of an exceptional language structure in older children and young adults. *Child Development, 43,* 121–130.

Kretschmer, E. (1951). *Korperbau and character.* Berlin, Germany: Springer-Verlag.

Kroh, O. (1944). *Entwicklungspsychologic des Grundschulkindes* (Developmental psychology of the elementary school child). Langensalza, Germany: Herman Beyer.

Labinowicz, E. (1980). *The Piaget primer.* Menlo Park, CA: Addison-Wesley.

Lahey, M. (1988). *Language disorders and language development.* New York: Macmillan.

Lahey, M. (1990). Who shall be called language disordered? Some reflections and one perspective. *Journal of Speech and Hearing Disorders, 55,* 612–620.

Lancaster, L., and Stillman, D. (2002). *When generations collide.* New York: HarperCollins.

Langdon, H.W. (2002). *Interpreters and translators in communication disorders: A practitioner's handbook.* Eau Claire, WI: Thinking Publications.

Langdon, H.W., and Cheng, L.-R.L. (2002). *Collaborating with interpreters and translators: A guide for communication disorders professionals.* Eau Claire, WI: Thinking Publications.

Lapadat, J. (1991). Pragmatic language skills of students with language and/or learning disabilities: A quantitative synthesis. *Journal of Learning Disabilities, 24*(3), 147–158.

Larson, M., and Dittman, F. (1975). *Compensatory education and early adolescence: Reviewing our national strategy.* Menlo Park, CA: Stanford Research.

Larson, V. Lord, and McKinley, N. (1985a). General intervention principles with language impaired adolescents. *Topics in Language Disorders, 5*(3), 70–77.

Larson, V. Lord, and McKinley, N. (1985b, November). *Innovative service delivery models for adolescents with language disorders.* Paper presented at the annual convention of the American Speech-Language-Hearing Association, Washington, DC.

Larson, V. Lord, and McKinley, N. (1987). *Communication assessment and intervention strategies for adolescents.* Eau Claire, WI: Thinking Publications.

Larson, V. Lord, and McKinley, N. (1988). Language disorders in the adolescent: Assessment. In D. Yoder and R. Kent (Eds). *Decision making in speech-language pathology* (pp. 46–47). Philadelphia: B.C. Decker.

Larson, V. Lord, and McKinley, N. (1990, November). *Adolescents with language disorders: An "action plan" for service delivery.* Poster session presented at the annual convention of the American Speech-Language-Hearing Association, Seattle, WA.

Larson, V. Lord, and McKinley, N. (1995). *Language disorders in older students: Preadolescents and adolescents.* Eau Claire, WI: Thinking Publications.

Larson, V. Lord, and McKinley, N. (1998). Adolescents conversations: A longitudinal study. *Clinical Linguistics and Phonetics, 12*(3), 183–203.

Larson, V. Lord, and McKinley, N. (2001, December). *Meeting the needs of adolescents with language disorders* [ASHA teleseminar]. Rockville, MD.

Larson, V. Lord, and McKinley, N. (2002, November). *Communication solutions for the older student.* Workshop presentation for Health Education Network, Rolling Meadows, IL.

Larson, V. Lord, and McKinley, N. (in press). Service delivery options for secondary students with language disorders. *Seminars in Speech-Language Pathology.*

Larson, V. Lord, McKinley, N., and Boley, D. (1993). Service delivery models for adolescents with language disorders. *Language, Speech, and Hearing Services in Schools, 24,* 36–42.

Lawson, A., and Wollman, W. (1976). Encouraging the transition from concrete to formal cognitive functioning—An experiment. *Journal of Research in Science Teaching, 13,* 413–430.

Leadbeater, B., and Dionne, J. (1981). The adolescent's use of formal operational thinking in solving problems related to identify resolution. *Adolescence, 16*(61), 111–121.

Leadholm, B.J., and Miller, J.F. (1992). *Language sample analysis: The Wisconsin guide.* Madison, WI: Wisconsin Department of Public Instruction.

Learning Disabilities Association of America (LDA). (1993). Inclusion: Position paper of the Learning Disabilities Association of America. Retrieved May 9, 2003, from http://www.ldanatl.org/positions/inclusion.html

Lee, L. (1974). *Developmental sentence analysis.* Evanston, IL: Northwestern University Press.

Leonard, L. (1991). Specific language impairment as a clinical category. *Language, Speech, and Hearing Services in Schools, 22,* 66–68.

Levine, J., and Sutton-Smith, B. (1973). Effects of age, sex, and task on visual behavior during dyadic interaction. *Developmental Psychology, 9,* 400–405.

Lewin, K. (1939). Field theory and experiment in social psychology concepts and methods. *American Journal of Sociology, 44,* 868–897.

Lewis, B., and Freebairn, L. (1992). Residual effects of preschool phonology disorders in grade school, adolescence, and adulthood. *Journal of Speech and Hearing Research, 35,* 819–831.

Lidz, C. (1991). *Practitioner's guide to dynamic assessment.* New York: Guilford Press.

Lipsitz, J. (1979). Adolescent development: Myths and realities. *Children Today, 8*(5), 2–7.

Lipsitz, J. (1980). *Growing up forgotten: A review of research and programs concerning early adolescence.* New Brunswick, NJ: Transaction.

Loban, W. (1976). *Language development: Kindergarten through grade twelve.* Urbana, IL: National Council of Teachers of English.

Logemann, J. (1994). Treatment efficacy and outcome: Everyone's job. *Asha, 36*(6/7), 3.

Logemann, J. (1998). Treatment outcomes and efficacy in the schools. *Language, Speech and Hearing Services in Schools, 29*(4), 243–244.

Logemann, J., and Baum, H. (1998). The need for epidemiologic studies in language. *Topics in Language Disorders, 19*(1), 27–30.

Lombardino, L., and Ahmed, S. (2000). Opinion pieces: What is the role of the speech-language pathologist in assessing and facilitating spelling skills? *Topics in Language Disorders, 20*(3), 83–93.

Long, S., Fey, M., and Channell, R. (2000). Computerized Profiling (CP; Version 9.26) [Computer software, Windows only]. Cleveland, OH: Case Western Reserve University. (Available as a free download at *http://www.cwru.edu/artsci/coisil/cp.htm*)

Long, S., and Masterson, J. (1993). Use in language analysis. *Asha, 35*(8), 40–41.

Lord, C., and Paul, R. (1997). Language and communication in autism. In D. Cohen and F. Volkmar (Eds.), *Handbook of autism and pervasive developmental disorders* (2nd ed.; pp. 195–225). New York: Wiley.

Lund, N., and Duchan, J. (1983). *Assessing children's language in naturalistic contexts.* Englewood Cliffs, NJ: Prentice-Hall.

Lunday, A.M. (1996). A collaborative communication skills program for job corps centers. *Topics in Language Disorders, 16*(3), 23–36.

Lutzer, V. (1988). Comprehension of proverbs by average children and children with learning disorders. *Journal of Learning Disabilities, 21,* 104–108.

Lyon, G.R. (1996). Special education for students with disabilities. *The Future of Children, 6,* 1–16.

MacLachlan, B., and Chapman, R. (1988). Communication breakdowns in normal and language learning-disabled children's conversation and narration. *Journal of Speech and Hearing Disorders, 53,* 2–7.

Maeroff, G. (1988). Withered hopes, stillborn dreams: The dismal panorama of urban schools. *Phi Delta Kappan, 69,* 632–638.

Malgady, R.G. (1977). Children's interpretation and appreciation of similes, *Child Development, 48,* 1734–1738.

Mandler, J., and Johnson, N. (1977). Remembrance of things parsed: Story structure and recall. *Cognitive Psychology, 9,* 111–151.

Mann, V., Cowin, E., and Schoenheimer, J. (1989). Phonological processing, language comprehension, and reading ability. *Journal of Learning Disabilities, 22,* 76–89.

Markgraf, B. (1966). An observational study determining the amount of time that students in the 10th and 12th grades are expected to listen in the classroom. In S. Duker (Ed.), *Listening readings* (pp. 90–101). New York: Scarecrow Press.

Marquis, M.A., and Addy-Trout, E. (1992). *Social communication: Activities for improving peer interactions and self-esteem.* Eau Claire, WI: Thinking Publications.

Martorano, S. (1977). A developmental analysis of performance on Piaget's formal operations tasks. *Developmental Psychology, 13*(6), 666–672.

Mason, W. (1976). Specific (developmental) dyslexia. *Developmental Medicine and Child Neurology, 9,* 183–190.

Masterson, J., and Apel, K. (2000). Spelling assessment: Charting to optimal intervention. *Topics in Language Disorders, 20*(3), 50–65.

Masterson, J., Apel, K., and Wasowicz, J. (2002). *SPELL: Spelling Performance Evaluation for Language and Literacy.* Chicago: Learning by Design.

Masterson, J., and Crede, L. (1999). Learning to spell: Implications for assessment and intervention. *Language, Speech, and Hearing Services in Schools, 30,* 243–254.

Mayo, P., and Waldo, P. (1994). Scripting: Social communication for adolescents (2nd ed.). Eau Claire, WI: Thinking Publications.

McCabe, A. (1995). Evaluation of narrative discourse skills. In K. Cole, P. Dale, and D. Thal (Eds.), *Assessment of communication and language* (pp. 121–141). Baltimore: Brookes.

McCarthy, D. (1930). *The language development of the preschool child* (Institute of Child Welfare Monograph Series No. 4). Minneapolis, MN: University of Minnesota Press.

McCray, A.D., Vaughn, S., and Neal, L.I. (2001). Not all students learn to read by third grade: Middle school students speak out about their reading disabilities. *The Journal of Special Education, 35*(1), 17–30.

McFadden, T. (1991). Narrative and expository language: A criterion-based assessment procedure for school-age children. *Journal of Speech-Language Pathology and Audiology, 15*(4), 57–63.

McGhee-Bidlack, B. (1991). The development of noun definitions: A metalinguistic analysis. *Journal of Child Language, 18,* 417–434.

McKinley, N., and Larson, V. Lord. (1983, November). *Adolescents' conversations with a friend and an unfamiliar adult.* Paper presented at the annual convention of the American Speech-Language-Hearing Association, Cincinnati, OH.

McKinley, N., and Larson, V. Lord. (1985). Neglected language disordered adolescents: A delivery model. *Language, Speech, and Hearing Services in Schools, 16,* 2–15.

McKinley, N., and Larson, V. Lord. (1989). Students who can't communicate: Speech-language services at the secondary level. *National Association of Secondary School Principals Curriculum Report, 19*(2), 1–8.

McKinley, N., and Larson, V. Lord. (1990). Language and learning disorders in adolescents. *Seminars in Speech and Language, 11,* 182–191.

McKinley, N., and Larson, V. Lord. (1991, November). *Seventh, eighth, and ninth graders' conversations in two experimental conditions.* Poster session presented at the annual convention of the American Speech-Language-Hearing Association, Atlanta, GA.

McKinley, N., and Larson, V. Lord. (1996, November). Adolescents' conversations: A longitudinal analysis. Paper presented at the annual convention of the American Speech-Language-Hearing Association. Seattle, WA.

545

McKinley, N., and Larson, V. Lord. (1998, November). *Assessing older students' communication/cognitive skills: Process over product outcomes.* Paper presented at the annual convention of the American Speech Language-Hearing Association. San Antonio, TX.

McKinley, N., and Larson, V. Lord. (1999, November). Advancing emotional intelligence in older students with language disorders. Poster session presented at the annual convention of the American Speech-Language-Hearing Association. San Francisco, CA.

McKinley, N., and Larson, V. Lord. (2000, November). *Connecting the disconnected: Adolescents with language disorders and the Internet.* Paper presented at the annual convention of the American Speech-Language-Hearing Association. Washington, DC.

McLaughlin, M. Smith, and Hazouri, S. Peyser. (1992), TLC: Tutoring, learning, cooperating. Minneapolis, MN: Educational Media.

McLean, J., and Snyder-McLean, L. (1978). *A transactional approach to early language training.* Columbus, OH: Merrill.

McLoyd, V.C. (1998). Changing demographics in the American population. In V.C. McLoyd and L. Steinberg (Eds.), *Studying minority adolescents: Conceptual, methodological, and theoretical issues* (pp. 251–278). Mahwah, NJ: Erlbaum.

Mead, M. (1950). *Coming of age in Samoa.* New York: New American Library.

Medrich, E. (2002). *School-to-work: A summary of progress measures and performance indicators 1996–2001.* Washington, DC: U.S. Department of Education.

Meece, J.L., and Kurtz-Costes, B. (2001). Introduction: The schooling of ethnic minority children and youth. *Educational Psychologist, 36*(1), 1–7.

Mehrabian, A. (1968). Communication without words. *Psychology Today, 2,* 51–52.

Mendelberg, H. (1984). Split and continuity in language use of Mexican-American adolescents of migrant origin. *Adolescence, 19*(73), 171–182.

Mentis, M. (1994). Topic management in discourse: Assessment and intervention. *Topics in Language Disorders, 14*(3), 29–54.

Menyuk, P. (1991). Metalinguistic abilities and language disorder. In J. Miller (Ed.), *Research on child language disorders: A decade of progress* (pp. 387–397). Austin, TX: Pro-Ed.

Menyuk, P., and Chesnick, M. (1997). Metalinguistic skills, oral language knowledge, and reading. *Topics in Language Disorders, 17*(3), 75–87.

Merritt, D., and Liles, B. (1987). Story grammar ability in children with and without language disorder: Story generation, story retelling, and story comprehension. *Journal of Speech and Hearing Research, 30,* 539–552.

Michaels, C. (1994). *Transition strategies for persons with learning disabilities.* San Diego, CA: Singular.

Miller, J. (1981). *Assessing language production in children: Experimental procedures.* Baltimore: University Park Press.

Miller, J., and Chapman, R. (2000). SALT: A Computer Program for the Systematic Analysis of Language Transcripts [Computer software]. Madison, WI: Language Analysis Laboratory, Waisman Center, University of Wisconsin.

Miller, J.F., Freiberg, C., Rolland, M., and Reeves, M. (1992). Implementing computerized language sample analysis in the public school. *Topics in Language Disorders, 12*(2), 69–82.

Miller, N., and Dollard, J. (1941). *Social learning and imitation.* New Haven, CT: Yale University Press.

Miller, P. (1989). Theories of adolescent development. In J. Worell and F. Danner (Eds.), *The adolescent as decision-maker: Applications to development and education* (pp. 13–49). San Diego, CA: Academic Press.

Minskoff, E., and Allsopp, D. (2003). *Academic success strategies for adolescents with learning disabilities and ADHD.* Baltimore: Brookes.

Mitchell, J. (1979). *Adolescent psychology.* Toronto, Canada: Holt, Rinehart and Winston.

Moats, L.C. (2000). *Speech to print: Language essentials for teachers.* Baltimore: Brookes.

Montague, M., and Lund, K. (1991). *Job-related social skills: A curriculum for adolescents with special needs.* Ann Arbor, MI: Exceptional Innovations.

Montemayor, R., and Eisen, M. (1977). The development of self-conceptions from childhood to adolescence. *Developmental Psychology, 13,* 314–319.

Montgomery, J., and Herer, G. (1994). Future watch: Our schools in the 21st century. *Language, Speech, and Hearing Services in Schools, 25,* 130–135.

Moore, M. (2001) *Transcript builder.* Eau Claire, WI: Thinking Pubilications.

Moore-Brown, B.J., and Montgomery, J.K. (2001). *Making a difference for America's children: Speech-language pathologists in public schools.* Eau Claire, WI: Thinking Publications.

Mordecai, D., Palin, M., and Palmer, C. (1982). Lingquest 1: Language Sample Analysis [Computer software]. Napa, CA: Lingquest Software.

Muma, J. (1978). *Language handbook: Concepts, assessment, intervention.* Englewood Cliffs, NJ: Prentice-Hall.

Muuss, R. (1975). *Theories of adolescence.* New York: Random House.

Myrick R., and Erney, T. (2000). Caring and sharing; Becoming a peer facilitator. Minneapolis, MN: Educational Media.

Nation, K., and Hulme, C. (1997). Phonemic segmentation, not onset-rime segmentation, predicts early reading and spelling skills. *Reading Research Quarterly, 32,* 154–167.

National Alliance of Business. (1996). Understanding the new economy. *Workforce Economics, 2*(2), 11.

National Center for Chronic Disease Prevention and Health Promotion. (2002, September 30). Summary results, 2001: United States. In *Data and statistics: Youth Risk Behavior Surveillance System: 2001 information and results.* Retrieved February 19, 2003, from http://www.cdc.gov/nccdphp/dash/yrbs/2001/summary_results/usa.htm

National Center for Educational Statistics. (1999). *Digest of educational statistics.* Washington, DC: U.S. *Department* of Education, Office of Educational Research and Improvement.

National Center for Educational Statistics. (2000a). *The condition of education, 2000.* Washington, DC: U.S. Department of Education, Office of Educational Research and Improvement.

National Center for Educational Statistics. (2000b). *National Assessment of Educational Progress (NAEP). 1999 long-term trend assessment.* Washington, DC: U.S. Department of Education, Office of Educational Research and Improvement.

National Center for Educational Statistics. (2002). *Student effort and educational progress.* Retrieved May 9, 2003, from http://nces.ed.gov//programs/coe/2002/section3/indicator20.asp

National Center on Education, Disability, and Juvenile Justice. (2002, January 25*).* Juvenile correctional education programs. In *Focus areas: Education programs.* Retrieved February 19, 2003, from http://www.edjj.org/education.html

National Institutes of Health. (1984). *Head injury: Hope through research.* (NIH Publication No. 84-2478, pp. 1–37). Bethesda, MD: Author.

National Institutes of Health. (2002). *Research in adolescent literacy.* Retrieved March 24, 2003, from http://grants.nih.gov/grants/guide/rfa-files/RFA-HD-03-012.html

National Joint Committee on Learning Disabilities. (1991). Learning disabilities: Issues on definition. *Asha, 33*(Suppl. 5), 18–20.

National Joint Committee on Learning Disabilities. (1996). Position paper. In *Topics in Language Disorders, 16*(3), 69–73.

National Research Council. (1997). The new Americans: Economic, demographic, and fiscal effects of immigration. Washington, DC: National Academy Press.

National Women's Health Information Center. (2000). What are the most pressing issues in adolescent health today? In *Frequently asked questions about women's health: Adolescent health: Overview.* Retrieved February 19, 2003, from http://www.4woman.gov/faq/adoles.htm#1

Neimark, E. (1979). Current status of formal operations research. *Human Development, 22,* 60–67.

Neimark, E. (1980). Intellectual development in the exceptional adolescent as viewed within a Piagetian framework. *Exceptional Education Quarterly, 1*(2), 47–56.

Nelsen, E.A., and Rosenbaum, E. (1972). Language patterns within the youth subculture: Development of slang vocabularies. Merrill-Palmer Quarterly, *18,* 273–285.

Nelson, N.W. (1984). Beyond information processing: The language of teachers and textbooks. In G. Wallach and K. Butler (Eds.), *Language learning disabilities in school-age children* (pp. 154–178). Baltimore: Williams and Wilkins.

Nelson, N.W. (1988). The nature of literacy. In M. Nippold (Ed.), *Later language development: Ages nine to nineteen* (pp. 11–28). Boston: Little, Brown.

Nelson, N.W. (1989). Curriculum-based language assessment and intervention. *Language, Speech, and Hearing Services in Schools, 20,* 170–184.

Nelson, N.W. (1992). Targets of curriculum-based language assessment. In J. Damico (Ed.), *Best practices in school speech-language pathology* (pp. 73–86). San Antonio, TX: Psychological Corporation.

Nelson, N.W. (1993). *Childhood language disorders in context: Infancy through adolescence.* New York: Macmillan.

Nelson, N.W. (1998). *Childhood language disorders in context: Infancy through adolescence* (2nd ed.). Boston: Allyn and Bacon.

Nelson, N.W. (2000). Basing eligibility on discrepancy criteria: A bad idea whose time has passed. *ASHA Special Interest Division I, Language Learning and Education, 7*(1), 8.

Nelson, N.W., and Friedman, K. (1988). *Development of the concept of story in narratives written by older children.* Unpublished paper, Western Michigan University, Kalamazoo.

Nelson, N.W., and Van Meter, A. (2002). Assessing curriculum-based reading and writing samples. *Topics in Language Disorders, 22*(2), 35–59.

Nichols, R., and Lewis, T. (1954). *Listening and speaking: A guide to effective oral communication.* Dubuque, IA: Wm. C. Brown.

Nichols, R., and Stevens, L. (1957). Listening to people. *Harvard Business Review, 35*(5), 85–92.

Nippold, M. (1985). Comprehension of figurative language in youth. *Topics in Language Disorders, 5*(3), 1–20.

Nippold, M. (1988a). Figurative language. In M. Nippold (Ed.), Later *language development: Ages nine through nineteen* (pp. 179–210). Boston: Little, Brown.

Communication Solutions
for Older Students

Nippold, M. (1988b). Introduction. In M. Nippold (Ed.), *Later language development: Ages nine to nineteen* (pp. 1–10). Boston: Little, Brown.

Nippold, M. (Ed.). (1988c). *Later language development: Ages nine through nineteen.* Boston: Little, Brown.

Nippold, M. (1988d). Linguistic ambiguity. In M. Nippold (Ed.), *Later language development: Ages nine to nineteen* (pp. 211–224). Boston: Little, Brown.

Nippold, M. (1988e). The literate lexicon. In M. Nippold (Ed.), *Later language development: Ages nine to nineteen* (pp. 29–48). Boston: Little, Brown.

Nippold, M. (1991). Evaluating and enhancing idiom comprehension in language disordered students. *Language, Speech, and Hearing Services in Schools, 22,* 100–106.

Nippold, M. (1993). Developmental markers in adolescent language: Syntax, semantics, and pragmatics. *Language, Speech, and Hearing Services in Schools, 24,* 21–28.

Nippold, M. (1994). Third-order verbal analogical reasoning: A developmental study of children and adolescents. *Contemporary Educational Psychology, 19,* 101–107.

Nippold, M. (1998). *Later language development: The school-age and adolescent years* (2nd ed.). Austin, TX: Pro-Ed.

Nippold, M. (2000). Language development during the adolescence years: Aspects of pragmatics, syntax, and semantics. *Topics in Language Disorders, 20*(2), 15–28.

Nippold, M., and Allen, M. (1998, November). Word knowledge and the development of proverb understanding in youth. Paper presented at the annual convention of the American Speech-Language-Hearing Association, San Antonio, TX.

Nippold, M., Cuyler, J., and Braunbeck-Price, R. (1988). Explanation of ambiguous advertisements: A developmental study with children and adolescents. *Journal of Speech and Hearing Research, 31,* 466–474.

Nippold, M., and Fey, M. (1983). Metaphoric understanding in preadolescents having a history of language acquisition difficulties. *Language, Speech, and Hearing Services in Schools, 14,* 171–180.

Nippold, M., Hegel, S., Uhden, L., and Bustamante, S. (1998). Development of proverb comprehension in adolescents: Implications for instruction. *Journal of Children's Communication Development, 19,* 49–55.

Nippold, M., and Martin, S. (1989). Idiom interpretation in isolation versus context: Developmental study with adolescents. *Journal of Speech and Hearing Research, 32,* 59–66.

Nippold, M., Martin, S., and Erskine, B. (1988). Proverb comprehension in context: A developmental study with children and adolescents. *Journal of Speech and Hearing Research, 31,* 19–28.

Nippold, M., Schwarz, I., and Undlin, R. (1992). Use and understanding of adverbial conjuncts: A developmental study of adolescents and young adults. *Journal of Speech and Hearing Research, 35,* 108–118.

Nippold, M.A., and Taylor, C.I. (2002). Judgments of idiom familiarity and transparency: A comparison of children and adolescents. *Journal of Speech, Language, and Hearing Research, 45,* 384–391.

Nippold, M.A., Uhden, L.D., and Schwarz, I. (1997). Proverb explanation through the lifespan: A developmental study of adolescents and adults. *Journal of Speech, Language, and Hearing Research, 40,* 245–253.

Nisbet, J., Zanella, K., and Miller, J. (1984). An analysis of conversations among handicapped students and a non-handicapped peer. *Exceptional Children, 51,* 156–162.

Noel, M. (1980). Referential communication abilities of learning disabled children. *Learning Disability Quarterly, 3,* 70–75.

O'Malley, R., and Bachman, J. (1983). Self-esteem: Change and stability between 13 and 23. *Developmental Psychology, 19,* 257–268.

O'Neil, J. (1992). Preparing for the changing workplace. *Educational Leadership, 49*(6), 6–9.

O'Toole, T., Baum, H., and Logemann, J. (1998). Issues in conducting language research in nontraditional settings. *Topics in Language Disorders, 19*(1), 44–53.

O'Toole, T., Logemann, J., and Baum, H. (1998). Conducting clinical trials in the public schools. *Language, Speech, and Hearing Services in Schools, 29,* 257–262.

Offer, D., Ostrov, E., Howard, K., and Atkinsen, R. (1988). *The teenage world: Adolescents' self-image in ten countries.* New York: Plenum.

Ogbu, J.U. (1992). Understanding cultural diversity and learning. *Educational Researcher, 21*(8), 5–14.

Olver, R., and Hornsby, J. (1966). On equivalence. In J. Bruner, R. Olver, and P. Greenfield (Eds.), *Studies in cognitive growth* (pp. 68–85). New York: Wiley.

Overton, W., and Meehan, A. (1982). Individual differences in formal operational thought: Sex role and learned helplessness. *Child Development, 53,* 1536–1543.

Owens, R., Jr. (1991). *Language disorders: A functional approach to assessment and intervention.* New York: Macmillan.

Owens, R., Jr. (2001). *Language development: An introduction* (5th ed.). Needham Heights, MA: Allyn and Bacon.

Pacheco, R. (1983). Bilingual mentally retarded children: Language confusion or real deficits? In D.R. Omark and J.G. Erickson (Eds.), *The bilingual exceptional child* (pp. 233–254). San Diego, CA: College-Hill.

Page, J., and Stewart, S. (1985). Story grammar skills in school-age children. *Topics in Language Disorders, 5*(2), 16–30.

Papalia, D., and Olds, S. (1975). *A child's world—Infancy through adolescence.* New York: McGraw-Hill.

Paratore, J. (1995). Assessing literacy: Establishing common standards in portfolio assessment. *Topics in Language Disorders, 16*(1), 67–82.

Parent Advocacy Coalition for Educational Rights. (1988). *The students in transition using planning teacher's manual.* Minneapolis, MN: PACER Center.

Pascual-Leone, J. (1980). Constructive problems for constructive theories: The current relevance of Piaget's work and a critique of information processing simulation psychology. In H. Speda and P. Kluwe (Eds.), *Psychological models of thinking* (pp. 176–203). New York: Academic Press.

Paul, Rhea. (2001). *Language disorders from infancy through adolescence: Assessment and intervention.* St Louis, MO: Mosby.

Paul, Richard. (1993). Critical thinking: Basic questions and answers. In R. Paul (Ed.), *Critical thinking: How to prepare students for a rapidly changing world* (pp. 91–100). Santa Rosa, CA: Foundation for Critical Thinking.

Paul, Richard, and Nosich, G. (1993). A model for the National Assessment of Higher Order Thinking. In R. Paul (Ed.), *Critical thinking: How to prepare students for a rapidly changing world.* Santa Rosa, CA: Foundation for Critical Thinking.

Paul, Richard, and Willsen, J. (1993). Critical thinking: Identifying the targets. In R. Paul (Ed.), *Critical thinking: How to prepare students for a rapidly changing world* (pp. 17–36). Santa Rosa, CA: Foundation for Critical Thinking.

Paulson, F., Paulson, P., and Meyer, C. (1991). What makes a portfolio a portfolio? *Educational Leadership, 48*(5), 60–63.

Peck, M. (1982). Youth suicide. *Death Education, 6,* 29–47.

Perera, K. (1986). Language acquisition and writing. In P. Fletcher and M. Garman (Eds.), *Language acquisition: Studies in first language acquisition* (2nd ed., pp. 494–519). New York: Cambridge University Press.

Phillips, P. (1990). A self-advocacy plan for high school students with learning disabilities: A comparative case study analysis of students' teachers' and parents' perceptions of program effects. *Journal of Learning Disabilities, 23,* 466–471.

Piaget, J. (1952). *The origins of intelligence in children.* New York: International Universities Press.

Piaget, J. (1959). *The language and thought of the child.* London: Routledge and Kegan Paul. (Original work published 1926).

Piaget, J. (1970). Piaget's theory. In P. Mussen (Ed.), *Carmichael's manual of child psychology* (Vol. 1, pp. 703–732). New York: Wiley.

Piaget, J., and Inhelder, B. (1969). *The psychology of the child.* New York: Basic Books.

Piaget, J., Montangero, J., and Billeter, J.B. (1977). La formation des correlats (The formation of correlations). In J. Piaget (Ed.), *Recherches sur l'abstraction relechissante: L'abstraction des relations logico-arithmetiques [Research on abstract thinking: The abstraction of logical-arithmetical relationships]* (pp. 115–129). Paris, France: Presses Universitaires de France.

Polanski, V.G. (1989). Spontaneous production of figures in writing of students. Grades four, eight, twelve and third year in college. *Education Research Quarterly, 13,* 47–55.

Pollacco, J. (2001, January 31–February 6). Old economy vs. new economy. *Business Times.* Retrieved from www.businesstimes.com.mt/2001/0131/focus.html

Prutting, C., and Kirchner, D. (1983). Applied pragmatics. In T. Gallagher and C. Prutting (Eds.), *Pragmatic assessment and intervention issues in language* (pp. 29–64). San Diego, CA: College-Hill.

Raffaelli, M., and Duckett, E. (1989). "We were just talking..." Conversations in early adolescence. *Journal of Youth and Adolescence, 18,* 567–582.

Rank, O. (1936). *Will therapy and truth and reality.* New York: Knopf.

Rankin, R. (1926). *The measurement of the ability to understand spoken language.* Unpublished doctoral dissertation, University of Michigan, Ann Arbor.

Rashotte, L.S. (2002). What does that smile mean? The meaning of nonverbal behaviors in social interaction. *Social Psychology Quarterly, 65*(1), 92–102.

Ratner, V., and Harris, L. (1994). *Understanding language disorders: The impact on learning.* Eau Claire, WI: Thinking Publications.

Reed, N. (1977). *An analysis of comprehension levels of an ask/tell syntactic structure in a group of adolescents, aged ten to eighteen years.* Unpublished master's thesis, University of Ohio, Cincinnati.

Reed, V. (1994). *An introduction to children with language disorders* (2nd ed.). New York: Macmillan.

Rees, N. (1974). The speech pathologist and the reading process. *Asha, 16,* 255–258.

Communication Solutions
for Older Students

Rees, N. and Wollner, S. (1982, February). *A taxonomy of pragmatic abilities.* (Teleconference program). Madison, WI: Educational Teleconferencing Network.

Rehabilitation Act of 1973, 29 U.S.C. § 794 *et seq.*

Remplein, H. (1956). *Die seelische entwicklung in der kindheit und reifezeit [The spiritual development in childhood and adolescence].* Munchen, Germany: Ernst Reinhard.

Retherford, K. (2000). *Guide to analysis of language transcripts* (3rd ed.). Eau Claire, WI: Thinking Publications.

Rhyner, P. (2000). From the editor. *ASHA Special Interest Division 1, it's on p. 267 Language Learning and Education, 7*(1), 1–2.

Rice, M. (1983). Contemporary accounts of the cognition/language relationship: Implications for speech-language clinicians. *Journal of Speech and Hearing Disorders, 48,* 347–359.

Riedlinger-Ryan, K., and Shewan, C. (1984). Comparison of auditory language comprehension skills in learning-disabled and academically achieving adolescents. *Language, Speech, and Hearing Services in Schools, 15,* 127–136.

Ritter, E. (1979). Social perspective taking ability, cognitive complexity and listener adapted communication in early and late adolescence. *Communication Monographs, 46*(1), 40–51.

Ritter, E. (1981). The social-cognitive development of adolescents: Implications for the teaching of speech. Communication *Education, 30*(1), 1–10.

Roberge, J.J., and Paulus, D.H. (1971). Developmental patterns for children's class and conditional reasoning abilities. *Developmental Psychology, 4,* 191–200.

Robinson, E. (1981). The child's understanding of inadequate messages and communication failure: A problem of ignorance or egocentrism? In W. Dickson (Ed.), *Children's oral communication skills* (pp. 167–187). New York: Academic Press.

Rosa-Lugo, L., Rivera, E., and McKeown, S. (1998). Meeting the critical shortage of speech-language pathologists to serve the public schools-collaborative rewards. *Language, Speech, and Hearing Services in Schools, 29,* 232–242.

Roseberry-McKibbin, C. (2002). *Multicultural students with special language needs* (2nd ed.). Oceanside, CA: Academic Communication Associates.

Rosenberg, M. (1979). *Conceiving the self.* New York: Basic Books.

Rosenberg, M. (1986). Self-concept from middle childhood through adolescence. In J. Suls and A.G. Greenwald (Eds.), *Psychological perspectives on the self* (Vol. 3, pp. 107–135). Hillsdale, NJ: Erlbaum.

Rosenthal, D. (1979). Language skills and formal operations. *Merrill-Palmer Quarterly, 25*(2), 133–143.

Rosenthal, I. (1992). Counseling the learning disabled late adolescent and adult: A self-psychology perspective. *Learning Disabilities Research and Practice, 7,* 217–225.

Roth, F. (2000). Narrative writing: Development and teaching with children with writing difficulties. *Topics in Language Disorders, 20*(4), 15–28.

Roth, F., and Spekman, N. (1986). Narrative disclosure: Spontaneously generated stories of learning disabled and normally achieving students. *Journal of Speech and Hearing Disorders, 51,* 8–23.

Rubin, D. (1987). Divergence and convergence between oral and written communication. *Topics in Language Disorders, 7*(4), 1–18.

Rumelhart, D. (1975). Notes on a schema for stories. In D. Bobrow and A. Collins (Eds.), *Representation and understanding: Studies in cognitive science* (pp. 211–236). New York: Academic Press.

Rutherford, R. (1976). Talk about pop. In S. Rogers (Ed.), *They don't speak our language: Essays on the language world of children and adolescents* (pp. 106–127). London: Arnold.

Rutherford, R., Freeth, M., and Mercer, E. (1969). *Topics of conversation in 15-year-old children.* London: The Nuffield Foundation.

Saenz, T., Wyatt, T., and Reinard, J. (1998). Increasing the recruitment and retention of historically underrepresented minority students in higher education: A case study. *American Journal of Speech-Language Pathology, 7*(3), 39–48.

Samovar, L., and Porter, R. (1991). *Communication between cultures.* Belmont, CA: Wadsworth.

Sanders, L. (1971). The comprehension of certain syntactic structures by adults. *Journal of Speech and Hearing Disorders, 14,* 739–745.

Sanger, D., Creswell, J., Dworak, J., and Schultz, L. (2000). Cultural analysis of communication patterns among juveniles in a correctional facility, *Journal of Communication Disorders, 33,* 31–57.

Sanger, D., Hux, K., and Belau, D. (1997). Oral language skills of female juvenile delinquents. *American Journal of Speech-Language Pathology, 6*(1), 70–76.

Sanger, D., Moore-Brown, B., and Alt, E. (2000). Advancing the discussion on communication and violence. *Communication Disorders Quarterly, 22,* 43–48.

Sanger, D., Moore-Brown, B., Magnuson, G., and Svoboda, N. (2001). Prevalence of language problems among adolescent delinquents: A closer look. *Communication Disorders Quarterly, 23*, 17–26.

Schlesinger, I. (1977). The role of cognitive development and linguistic input in language acquisition. *Journal of Child Language, 4*, 153–169.

Schooling, T. (2000). NOMS bears fruit: Clinicians collect treatment outcomes data. *The ASHA Leader, 5*(10), 4–5.

School-to-Work Opportunities Act of 1994, 20 U.S.C. § 6101 *et seq.*

Schory, M. (1990). Whole language and the speech-language pathologist. *Language, Speech, and Hearing Services in Schools, 21*, 206–211.

Schreiber, L., and McKinley, N. (1987). *Make-it-yourself barrier activities: Barrier activities for speakers and listeners.* Eau Claire, WI: Thinking Publications.

Schreiber, L., and McKinley, N. (1995). *Daily communication: Strategies for the language disordered adolescent* (2nd ed.). Eau Claire, WI: Thinking Publications.

Schubert, R., and Gates, M. (1990). *Making the grade: A report card on American youth.* Washington, DC: National Collaboration for Youth.

Schuele, C., and van Kleeck, A. (1987). Precursors to literacy: Assessment and intervention. *Topics in Language Disorders, 7*(2), 32–44.

Schumaker, J., and Hazel, J. (1984). Social skills assessment and training for the learning disabled: Who's on first and what's on second? Part II. *Journal of Learning Disabilities, 17*(8), 492–499.

Schumaker, J., Sheldon-Wildgen, J., and Sherman, J. (1980). An observational study of the academic and social behavior of learning disabled adolescents in the regular classroom (Research Report 22). Lawrence, KS: University of Kansas, Institute for Research in Learning Disabilities.

Schwartz, A. (1985). Microcomputer-assisted assessment of linguistic and phonological processes. *Topics in Language Disorders, 6*(1), 26–40.

Scott, C. (1988). Spoken and written syntax. In M. Nippold (Ed.), *Later language development: Ages nine through nineteen* (pp. 49–96). Boston: Little, Brown.

Scott, C. (1999). Learning to write. In Catts and Kamhi, (Eds.), *Language and reading disabilities* (pp. 224–258). Boston: Allyn and Bacon.

Scott, C., and Erwin, D.L. (1992). Descriptive assessment of writing: Process and products. In W. Secord and J. Damico (Eds.), *Best practices in school speech-language pathology* (pp. 87–98). San Antonio, TX: Psychological Corporation.

Scott, C., and Stokes, S. (1995). Measures of syntax in school-age children and adolescents. *Language, Speech, and Hearing Services in Schools, 26*, 309–317.

Searle, J. (1965). What is a speech act? In M. Black (Ed.), *Philosophy in America* (pp. 221–239). New York: Allen and Union, Cornell University Press.

Seidenberg, P. (1988). Cognitive and academic instructional intervention for learning-disabled adolescents. *Topics in Language Disorders, 8*(3), 56–71.

Selman, R.L., Beardslee, W., Schultz, L.H., Krupa, M., and Podorefsky, D. (1986). Assessing adolescent interpersonal negotiation strategies: Toward the integration of structural and functional models. *Developmental Psychology, 19*, 82–102.

Shantz, C. (1981). The role of role-taking in children's referential communication. In W. Dickson (Ed.), *Children's oral communication skills* (pp. 85–102). New York: Academic Press.

Shaywitz, S., Fletcher, J., and Shaywitz, B. (1994). Issues in the definition and classification of attention deficit disorder. *Topics in Language Disorders, 14*(4), 1–25.

Sheehy, G. (1981). *Pathfinders: Overcoming the crises of adult life and finding your own path to well-being.* New York: Bantam Books.

Sheehy, G. (1995). *New passages: Mapping your life across time.* New York: Random House.

Sheldon, A. (1977). On strategies for processing relative clauses: A comparison of children and adults. *Journal of Psycholinguistic Research, 6*, 305–318.

Shelton, T., and Barkley, R. (1994). Critical issues in the assessment of attention deficit disorders in children. *Topics in Language Disorders, 14*(4), 26–41.

Shultz, T.R., and Pilon, R. (1973). Development of the ability to detect linguistic ambiguity. *Child Development, 44*, 728–733.

Siegal, M. (1980). Kohlberg versus Piaget: To what extent has one theory eclipsed the other? *Merrill-Palmer Quarterly, 26*(4), 285–297.

Siegel, L., and Ryan, E. (1988). Development of grammatical-sensitivity, phonological, and short-term memory skills in normally achieving and learning disabled children. *Developmental Psychology, 2*(1), 28–37.

Sikes, A., and Pearlman, E. (2000). *Fast forward: America's leading experts reveal how the Internet is changing your life.* New York: Morrow.

Communication Solutions
for Older Students

Silliman, E., Ford, C., Beasman, J., and Evans, D. (1999). An inclusion model for children with language learning disabilities: Building classroom partnerships. *Topics in Language Disorders, 19*(3), 1–18.

Silliman, E., Wilkinson, L., and Hoffman, L. (1993). Documenting authentic progress in language and literacy learning: Collaborative assessment in classrooms. *Topics in Language Disorders, 14*(1), 58–71.

Siltanen, S.A. (1981). *Apple noses and popsicle toeses: A developmental investigation of metaphorical comprehension.* Unpublished doctoral dissertation, Ohio State University, Columbia, OH.

Simmons, R., Blyth, D., Van Cleave, E., and Bush, D. (1979). Entry into early adolescence: The impact of school structure, puberty, and early dating on self-esteem. *American Sociological Review, 44,* 948–967.

Simon, C. (1979). *Communicative competence: A functional-pragmatic approach to language therapy.* Tucson, AZ: Communication Skill Builders.

Simon, C. (1981, November). *After is verbing: Then what?* Paper presented at the annual convention of the American Speech-Language-Hearing Association Convention. Los Angeles, CA.

Simon, C. (1994). *Evaluating communicative competence: A language sampling procedure* (Rev. 2nd ed.). Tempe, AZ: Communi-Cog.

Simon, C., and Myrold-Gunyuz, P. (1990). *Into the classroom: The SLP in the collaborative role.* Tucson, AZ: Communication Skill Builders.

Simon, J. (2001). Legal issues in serving postsecondary students with disabilities. *Topics in Language Disorders, 21*(2), 1–16.

Sipe, R., Walsh, J., Reed-Nordwall, K., Putnam, D., and Rosewarne, T. (2002). Supporting challenged spellers. *Voices from the Middle, 9*(3), 23–32.

Sizer, T. (1991). No pain, no gain. *Educational Leadership, 48*(8), 32–34.

Skinner, B. (1957). *Verbal behavior.* New York: Appleton-Century Crofts.

Slater, S., and Baum, H. (1998). Research methodologies in language treatment research. *Topics in Language Disorders, 19*(1), 31–43.

Slaughter-Defoe, D.T., and Rubin, H. (2001). A longitudinal case study of Head Start eligible children: Implications for urban education. *Educational Psychologist, 36*(1), 31–44.

Smith, S., Mann, V., and Shankweiler, D. (1986). Spoken sentence comprehension by good and poor readers: A study with the Token Test. *Cortex, 22,* 627–632.

Snyder, L., and Downey, D. (1991). The language-reading relationship in normal and reading-disabled children. *Journal of Speech and Hearing Research, 34,* 129–140.

Snyder, L., and Godley, D. (1992). Assessment of word-finding disorders in children and adolescents. *Topics in Language Disorders, 13*(1), 15–32.

Sparks, S. (1993). *Children of prenatal substance abuse.* San Diego, CA: Singular.

Spekman, N. (1981). A study of the dyadic verbal communication abilities of learning disabled and normally achieving 4th and 5th grade boys. *Learning Disability Quarterly, 4,* 139–151.

Spencer, M.B., Noll, E., Stoltzfus, J., and Harpalani, V. (2001). Identity and school adjustment: Revisiting the "acting White" assumption. *Educational Psychologist, 36*(2), 21–30.

Spor, M.W., and Schneider, B.K. (1999). Content reading strategies: What teachers know, use, and want to learn. *Reading Research and Instruction, 33,* 221–231.

Spranger, E. (1955). *Psychologie des jugendalters [Adolescent psychology]* (24th ed.). Heidelberg, Germany: Quelle and Meyer.

Steele, C. (1992). Race and the schooling of Black America. *Atlantic Monthly, 269*(4), 68–78.

Stein, N., and Glenn, C. (1979). An analysis of story comprehension in elementary school children. In R. Freedle (Ed.), *New directions in discourse processing* (Vol. 2, pp. 53–120). Norwood, NJ: Ablex.

Stemmer, P., Brown, B., and Smith, C. (1992). The employability skills portfolio. *Educational Leadership, 49*(6), 32–35.

Sternberg, R. (1985). *Beyond IQ: A triarchic theory of human intelligence.* New York: Cambridge University Press.

Sternberg, R.J. (1979). Developmental patterns in the encoding and combination of logical connectives. *Journal of Experimental Child Psychology, 28,* 469–498.

Sternberg, R.J. (1980). The development of linear syllogistic reasoning. *Journal of Experimental Child Psychology, 29,* 340–356.

Sternberg, R.J., and Nigro, G. (1980). Developmental patterns in the solution of verbal analogies. *Child Development, 51,* 27–38.

Stockman, I. (1996). The promises and pitfalls of language sample analysis as an assessment tool for linguistic minority children. *Language, Speech, and Hearing Services in Schools, 27,* 355–366.

Stone, C.A., and Forman, E.A. (1988). Differential patterns of approach to a complex problem-solving task among learning disabled adolescents. *Journal of Special Education, 22*(2), 167–185.

Stothard, S., Snowling, M., Bishop, D., Chipchase, B., and Kaplan, C. (1998). Language-impaired preschoolers: A follow-up into adolescence. *Journal of Speech, Language, and Hearing Research, 41,* 407–418.

Strain, P., Guralnick, M., and Walker, H. (Eds.). (1986). Children's social behavior: Development, assessment, and modification. New York: Academic Press.

Street, C. (2002). Expository text and middle school students: Some lessons learned. *Voices from the Middle, 9*(4), 33–38.

Strominger, A., and Bashir, A. (1977, November). *A nine-year follow-up of language-delayed children.* Paper presented at the annual convention of the American Speech and Hearing Association, Chicago, IL.

Strong, C. (1998). *Strong Narrative Assessment Procedure.* Eau Claire, WI: Thinking Publications.

Strong, C., and North, K. Hoggan. (1996). *The Magic of stories: Literature-based language intervention.* Eau Claire, WI: Thinking Publications.

Sturm, J., and Koppenhaver, D. (2000). Supporting writing development in adolescents with developmental disabilities. *Topics in Language Disorders, 20*(2), 73–92.

Sturomski, N. (1996). The transition of individuals with learning disabilities into the work setting. *Topics in Language Disorders, 16*(3), 37–51.

Sue, D. (1981). *Counseling the culturally different: Theory and practice.* New York: Wiley.

Suls, J. (1989). Self-awareness and self-identity in adolescence. In J. Worrell and F. Danner (Eds.), *The adolescent as decision maker: Applications to development and education* (pp. 144–179). San Diego, CA: Academic Press.

Sum, A. (1999). Literacy in the labor force: Results from the National Adult Literacy Survey. *Education Statistics Quarterly, 1*(4), 95–98.

Tanner, J. (1974). Sequence and tempo in the somatic changes in puberty. In M. Grumbach, G. Grave, and F. Mayer (Eds.), *Control of the onset of puberty* (pp. 448–470). New York: Wiley.

Taplin, J.E., Staudenmayer, H., and Taddonio, J.L. (1974). Developmental changes in conditional reasoning: Linguistic or logical? *Journal of Experimental Child Psychology, 17,* 360–373.

Tattershall, S. (2002). *Adolescents with language and learning needs: A shoulder-to-shoulder collaboration.* Albany, NY: Singular/Thomson Learning.

Taylor, D. (1988). Ethnographic educational evaluation for children, families, and schools. *Theory into Practice, 27*(1), 108, 939.

Taylor, J. (1969). *The communicative abilities of juvenile delinquents: A descriptive study.* Unpublished doctoral dissertation, University of Missouri, Columbia.

Taylor, O., and Peters, C. (1982). Sociolinguistics and communication disorders. In N. Lass, L. McReynolds, J. Northern, and D. Yoder (Eds.), *Speech, language, and hearing: Vol. II: Pathologies of speech and language* (pp. 802–818). Philadelphia: W.B. Saunders.

Teale, W., and Sulzby, E. (1986). Introduction: Emergent literacy as a perspective for examining how young children become writers and readers. In W. Teale and E. Sulzby (Eds.), *Emergent literacy: Writing and reading* (pp. vii–xxv). Norwood, NJ: Ablex.

Thomas, E., and Walmsley, S. (1976, August). *Some evidence of continuing linguistic acquisition in learning disabled adolescents.* Paper presented at the International Federation of Learning Disabilities Third International Scientific Conference, Montreal, Canada.

Thorndyke, P. (1977). Cognitive structures in comprehension and memory of narrative discourse. *Cognitive Psychology, 9,* 77–110.

Turner, J., and Helms, D. (1979). *Life span development.* Philadelphia: W.B. Saunders.

Tyack, D., and Gottsleben, R. (1974). *Language sampling, analysis, and training: A handbook for teachers and clinicians.* Palo Alto, CA: Consulting Psychologists Press.

U.S. Census Bureau. (2001). *Overview of race and Hispanic origin.* Retrieved May 9, 2003, from http://www.census.gov/prod/2001pubs/c2kbr01-1.pdf

U.S. Department of Education. (1996). *National assessment of educational progress.* Washington, DC: Author.

U.S. Department of Education. (1998). *National assessment of educational progress.* Washington, DC: Author.

U.S. Department of Education. (2000). *A back to school report.* Washington, DC: Author.

U.S. Department of Education, Office of Special Education. (1999). *Twenty-first annual report to Congress on the implementation of the Individuals with Disabilities Education Act.* Washington, DC: Author.

U.S. Department of Education, Office of Special Education. (2000). *Twenty-second annual report to Congress on the implementation of the Individuals with Disabilities Education Act.* Washington, DC: Author.

Vacca, R. (2002). From efficient decoders to strategic readers. *Educational Leadership, 60*(3), 6–11.

Valletutti, P., and Bender, M. (1982). *Teaching interpersonal and community living skills: A curriculum model for handicapped adolescents and adults.* Baltimore: University Park Press.

van Kleeck, A. (1987). Foreword. The metas: Implications for the language impaired. *Topics in Language Disorders, 7*(2), vi–vii.

553

Communication Solutions
for Older Students

Van Reusen, A., Bos, C., Schumaker, J., and Deshler, D. (1987). *The education planning strategy: I PLAN*. Lawrence, KS: Excell Enterprises.

Velluntino, F. (1978). Toward an understanding of dyslexia: Psychological factors in specific reading disability. In A. Benton and D. Pearl (Eds.), *Dyslexia: An appraisal of current knowledge* (pp. 61–111). New York: Oxford University Press.

Vetter, D.K. (1985). Evaluation of clinical intervention: Accountability. *Seminars in Speech and Language, 6*(1), 55–64.

Vetter, D.K. (1991). Needed: Intervention research. In J. Miller (Ed.), *Research on child language disorders: A decade of progress* (pp. 243–252). Austin, TX: Pro-Ed.

Vogel, S. (1974). Syntactic abilities in normal and dyslexic children. *Journal of Learning Disabilities, 7*, 47–53.

Vygotsky, L. (1962). *Thought and language*. Cambridge, MA: MIT Press.

Walker, H., Schwarz, I., Nippold, M., Irvin, L., Noell, J. (1994). Social skills in school-age children and youth: Issues and best practices in assessment and intervention. *Topics in Language Disorders, 14*(3), 70–82.

Wallach, G. (1990). Magic buries Celtis: Looking for broader interpretations of language learning and literacy. *Topics in Language Disorders, 10*(2), 63–80.

Wallach, G., and Miller, L. (1988). *Language intervention and academic success*. Boston: Little, Brown.

Weaver, H. (1972). *Human listening: Processes and behavior*. Indianapolis, IN: Bobbs-Merrill.

Weaver, P., and Dickinson, D. (1982). Scratching below the surface structure: Exploring the usefulness of story grammars. *Discourse Processes, 5*, 225–243.

Weiner, F. (1984). Computerized Language Sample Analysis (Computer software). State College, PA: Parrot Software.

Weiner, F. (1985). The value of follow-up studies. *Topics in Language Disorders, 5*(3), 78–92.

Weiner, F. (1988). Parrot Easy Language Sample Analysis (Computer software). State College, PA: Parrot Software.

Weiss, R., Hansen, K., and Heubelein, T. (1979, November). *Pragmatic psycholinguistic therapy for language disorders in early childhood*. Short course presented at the annual convention of the American Speech-Language-Hearing Association, Atlanta, GA.

Wellington, J. Brice. (1994, September). *Reflections of a juvenile court judge: Problems and prospects*. Paper presented at the International Adolescent Conference, Miami, FL.

Werner, E. (1975). *A study of communication time*. Unpublished master's thesis, University of Maryland, College Park.

Westby, C. (1984). Development of narrative language abilities. In G. Wallach and K. Butler (Eds.), *Language learning disabilities in school-age children* (pp. 103–127). Baltimore: Williams and Wilkins.

Westby, C. (1989). Assessing and remediating text comprehension problems. In A. Kamhi and H. Catts (Eds.), *Reading disabilities: A developmental language perspective* (pp. 199–259). Austin, TX: Pro-Ed.

Westby, C. (1990). The role of the speech-language pathologist in whole language. *Language, Speech, and Hearing Services in Schools, 21*, 228–237.

Westby, C. (1991a). Learning to talk—talking to learn: Oral-literate language differences. In C. Simon (Ed.), *Communication skills and classroom success: Assessment and therapy methodologies for language and learning disabled students* (pp. 334–357). Eau Claire, WI: Thinking Publications.

Westby, C. (1991b). *Steps to developing and achieving language-based curriculum in the classroom*. Rockville, MD: American Speech-Language-Hearing Association.

Westby, C. (1998a). Communicative refinement in school age and adolescence. In W. Hayes and B. Shulman (Eds.), *Communication development: Foundations, processes, and clinical applications* (pp. 311–360). Baltimore: Williams and Wilkins.

Westby, C. (1998b). Social-emotional bases of communication development. In W. Hayes and B. Shulman (Eds.), *Communication development: Foundations, processes, and clinical applications* (pp. 165–204). Baltimore: Williams and Wilkins.

Westby, C. (1999). Assessing and facilitating text comprehension problems. In H. Catts and A. Kamhi (Eds.), *Language and reading disabilities* (pp. 154–223). Boston: Allyn and Bacon.

Westby, C., and Clauser, D. (1999). The right stuff for writing: Assessing and facilitating written language. In H. Catts and A. Kamhi (Eds.), *Language and reading disabilities* (pp. 259–324). Needham Heights: Allyn and Bacon.

Westby, C., and Cutler, S. (1994). Language ADHD: Understanding the bases and treatment of self-regulatory deficits. *Topics in Language Disorders, 14*(4), 58–76.

Westby, C., and Erickson, J. (1992). Prologue. *Topics in Language Disorders, 12*(3), v–viii.

Whitmire, K. (2000). Adolescence as a developmental phase: A tutorial. *Topics in Language Disorders, 20*(2), 1–14.

Whitmire, K. (2002). The evolution of school-based speech-language services: A half century of change and a new century of practice. *Communication Disorders Quarterly, 23*, 68–76.

Wiggins, G. (1989). Teaching to the (authentic) test. *Educational Leadership, 46*(7), 41–47.

Wiig, E. (1982, May). *Identifying language disorders in adolescents*. Oral presentation at Gunderson Clinic, La Crosse, WI.

Wiig, E. (1983, October/November). *Assessment and development of social communication skills in adolescents with language-learning disabilities.* Madison, WI: Educational Teleconferencing Network.

Wiig, E., and Becker-Caplan, L. (1984). Linguistic retrieval strategies and word-finding difficulties among children with language disabilities. *Topics in Language Disorders, 4*(3), 1–18.

Wiig, E., and Harris, S. (1974). Perception and interpretation of nonverbally expressed emotions by adolescents with learning disabilities. *Perceptual and Motor Skills, 38,* 239–245.

Wiig, E., Kutner, S., Florence, D., Sherman, B., and Semel, E. (1977). Perception and interpretation of explicit negations by learning-disabled children and adolescents. *Perceptual and Motor Skills, 44,* 1251–1257.

Wiig, E., and Larson, V. Lord. (in press). *Structured-multidimensional assessment profiles (S-MAPs) for curriculum-based assessment and intervention.* Eau Claire, WI: Thinking Publications.

Wiig, E., and Secord, W. (1992a). From word knowledge to world knowledge. *The Clinical Connection, 6*(3), 12–14.

Wiig, E., and Semel, E. (1975). Productive language abilities in learning disabled adolescents. *Journal of Learning Disabilities, 8*(9), 45–53.

Wiig, E., and Semel, E. (1976). *Language disabilities in children and adolescents.* Columbus, OH: Merrill.

Wiig, E., and Semel, E. (1980). *Language assessment and intervention for the learning disabled.* Columbus, OH: Merrill.

Wiig, E., and Wilson, C. (2001*). Map it out: Visual tools for thinking, organizing, and communicating.* Eau Claire, WI: Thinking Publications.

Wiig, E., and Wilson, C. (2002). *The learning ladder: Assessing and teaching text comprehension.* Eau Claire, WI: Thinking Publications.

Williams, J. (1992). What do you know? What do you need to know? *Asha, 34*(6/7), 54–61.

Wilson, G. (1994). Self-advocacy skills. In Michaels, C. (Ed.). *Transition strategies for persons with learning disabilities.* San Diego, CA: Singular.

Wolf, D. (1989). Portfolio assessment: Sampling student work. *Educational Leadership, 46*(7), 35–39.

Wolff, F., and Marsnik, N. (1992). *Perceptive listening* (2nd ed.). New York : Harcourt, Brace, Jovanovich.

Wolff, F., Marsnik, N., Tacey, W., and Nichols, R. (1983). *Perceptive listening.* Chicago: Holt, Rinehart and Winston.

Wong, B. (Ed.). (1991). *Learning about learning disabilities.* San Diego, CA: Academic Press.

Wong, C.A., and Rowley, S.J. (2001). The schooling of ethnic minority children: Commentary. *Educational Psychologist, 36,* 57–66.

Worden, P., Malmgren, I., and Gabourie, P. (1982). Memory for stories in learning disabled adults. *Journal of Learning Disabilities, 15*(3), 145–152.

Worden, P., and Nakamura, G. (1982). Story comprehension and recall in learning-disabled versus normal college students. *Journal of Educational Psychology, 74*(5), 633–641.

Work, R., Cline, J., Ehren, B., Keiser, C., and Wujek, C. (1993). Adolescent language programs. *Language, Speech and Hearing Services in Schools, 24*(1), 43–53.

World Health Organization. (n.d.). *World Health Organization (WHO) approach to adolescents.* Retrieved May 8, 2003, from http://www.un.org.in/Jinit/who.pdf

Worthen, B., and Spandel, V. (1991). Putting the standardized test debate in perspective. *Educational Leadership, 48*(5), 65–69.

Ylvisaker, M., and DeBonis, D. (2000). Executive function impairment in adolescence: TBI and ADHD. *Topics in Language Disorders, 20*(2), 29–57.

Ylvisaker, M., and Feeney, T. (1995). Traumatic brain injury in adolescence: Assessment and integration. *Seminars in Speech and Language, 16*(1), 32–44.

Zeller, W. (1952). *Konstitution und entwicklung [Formation and development].* Gottingen, Germany: Psychologische Rundschau.

Indexes

Author Index

Subject Index